Principles of Orthopedic Pra
Providers

Jeffrey N. Katz • Cheri A. Blauwet
Andrew J. Schoenfeld

Editors

Principles of Orthopedic Practice for Primary Care Providers

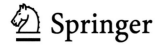 Springer

Editors
Jeffrey N. Katz
Department of Orthopedic Surgery
Brigham and Women's Hospital,
Harvard Medical School
Boston, MA, USA

Andrew J. Schoenfeld
Department of Orthopedic Surgery
Brigham and Women's Hospital,
Harvard Medical School
Boston, MA, USA

Cheri A. Blauwet
Departments of Physical Medicine and
Rehabilitation and Orthopedic Surgery
Brigham and Women's Hospital/
Spaulding Rehabilitation Hospital,
Harvard Medical School
Boston, MA, USA

ISBN 978-3-319-68660-8   ISBN 978-3-319-68661-5   (eBook)
https://doi.org/10.1007/978-3-319-68661-5

Library of Congress Control Number: 2017960169

Printed on acid-free paper

This Springer imprint is published by Springer Nature
The registered company is Springer International Publishing AG
The registered company address is: Gewerbestrasse 11, 6330 Cham, Switzerland

Foreword

More than a third of symptoms and complaints reported to primary care physicians are musculoskeletal in nature. Therefore, primary care providers are the frontline clinicians for most orthopedic and musculoskeletal disorders. The basic premise of this book *Principles of Orthopedic Practice for Primary Care Providers*, edited by Drs. Katz, Blauwet, and Schoenfeld, is to provide a concise educational tool and quick reference to primary care providers in order to give them a framework for diagnosis and early treatment of common musculoskeletal disorders. The editors have put together a comprehensive collection of chapters that provide an overview of the most common disorders that affect the upper and lower extremities as well as the spinal column. A primer on basic physical examination of the various musculo-skeletal systems and imaging guidelines are nicely organized and presented for practical application. The general practitioner should be able to develop a differential diagnosis quickly and then determine when a referral to a specialist may be indicated for more definitive treatment.

One unique feature of this book is that all the senior authors are faculty of the Brigham and Women's Hospital and Harvard Medical School. Most of the senior authors are nationally and internationally acclaimed experts in orthopedic surgery, physical medicine and rehabilitation, and rheumatology. The interdisciplinary nature of this book by the surgical and nonoperative experts in musculoskeletal medicine should provide a balanced approach to these common entities for which our patients seek care. This book should help fulfill our goal of providing the highest quality patient care as all health care providers become more educated and efficient in the way they handle patients with musculoskeletal disorders.

Boston, MA, USA   James D. Kang

Preface

Musculoskeletal disorders are prevalent, disabling, and costly. In fact, the direct medical and disability costs associated with musculoskeletal disorders exceed 3% of the gross domestic product in the USA, with similar impacts in other Western countries. These disorders occur in people of all ages, races, and ethnicities, lasting days in some instances and a lifetime in others.

Our capacity to diagnose these conditions accurately and treat them effectively has expanded dramatically over the last several decades with the use of advanced imaging and sophisticated rehabilitative and surgical approaches. Technological advances notwithstanding, the foundation of quality musculoskeletal care remains to be careful history taking and physical examination coupled with an understanding of the differential diagnosis and natural history of common musculoskeletal disorders and the circumstances in which referral to musculoskeletal specialists is appropriate.

Patients with musculoskeletal problems generally seek care from their primary care providers, who must make the critical initial assessment of the diagnosis, treatment pathway, and necessity for further testing and referral. This is a tall order. We are musculoskeletal specialists who work closely with our community of primary care providers. We created this book to help primary care providers everywhere develop greater comfort with the recognition and early management of the more prevalent musculoskeletal disorders. The chapter authors are active clinicians with practices based at Brigham and Women's Hospital in Boston.

The book includes chapters on disorders affecting the spine, the upper extremities, and the lower extremities. Within each of these broad anatomic categories, individual chapters focus on one or a cluster of related entities. Each chapter covers the clinical presentation of the problem(s), differential diagnosis, indications for diagnostic testing, evidence-based recommendations for initial nonoperative treatment, and indications for surgical referral.

We are privileged to work with and learn daily from a community of dedicated primary care providers and of superb musculoskeletal specialists, many of whom are chapter authors of this volume. We are further privileged to care for a vibrant community of patients in the Boston area, who teach us more about musculoskeletal disorders each day. Finally, we are privileged to have the support of our loving families and in particular of our spouses—Susan Zeiger, Erin Schoenfeld, and Eli Wolff.

Boston, MA   Jeffrey N. Katz
Boston, MA   Cheri A. Blauwet
Boston, MA   Andrew J. Schoenfeld

Contents

Part XI   Foot and Ankle

Part XII   Bone Stress Injuries

Contributors

Editors

Jeffrey N. Katz, MD, MSc Department of Orthopedics Surgery, Brigham and Women's Hospital, Harvard Medical School, Boston, MA, USA

Cheri A. Blauwet, MD Department of Physical Medicine and Rehabilitation, Brigham and Women's Hospital/Spaulding Rehabilitation Hospital, Harvard Medical School, Boston, MA, USA

Andrew J. Schoenfeld, MD, MSc Department of Orthopedic Surgery, Brigham and Women's Hospital, Harvard Medical School, Boston, MA, USA

Authors

Arnold B. Alqueza, MD Department of Orthopedics, Brigham and Women's Hospital, Harvard Medical School, Boston, MA, USA

Amandeep Bhalla, MD Department of Orthopedic Surgery, Brigham and Women's Hospital, Harvard Medical School, Boston, MA, USA

Philip E. Blazar, MD Department of Orthopedic Surgery: Hand and Upper Extremity, Brigham and Women's Hospital, Boston, MA, USA

Eric M. Bluman, MD, PhD Department of Orthopedic Surgery, Brigham and Women's Hospital, Boston, MA, USA

Christopher M. Bono, MD Department of Orthopaedic Surgery, Harvard Medical School, Brigham and Women's Hospital, Boston, MA, USA

Emily M. Brook, BA Department of Orthopedic Surgery, Brigham and Women's Hospital, Boston, MA, USA

Christopher P. Chiodo, MD Department of Orthopedic Surgery, Brigham and Women's Hospital, Boston, MA, USA

Courtney Dawson, MD Orthopedic Surgeon, Sports Medicine and Orthopedic Surgery, Brigham and Women's Hospital, Boston, MA, USA

George S.M. Dyer, MD Department of Orthopedic Surgery, Brigham and Women's Hospital, Boston, MA, USA

Brandon E. Earp, MD Department of Orthopedic Surgery, Brigham and Women's Faulkner Hospital, Boston, MA, USA

Marco L. Ferrone, MD, FRCSC Department of Orthopaedic Surgery, Brigham and Women's Hospital/Dana Farber Cancer Institute, Harvard Medical School, Boston, MA, USA

Andreas H. Gomoll, MD Department of Orthopedic Surgery, Brigham and Women's Hospital, Boston, MA, USA

Mitchel B. Harris, MD FACS Department of Orthopaedic Surgery, Brigham and Women's Hospital, Harvard Medical School, Boston, MA, USA

Laurence D. Higgins, MD, MBA Sports Medicine and Shoulder Service, Brigham and Women's Hospital, Harvard Medical School, Boston, MA, USA

James P. Ioli, DPM Department of Orthopedics, Brigham and Women's Hospital, Harvard Medical School, Boston, MA, USA

James D. Kang, MD Department of Orthopaedic Surgery, Brigham and Women's Hospital, Harvard Medical School, Boston, MA, USA

Stella J. Lee, MD Department of Orthopaedic Surgery, Brigham and Women's Hospital, Boston, MA, USA

Scott D. Martin, MD Department of Orthopaedic Surgery, Massachusetts General Hospital and Brigham and Women's Hospital, Harvard Medical School, Boston, MA, USA

Elizabeth Matzkin, MD Department of Orthopaedic Surgery, Brigham and Women's Hospital, Boston, MA, USA

Michael J. Messina, MD Sports Medicine and Shoulder Service, Brigham and Women's Hospital, Harvard Medical School, Boston, MA, USA

Tom Minas, MD, MS Cartilage Repair Center, Brigham and Women's Hospital, Chestnut Hill, MA, USA

Ariana N. Mora, BA Department of Orthopedic Surgery: Hand and Upper Extremity, Brigham and Women's Hospital, Boston, MA, USA

Brian Mosier, MD Department of Orthopaedic Surgery, Brigham and Women's Hospital, Boston, MA, USA

Eziamaka C. Obunadike, MD Department of Physical Medicine and Rehabilitation, Spaulding Rehabilitation Hospital/Brigham and Women's Hospital, Harvard Medical School, Boston, MA, USA

Barry P. Simmons, MD Hand and Upper Extremity Service, Department of Orthopedic Surgery, Brigham and Women's Hospital, Boston, MA, USA

Jeremy T. Smith, MD Department of Orthopedic Surgery, Brigham and Women's Hospital, Harvard Medical School, Boston, MA, USA

Robert C. Spang III, MD, BA Orthopedic Surgeon, Sports Medicine and Orthopedic Surgery, Brigham and Women's Hospital, Boston, MA, USA

Harvard Combined Orthopaedic Residency Program, Boston, MA, USA

Adam S. Tenforde, MD Department of Orthopedics and Physical Medicine and Rehabilitation, Brigham and Women's Hospital, Spaulding Rehabilitation Hospital, Cambridge, MA, USA

Thomas S. Thornhill, MD Department of Orthopedics Surgery, Brigham and Women's Hospital, Harvard Medical School, Boston, MA, USA

Beverlie L. Ting, MD Seattle Hand Surgery Group, Seattle, WA, USA

Daniel G. Tobert, MD Department of Orthopaedic Surgery, Brigham and Women's Hospital, Harvard Medical School, Boston, MA, USA

Marie E. Walcott, MD Department of Orthopedics, Brigham and Women's Hospital, Harvard Medical School, Boston, MA, USA

Michael J. Weaver, MD Department of Orthopaedic Surgery, Brigham and Women's Hospital, Harvard Medical School, Boston, MA, USA

Kaitlyn Whitlock, PA-C Department of Orthopaedic Surgery, Brigham and Women's Hospital, Boston, MA, USA

Jay M. Zampini, MD Department of Orthopaedic Surgery, Brigham and Women's Hospital, Harvard Medical School, Boston, MA, USA

Part I
Axial Spine

Chapter 1
Axial Neck and Back Pain

Jay M. Zampini

Abbreviations

AP	Anteroposterior
ASIS	Anterior-superior iliac spine
CT	Computed tomography
FABER	Flexion-abduction-external rotation
MRI	Magnetic resonance imaging
SI	Sacroiliac
SPORT	Spine Patient Outcomes Research Trials.
PT	Physical therapy

Introduction

Greater than 80% of all adults will, at one time or another, experience back pain debilitating enough to impair activities of daily living, occupational performance, or quality of life. Although the lumbar spine is affected more frequently than the cervical or thoracic regions, pain that affects any segment of the spine can be termed "axial spinal pain" and should be distinguished from conditions with neurogenic pain such as neurogenic claudication and radiculitis. The pathophysiology and treatment of axial spinal pain differ from that of the neurogenic conditions, though the two may be present concomitantly. This chapter will review the pathophysiology, evaluation, and treatment of axial pain in the neck, the back, and the sacroiliac (SI) joints. The term "axial pain" will be used when referring generically to any segment of the spine. "Neck pain," "back pain," or "SI pain" will be used when referring specifically to the neck, back, or SI joints, respectively.

J.M. Zampini (✉)
Department of Orthopaedic Surgery, Brigham and Women's Hospital
Harvard Medical School, Boston, MA, USA
e-mail: jzampini@partners.org

© Springer International Publishing AG 2018
J.N. Katz et al. (eds.), *Principles of Orthopedic Practice for Primary Care Providers*, https://doi.org/10.1007/978-3-319-68661-5_1

3

Definition and Epidemiology

Axial pain is defined as pain localized to one or more regions of the spine and/or SI joints without radiation into the lower extremities. It typically is present at all times and not necessarily aggravated by ambulation or activity. Pain may be lessened with rest or lying flat, but this does not have to be the case and is not required for a diagnosis. There are a number of factors that may be responsible for axial pain including joint dysfunction, degenerative changes, trauma, tumor or infection, myofascial structures, and nonorganic pain generators.

With greater than 80% of the adult population experiencing axial spinal pain at some point in life, and many not seeking medical care, it is difficult to make conclusive epidemiologic statements about populations at risk. It can almost be stated that anyone who lives long enough is at risk for back pain. Certain factors are known to associate with a higher risk of chronic axial pain, including obesity, tobacco use, total body vibration as may occur in long-distance truck driving or use of a jackhammer, and repetitive hyperextension activities of the lumbar spine.

Clinical Presentation

Pain History

The evaluation of axial spinal pain is no different than any other pain evaluation and should include the time of onset, location of maximal pain, duration, severity, and associated symptoms. An inciting event should be noted if possible. A patient should be asked to consider events in the 2–3 days preceding the onset of pain since the inflammation which often causes axial spinal pain will increase over this time period. Body positions or maneuvers that exacerbate or alleviate the pain should be sought as should other associated symptoms. Patients should also be queried as to whether similar symptoms have presented in the past.

A thorough axial pain evaluation is then performed, with consideration given to the structures that may be pain generators. All spinal structures can potentially cause pain. These structures include the vertebral body and disc in the anterior spine; facet joints, other bony processes, interspinous and supraspinous ligaments, and SI joints posteriorly; as well as the myofascial tissue in all spinal regions (Fig. 1.1). As these structures each perform a unique function, they also possess characteristic patterns of pain that may be elucidated through the history and physical exam. The pain patterns typically associated with dysfunction of each key spinal structure are summarized in Table 1.1.

The history of axial pain should clearly document the presence or absence of any "red flag," signs, and symptoms. A history of acute, high-energy trauma, such as car accidents or falls from greater than standing height, would suggest the need for emergent evaluation. Constitutional symptoms such as unintended weight loss in

Fig. 1.1 Schematic of the human spine. The spine contains four zones: cervical, thoracic, lumbar, and sacrum

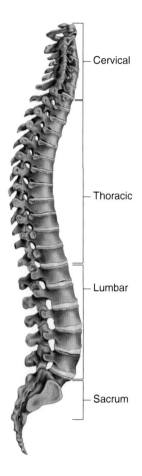

— Cervical

— Thoracic

— Lumbar

— Sacrum

excess of 10% of body weight or unexplained fevers or chills would suggest the need for a neoplastic or infectious workup. Other neurologic "red flags," such as bowel or bladder retention or incontinence, should be sought to identify potential neurologic emergencies.

Physical Examination

A specific diagnosis of axial pain can be made most often by the history alone. The physical examination serves to confirm the expected diagnosis. For most patients it is useful to examine all aspects of the spine not expected to be painful before focusing on the structure anticipated to be the pain generator since the examination is sure to exacerbate the pain at least temporarily. Any involuntary guarding associated with increased pain can obscure other aspects of the evaluation such as the neurologic examination. Examination of the sensory, motor, and reflex functions can

Table 1.1 Pain patterns typically associated with dysfunction of key spinal structures

	Myofascial	Fracture	Discogenic	Facetogenic	Sacroiliac
Injury identified	No	Yes	No	No	No
Tenderness	Trigger point	Focal	No	Focal	Focal
Exacerbating factors	Muscle stretch or activation	Spinal motion	Prolonged sitting or standing	Spinal hyperextension	Forced SI joint motion
Alleviating factors	Muscle rest	Immobilization	Recumbency	Recumbency	Recumbency
Neurologic symptoms	None	Possible	Possible	Possible	None
Referred pain[a]	None	Possible	Possible	Possible	Possible

[a]Cervical spine conditions can cause referred pain between the occiput and the lower scapulae, depending on the spinal level of the condition. Lumbar conditions can cause referred pain to the buttock and posterior thighs

often be performed first and without any additional discomfort to the patient. This should be followed by a standing examination of the spine. Spinal curvature and posture should be evaluated with attention to shoulder height, pelvic obliquity, and any deviation of spinal balance. Spinal balance generally means that the patient's head is centered over the pelvis in both the sagittal and coronal planes. Gait should be examined from this position as well; attention should be paid to voluntary and involuntary alteration of gait to avoid pain and to any assistance device required for mobility. In the standing position, the spine should be palpated in the midline to determine if any bony tenderness is present. The musculature should be palpated next, again focusing on areas not expected to be tender before palpating potentially painful muscles. Spinal motion should be assessed last as this is often most painful for the patient. Objective measurements of spinal flexion, extension, lateral bending, and rotation, while valuable to document objective responses to treatment, are typically not as helpful for diagnostic purposes.

Next, provocative maneuvers should be performed for diagnostic confirmation if necessary. For axial spinal pain, provocative maneuvers are most useful for confirming the SI joint as the source of pain. A patient should be supine for most of these tests. One sensitive test of the SI joint is performed by passively flexing the hip on the painful side and then abducting and externally rotating the hip while the contralateral leg remains on the examination table. This maneuver—flexion-abduction-external rotation (FABER) test—compresses the ipsilateral SI joint and reproduces pain as a result. The test is positive if pain near the SI joint is reproduced. The test is nonspecific, however, since several structures are manipulated simultaneously (the hip joint, SI joint, lumbar spine, musculature) and should be followed by other confirmatory tests. If pain at the SI joint can be reproduced by compressing the pelvis either by using bilateral, posteriorly directed pressure on the anterior-superior iliac spines (ASIS) in the supine position—the AP pelvic compression test—or by pressure on the greater trochanter with the patient in the lateral decubitus position (the lateral pelvic compression test), then the painful structure can be confirmed to be the SI joint. Additionally, the SI joint can be examined by sliding the supine patient to the side of the exam table, flexing the hip on the non-painful side, and hyperextending the hip on the painful side in what is called a Gaenslen's maneuver. Reproduction of pain is a positive finding. A final aspect of the physical examination includes evaluation of other potentially painful joints in the upper or lower extremities.

One further consideration in the examination of a patient with axial pain is the impact of psychological somatization and symptom magnification. These patients will perceive pain that is either present without any physical disruption of a spinal structure or out of proportion to what would be expected by the physical condition. To make this determination requires a nuanced approach to patient evaluation; several classic findings, termed Waddell's findings, have been reported to correlate with somatization and symptom magnification. Gentle downward compression of a patient's head does not cause any motion of the lumbar spine and should, therefore, cause no low back pain. Similarly, if spinal motion is simulated—with rotation of the shoulders, back, and pelvis at the same time—the spine itself is not affected and no pain should be experienced. Finally, light touch of the skin overlying the spine should not produce pain. Observation of pain with any of these maneuvers should alert the clinician that nonorganic factors are contributing to the patient's pain and should be taken into account when planning further evaluation and treatment.

Differential Diagnosis and Diagnostic Testing

Myofascial Pain

Muscles are the structures most susceptible to fatigue and overuse injury as well as to injuries resulting from acute demand exceeding muscle capacity. These injuries collectively comprise the most common cause of spinal pain and are generically called strains. Activation or passive stretch of the injured muscle will exacerbate the pain. Palpation will reveal focal, typically unilateral tenderness at the site of muscle injury. Multiple painful triggers may be encountered in the paraspinal musculature of patients with myofascial pain syndromes, such as fibromyalgia. Imaging does not help confirm a diagnosis, but does rule out other potential etiologies as a cause of the pain.

Pain Associated with Fractures and Ligamentous Injuries

In both young and old patients, referred pain can be felt in a pattern characteristic of the level of injury. Injuries close to the upper cervical spine will have referred pain to the occiput; injuries of the lower cervical spine will have referred pain even as far distally as the lower aspect of the scapulae. Similarly, lumbar fracture patients can complain of referred pain to the buttocks or upper thighs. Dermatomal symptoms to the hands or feet do not represent referred pain and suggest that a full neurologic exam should be included. Palpation reveals focal tenderness at the sight of injury. Plain film or computed tomographic (CT) imaging is used to diagnose or confirm a fracture. Magnetic resonance imaging (MRI) may be required if these initial studies are negative, to evaluate for concomitant disc or ligamentous injury, or to assess the acuity of a particular fracture.

Discogenic Pain

Several painful conditions have been shown to localize to the disc: tears of the annulus, herniated discs, and degenerative disc disease (Fig. 1.2). With an annular tear, patients complain of axial pain deep inside the spine and focally at or near the injury site. Pain is typically increased with lumbar flexion or sitting and relieved with lumbar extension or lying flat. Plain film images may be read as negative depending on the extent of degenerative changes involving the disc space (Fig. 1.3). MRI is the diagnostic test of choice and will accurately display the amount of disc degeneration at various levels within the spine (Fig. 1.4). As a result, this imaging modality is nonspecific and cannot identify which, if any of the degenerative discs identified, is the cause of a patient's axial pain.

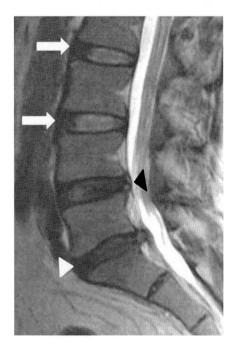

Fig. 1.2 This sagittal, T2-weighted MRI of the lumbar spine shows normal (*white arrow*) and degenerative discs. The degenerative discs show decreased disc height and low disc signal from loss of disc hydration (*white arrow head*) and annular tearing (*black arrow head*)

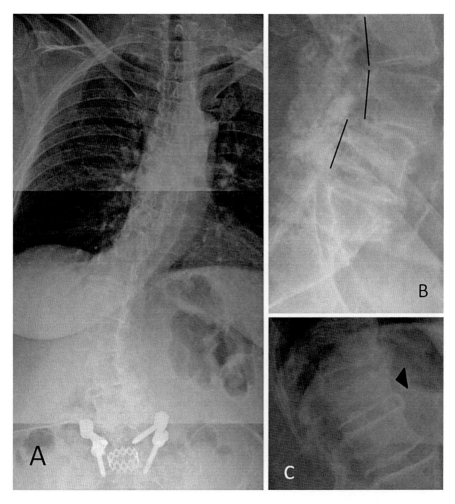

Fig. 1.3 Planar radiographs of the lumbar spine are ideal to identify and monitor scoliosis (**a**), spondylolisthesis (**b**), and compression fractures (**c**)

Facetogenic Pain

Patients with painful, degenerative facet joints will complain of morning pain and stiffness of the back. Spinal extension increases the load borne by the facet joints, and patients will complain that this maneuver exacerbates the pain. Referred pain is often present with painful facets: upper cervical facet referred pain may be perceived along the occiput with lower cervical referred pain felt in the shoulders or scapulae. Lumbar referred pain is perceived within the buttocks, pelvis, or posterior thighs. Spinal extension may increase the sensation of referred pain. It should be noted that the discs and facet joints age or degenerate concomitantly and may be

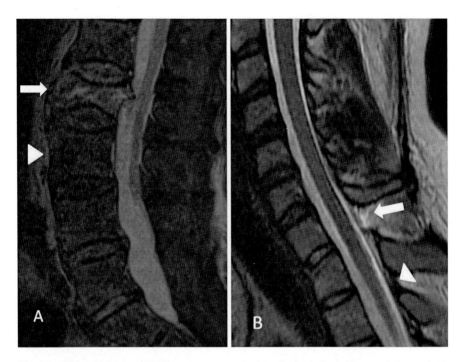

Fig. 1.4 MRI is useful for identifying the source of axial spinal pain including occult fractures (**a**) and ligament sprains (**b**). The occult fracture (**a**) is identified by the high STIR signal in the vertebral body (*arrow*) compared to low signal in an uninjured vertebra (*arrow head*). The ligament injury (**b**) is shown at the arrow compared to a normal-appearing ligamentum flavum seen at the level below (*arrow head*).

symptomatic simultaneously. These patients will note that prolonged sitting and standing both exacerbate pain. Plain film, CT, and MR imaging can all demonstrate evidence of facet arthrosis, although none of these imaging modalities are considered a specific test.

Sacroiliac Pain

The SI joints form the link between the spine and pelvis. The joints are extremely stable as a result of strong ligaments on both the posterior and anterior aspects of the joint. Patients with painful sacroiliac joints complain of pain just medial to the posterior superior iliac spines, the bony prominences at the top of the buttocks. Patients may experience pain with lumbosacral range of motion, ambulation, or single-leg stance. The unique location and function of the SI joints allows for a somewhat more focused examination than for other degenerative spinal conditions. At least three other provocative maneuvers (FABER test, thigh thrust, Gaenslen's test, and/or pelvic compression) should be positive to confirm SI pain with relative certainty. Plain film images and CT scans may show joint degeneration, while active inflammation or synovitis can be appreciated on MRI. The extent of findings localized to the SI joint does not necessarily correlate with the degree of a patient's SI-related pain.

Conditions Causing Referred Pain to the Spine

All evaluations of axial spinal pain should consider non-spinal sources as well. Visceral, vascular, autoimmune, neoplastic, and infectious conditions are responsible for 2–3% of all axial spinal pain. These conditions often cause nonmechanical pain or pain that does not change with spinal motion. Patients will report that they "just can't get comfortable in any position." Red flag signs and symptoms should be sought in these patients with a concomitant vascular examination as deemed necessary.

Nonoperative Management

A large majority of patients with newly diagnosed axial pain will return to their baseline state of spinal health within 4–6 weeks, oftentimes with little to no treatment. For this reason, noninvasive, nonoperative modalities are the preferred choice for the treatment of axial spinal pain.

For patients with acute spinal pain—whatever the underlying origin—a short period of rest from aggravating maneuvers is indicated. A patient should not be placed on complete bed rest for more than 1–2 days. After even a few days of bed rest, the musculature of the entire body including the paraspinal muscles will begin to atrophy, making effective rehabilitation a challenge. The patient should be advised to return to activity as soon as possible with avoidance of the most painful activities. Additionally, nonsteroidal anti-inflammatory drugs should be prescribed at an appropriate dose for the purposes of pain relief. An oral steroid taper can also be used but should be used with caution, as several reports have suggested that oral steroids may reduce the efficacy of later, more invasive treatments such as injections.

By 2–4 weeks following symptom onset, most patients will have recovered sufficiently to resume most activities of daily living and even more strenuous activities such as exercise. It is at this point that physical therapy (PT) can be helpful to further reduce pain and to begin rehabilitation and prevention of future exacerbations. Therapists can perform pain-relieving treatments including massage, stretch, and spinal manipulation to accelerate pain reduction. This phase of treatment may also include chiropractic care and acupuncture. The long-term goals of PT should focus on improving muscle strength. Patients with muscle strains require strengthening of the injured muscle and all muscles that support the spine (known as the "core" musculature) to become better able to participate in the activities that initially precipitated the pain. Even patients with annular tears, herniated discs, and degenerative conditions can benefit from the trunk stability provided by strengthening the paraspinal musculature. Using one or more of these three noninvasive treatments, greater than 90% of patients should experience relief of acute axial pain, and many should experience long-term maintenance of spinal health.

Patients who fail to achieve relief of axial spinal pain through activity modification, oral agents, and therapy often can be treated with spinal injections. Injection techniques vary and are chosen for the specific pathology to be treated. Chronic muscle strains or muscle spasm may benefit from trigger point injections at the point(s) of maximal muscle tenderness. Recalcitrant cases of muscle spasm, particularly with cervical torticollis, are sometimes treated with injection of botulinum toxin (Botox, Allergan, Dublin, Ireland).

Axial pain thought to result from the disc or facet joints can be treated with epidural and perifacet injections, respectively. Epidural injections typically involve localization of the affected spinal level on fluoroscopy followed by injection of lidocaine and a corticosteroid. Immediate reduction of the pain with the effect of the topical anesthetic agent confirms the target as a pain generator. Epidural injections are best reserved for pathology within the spinal canal—disc herniations and occasionally annular tears. Patients with facet pathology benefit from perifacet injections. These injections can be placed directly into the facet capsule; however, most pain specialists now inject anesthetic cranially and caudally to the facet to block the medial branch of the dorsal primary ramus of the nerve root, the main innervation of the joint. These medial branch blocks have been found to be safer and more effective for reduction in pain emanating from the facets. Additionally, medial branch blocks can be used to plan radiofrequency denervation of the facet joint, a technique that offers longer-term relief of facet-based pain in well-selected patients.

For individuals with painful SI joint dysfunction, injections directly into the joint may be beneficial. A pain specialist or interventional radiologist will identify the SI joint on fluoroscopy and advance a needle into the joint. Following fluoroscopic confirmation, a topical anesthetic agent and a corticosteroid are injected. In 80–90% of cases, well-selected patients will experience some degree of pain relief following the injection.

Aside from pain relief, two other benefits are provided through spinal injections. First, if a patient experiences partial relief with the injection, he or she may be better able to participate in therapy. The two modalities can then work synergistically to accelerate a patient's recovery. Second, the application of a topical anesthetic agent or corticosteroid can help to predict if a patient will respond favorably to surgery. Temporary but substantial relief of symptoms implies that a more permanent treatment option, namely, surgery, could be considered.

Indications for Surgery

Surgery is not indicated for the vast majority of patients with axial neck and back pain for several reasons: the condition is often not amenable to surgery (e.g., muscle strain, ligament sprain), the condition is stable and self-limited (e.g., most compression fractures and nearly all spinous process and transverse process fractures), or imaging findings are too diffuse to determine which process represents the main pain generator (e.g., multilevel degeneration with axial pain). Surgical treatment of axial pain is currently well indicated for patients with scoliosis and kyphosis, spondylolisthesis, and spinal instability resulting from fractures and dislocations. Surgical intervention for degenerative disease with axial pain in the absence of neurogenic symptoms is rarely indicated and only if the degeneration is localized, patients have failed to achieve sustained pain relief with nonoperative modalities, and significant clinical information can confirm that the degenerative conditions identified are the sole pain generators. The clinical information best able to predict a positive outcome following surgery is the observation of complete (or near-complete) resolution of axial pain with focal spinal injections coupled with consistent, reproducible physical examination findings pointing to the degenerative structures as pain generators. Additionally, the patient's history should be free of other psychosocial factors that could confound treatment. These factors include psychiatric conditions with predominant somatization symptoms, presence of active litigation related to an injury associated with the pain (e.g., car accidents, work-related injuries), and the presence of an active worker's compensation claim.

Operative Management

One of the most compelling reasons to avoid surgery for axial pain, if at all possible, is that fusion-based procedures are the primary treatment for these conditions. The main rationale for fusion follows the logic that pain from a moving structure can be controlled by eliminating motion at the structure. In all segments of the spine and SI joints, fusion involves preparing the environment surrounding two bones to be conducive for the growth of new bone. The bridging bone will then join the two initially independent segments into a single structure.

Anterior Spinal Fusion

Spinal fusion can be performed from an anterior approach to the disc space between the vertebral bodies. These operations are termed "interbody," or "intervertebral," fusions for this reason. The technique is most often used for anterior cervical spine surgery and in the lumbar spine for discogenic back pain. Anterior fusion enjoys the advantage of a large space for placement of bone graft for fusion between the well-vascularized vertebral bodies. Cervical spine surgery is readily accomplished in this manner with a relatively minimally invasive approach that exploits natural anatomic planes between the trachea, esophagus, and major neurovascular structures in the neck. Thoracolumbar surgery, however, has the disadvantage of requiring exposure through the thoracic and abdominal cavities with attendant risk of injury to the visceral and vascular structures contained therein. Bone graft, either from a cadaveric donor or harvested from the anterior iliac crest, is impacted into the space previously occupied by the intervertebral disc to achieve the fusion. This is typically stabilized using a metal plate affixed to the anterior aspect of the vertebrae with bone screws, as such instrumentation has been shown to provide more immediate stability and enhance the likelihood of fusion.

Postoperatively, patients often use a cervical collar or brace to protect the spine until pain begins to resolve. The fusion site will heal over the course of several months and is monitored using periodic radiographs. Visualization of bone bridging between the intended vertebrae signifies complete healing of the fusion.

Posterior Spinal Fusion

Thoracolumbar fusion is most commonly performed using a posterior approach. The advantage of the posterior approach in the thoracic and lumbar regions is that long segments of the spine can be accessed without violating the thoracic and abdominal cavities and complication rates are reduced as a result. Fusion can be achieved by placing an interbody graft using carbon fiber or titanium cages, cadaver bone, or autograft from the iliac crest or elsewhere. Stabilization is achieved via bone screws anchored to the vertebrae through channels created in the pedicles and connected by rods. Patients may be given a back brace to assist mobilization after thoracolumbar posterior fusion. The brace is typically used only until a patient's pain resolves and the muscles once again become able to assist stability. In patients with osteopenia or osteoporosis, a rigid brace may be prescribed for use until the fusion site shows signs of consolidation on radiographs.

SI Joint Fusion

Fusion of the SI joint requires debridement of the cartilage of the joint with replacement of the cartilage with bone graft. The SI joint can be accessed anteriorly or posteriorly with bone graft taken directly from the ilium. Stabilization is achieved using a plate bridging from the sacrum to the ilium or via percutaneously placed screws that span the joint space.

After SI fusion, patients are instructed to use crutches or a walker to assist in mobilization. Weight bearing on the operative limb is restricted to the so-called "toe-touch," or "touchdown," weight bearing for several weeks following surgery.

Expected Outcomes

The vast majority of patients (upward of 90%) with acute axial pain can be expected to experience pain relief within 6 weeks of symptom onset. Patients with initial episodes of pain can, therefore, be reassured that the pain will resolve and not result in a chronic condition. In general, the longer a patient experiences activity-limiting axial pain, the longer treatment will take to relieve the pain and the less likely he or she will be to experience complete pain relief. This observation was recently confirmed in an analysis of the multicenter Spine Patient Outcomes Research Trials (SPORT). Patients with lumbar disc herniations who experienced functional limitations for greater than 6 months were found to have inferior results, irrespective of treatment, as compared to patients in pain for less than 6 months. It is unclear if this finding suggests that patients developed chronic pain syndromes independent of the initial pain generator or if permanent structural damage to the spine was responsible.

If a patient is unable to achieve satisfactory relief through nonoperative measures, fusion-based procedures have been shown to result in long-term reductions in pain and improvement in function for only 60–70% of well-selected patients with axial neck and back pain. Reports of randomized trials and observational studies have shown that some well-selected patients could achieve pain relief and functional improvement following surgery. The selection process must be rigorous, however, in order to assure the best outcome possible. Ideally, patients should be free from nicotine products and should not be involved in litigation over the cause of pain to assure optimal outcomes. Patients must additionally be prepared to expect that no treatment will completely eliminate back pain. They should be counseled that pain reduction will approximate what was achieved with spinal injections and should be willing to accept that a 50% reduction in pain may be the best that can be achieved. Patients expecting full alleviation of pain following surgery should have their expectations appropriately adjusted through counseling from primary care physicians and surgeons prior to agreeing to any procedure.

Table 1.2 shows a summary of axial neck and back pain disorders with synopsis of presentation, diagnostic testing, and suggested management options.

Table 1.2 Summary of axial neck and back pain disorders with synopsis of presentation, diagnostic testing, and suggested management options

Clinical entity	Presentation	Diagnostic testing	Conservative management	Surgical indications and operative management
Myofascial pain	– Trigger point tenderness – Limited or no focal pain	– Primarily clinical	– Rest, ice, NSAIDS – PT – Trigger point injection	N/A
Fracture/ Ligamentous Injury	– History of trauma – Focal tenderness to palpation over injured region	– Plain films/ CT – MRI—if there is concern for ligamentous injury	– Rest, ice, NSAIDS – PT – Spinal bracing	– Spinal instability or failure of non-operative management with persistent pain – Spinal stabilization procedures often require instrumented fusion
Discogenic back pain	– Pain worse with sitting or standing – Forward flexion exacerbates the pain	– MRI—degenerative changes involving the discs (may not be diagnostic)	– NSAIDS – PT – Spinal injections	– Reserved for select cases where non-operative treatment fails – Fusion-based procedure
Facetogenic pain	– Pain worse with standing and ambulation – Extension exacerbates the pain	– MRI—degenerative changes involving the facet joints (may not be diagnostic)	– NSAIDS – PT – Facet injections, radiofrequency lesioning, rhizotomy	– Reserved for select cases where non-operative treatment fails – Fusion-based procedure
Sacroiliac pain	– Pain with single leg stance and ambulation – Positive provocative tests: FABER, Gaenslen's and/or pelvic compression	– Plain film/CT/ MRI—findings may not be diagnostic	– NSAIDS – PT – Sacroiliac injections, radiofrequency lesioning, rhizotomy	– Reserved for select cases where non-operative treatment fails – Fusion-based procedure

PT physical therapy, *CT* computed tomography, *MRI* magnetic resonance imaging, *NSAIDs* nonsteroidal anti-inflammatory drugs

Suggested Reading

Deyo RA, Weinstein JN. Low back pain. N Engl J Med. 2001;344(5):363–70.

Fritzell P, Hagg O, Wessberg P, Nordwall A. 2001 Volvo award winner in clinical studies: lumbar fusion versus nonsurgical treatment for chronic low back pain: a multicenter randomized controlled trial from the Swedish Lumbar Spine Study Group. Spine (Phila Pa 1976). 2001;26(23):2521–32.

Kaye AD, Manchikanti L, Abdi S, et al. Efficacy of epidural injections in managing chronic spinal pain: a best evidence synthesis. Pain Physician. 2015;18(6):E939–1004.

Pearson AM, Lurie JD, Tosteson TD, Zhao W, Abdu WA, Weinstein JN. Who should undergo surgery for degenerative spondylolisthesis? Treatment effect predictors in SPORT. Spine (Phila Pa 1976). 2013;38(21):1799–811.

Riew KD, Ecker E, Dettori JR. Anterior cervical discectomy and fusion for the management of axial neck pain in the absence of radiculopathy or myelopathy. Evid Based Spine Care J. 2010;1(3):45–50.

Part II
Cervical Spine

Chapter 2
Cervical Radiculopathy and Myelopathy

Amandeep Bhalla and James D. Kang

Abbreviations

CSM   Cervical spondylotic myelopathy
CT   Computed tomography
MRI   Magnetic resonance imaging

Cervical Radiculopathy

Definition and Epidemiology

Cervical radiculopathy represents dysfunction of the cervical nerve root that typically presents with radiating pain in the upper extremity and varying degrees of sensory loss, motor weakness, and reflex changes. Population-based studies have shown an annual incidence of 107/100,000 men and 64/100,000 women, with a peak incidence in the sixth decade of life. About 15% of patients report an antecedent episode of physical exertion or trauma that precedes symptom onset. The majority of the cases stem from compression of nerve roots in the lower cervical spine (C4-T1), likely due to greater segmental mobility and smaller neuroforamina in this region.

A. Bhalla (✉)
Department of Orthopaedic Surgery, Brigham and Women's Hospital, Harvard Medical School, 75 Francis St, Boston, MA 02115, USA

Department of Orthopaedic Surgery, Harbor-UCLA Medical Center, 1000 West Carson Street, Box 422, Torrance, CA 90509, USA
e-mail: amandeep.bhalla@gmail.com

J.D. Kang
Department of Orthopaedic Surgery, Brigham and Women's Hospital, Harvard Medical School, 75 Francis St, Boston, MA 02115, USA
e-mail: jdkang@partners.org

© Springer International Publishing AG 2018
J.N. Katz et al. (eds.), *Principles of Orthopedic Practice for Primary Care Providers*, https://doi.org/10.1007/978-3-319-68661-5_2

Clinical Presentation

Cervical radiculopathy is usually the result of neuroforaminal stenosis due to herniated disc material or overgrowth of the uncovertebral joints anteriorly or facet joints posteriorly. It can manifest with pain, sensory disturbances, diminished reflexes, and muscle weakness that correspond to the affected nerve root. A general understanding of the myotomes and dermatomes of the cervical spine aids in the diagnosis (Fig. 2.1). However, radicular symptoms do not always follow a predictable pattern of the affected root, and the type and intensity of symptoms vary widely. Some patients complain of less specific upper trapezial and interscapular pain or discomfort about the shoulder girdle. There may also be more than a single nerve root involved, or anatomic variations in innervation, such that symptoms seem to cross over dermatomes and/or myotomes. Radiculopathy may also be present in the bilateral upper extremities and can exist concurrently in patients with myelopathy.

The physical exam, performed in a systematic root-specific manner, can elucidate sensory disturbances, motor deficits, and diminished reflexes. Pain and sensory changes in the affected root distribution are more commonly seen, while motor

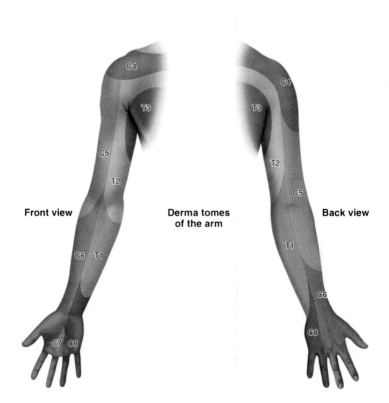

Fig. 2.1 Map of the most common anatomic distribution of cervical dermatomes and myotomes in the arm. The C5 through C8 levels are most frequently affected by radiculopathy

weakness and reflex changes are encountered less often. The examiner can sometimes reproduce radicular pain by performing the Spurling's test, where the patient extends the neck and bends it toward the affected side. This maneuver narrows the neuroforamina and causes root impingement. As a corollary, patients often endorse relief of radicular symptoms when they sleep with their arm overhead, which enlarges the neuroforamina and decreases root compression. One must examine the shoulder with various maneuvers (refer to shoulder chapter) to rule out intrinsic shoulder pathology which can mimic or coexist with cervical radiculopathy. Shoulder pain that seems to localize anteriorly is generally intrinsic to that joint, but shoulder pain that localizes to the posterior scapular region is typically referred from the cervical spine.

For any patient presenting with cervical radiculopathy, care must be taken to screen for concurrent myelopathy. Part of the history should include inquiry about changes in gait, manual dexterity while performing fine motor tasks, and bowel and bladder incontinence. Screening for myelopathy should also include an examination for the presence of long tract signs, including tests for positive Hoffman or Babinski signs, as well as clonus or an inverted brachioradialis reflex. A more detailed discussion of the evaluation for myelopathy will be discussed in a later section.

Differential Diagnosis and Diagnostic Testing

The diagnosis of cervical radiculopathy is typically made using clinical history and physical exam alone, without the need for imaging or special tests. The differential diagnosis for radicular symptomatology includes peripheral nerve entrapment, brachial plexus injury, and tendinopathies (shoulder and elbow) of the upper extremity. Some patients will present with a neck-shoulder syndrome where pathology coexists at both anatomic locations. Hence they will have both radicular features and intrinsic shoulder pain (rotator cuff pathology) with certain maneuvers and therefore can often be confusing to the clinician. Patients should also be screened for "red flags," such as unexplained weight loss, fever, intravenous drug abuse, and history of previous cancer, which may suggest the possibility of infection or tumor.

Cervical radiculopathy can exist concurrently with peripheral neuropathy, a so-called double crush syndrome, where there is pathologic compression at more than one location along the course of a peripheral nerve. This may present a diagnostic challenge. For example, a patient with carpal tunnel syndrome may also have a C6 radiculopathy, both of which might result in a similar distribution of numbness and sensory deficits. In patients with carpal tunnel syndrome, it is helpful to inquire if symptoms radiate from the neck and to perform a provocative Spurling's test to assess for radiculopathy. By screening patients in this manner, fewer cases of double crush syndrome would go undiagnosed, and patients would benefit from timely treatment of both the cervical radiculopathy and peripheral nerve compression. Interestingly, the diagnosis of double crush syndrome is often made when patients are dissatisfied with the outcomes of a carpal tunnel release, presumably because of coexisting C6 radiculopathy.

Because the diagnosis is reliably made clinically and the natural history is usually self-limiting, it is reasonable to limit the use of diagnostic imaging until patients have been symptomatic for 4–6 weeks. The imaging helps to confirm the diagnosis and to facilitate treatment. Of course, if there is a concern for infection or tumor, diagnostic imaging should be obtained expeditiously. Plain anteroposterior and lateral cervical radiographs are of limited diagnostic value, but they do demonstrate overall cervical alignment and the extent of degeneration as evidenced by intervertebral disc height loss and osteophyte formation. Magnetic resonance imaging (MRI) is the study of choice for cervical radiculopathy. MRI provides detail of the neural elements and surrounding soft tissue structures (Fig. 2.2a, b). When an MRI is contraindicated, a computed tomography (CT)-myelogram can be useful to show focal areas of compression.

Results from MRI should be interpreted cautiously given the high sensitivity for detecting abnormalities. It is well established that asymptomatic patients have a high incidence of positive MRI findings, so areas of nerve root compression must be correlated with clinical findings. From a surgeon's perspective, it is ideal when there is correlation between anatomic abnormalities on neuroradiographic studies, patients' symptoms, and physical exam findings. In cases where imaging studies are equivocal, selective nerve root injections at the suspected level of involvement can be both diagnostic and therapeutic. Furthermore, electromyography studies and nerve conduction tests can be used adjunctively when patient's history and physical exam are inadequate to differentiate cervical radiculopathy from other neurologic causes of pain. For example, the presence of abnormal insertional activity in the paraspinal musculature can differentiate cervical radiculopathy from brachial plexopathy. These studies should be interpreted in the context of the clinical exam and radiographic findings and can effectively rule out other sites of compression. When concomitant shoulder pain coexists and the clinical exam would suggest an intrinsic shoulder problem, an MRI of the shoulder may also be considered to clarify the diagnosis.

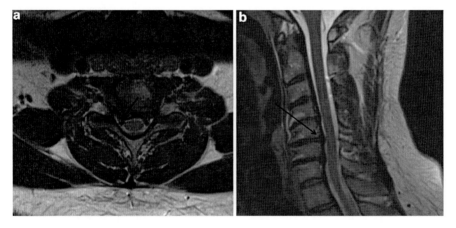

Fig. 2.2 Axial (**a**) and sagittal (**b**) magnetic resonance images (MRI) of a disc process at C5–C6 causing a right-sided radiculopathy (*black arrows*)

Nonoperative Management

Nonsurgical management is the mainstay of treatment for cervical radiculopathy. There is a lack of well-established nonsurgical treatment guidelines based on high-quality scientific evidence, and much of conservative treatment is centered on anecdotal experience. In the setting of herniated disc material, chemical inflammatory mediators are thought to significantly contribute to radicular pain. These properties make oral anti-inflammatory medications an efficacious first-line treatment. Narcotics should rarely be prescribed for routine analgesia but can be considered on occasion for breakthrough pain or in patients who cannot tolerate NSAIDs. Some patients benefit from a multimodal analgesic regimen, which may include muscle relaxants, antidepressants, and gabapentin. For symptoms that are unresponsive to anti-inflammatories, in patients without medical contraindications, an oral tapered steroid regimen may also be prescribed.

Postural education, improved ergonomics, and lifestyle modification help to improve functional capacity. Patients are encouraged to mobilize early and to participate in physical therapy once pain has subsided. There is no proven role for immobilization or bed rest. Nonimpact aerobic exercises such as stationary biking can help relieve symptoms and maintain fitness. Some patients also derive temporary relief from intermittent home traction, which temporarily enlarges the neuroforamina and decompresses the exiting roots. Traction is not advised in patients with myelopathy, since lengthening the spinal column across an area of cord compression can be dangerous.

For persistent symptoms that have not been adequately relieved by oral analgesics and functional rehabilitation, epidural corticosteroid injections can be considered. Epidural corticosteroid injections offer a powerful, locally concentrated anti-inflammatory effect. Selective nerve root blocks more specifically target the perineural space surrounding the affected root and avoid the spinal canal. Although relatively safe, epidural injections are invasive and come with risks, which include but are not limited to dural puncture, epidural hematoma, and epidural abscess. Conservative management should be continued for 6–8 weeks since the natural history of most cervical radiculopathy is for spontaneous pain resolution within 80–90% of patients.

Indications for Surgery

While conservative management is the predominant treatment for this typically self-limiting condition, there are cases where surgery is warranted and largely beneficial. Ideal surgical candidates have neuroradiographic evidence of root impingement, with corresponding root dysfunction, and persistence of symptoms despite several months of conservative care. Functionally significant motor deficits and debilitating radicular symptoms not responsive to conservative measures are indications for earlier surgical intervention. Subtle motor weakness which can be seen in early acute radiculopathy is often due to inflammation and pain and should spontaneously resolve with conservative management. However, if the weakness persists or progresses and leads to early muscle atrophy, the patient should be referred to a spine specialist for closer surveillance.

Operative Management and Expected Outcomes

Anteriorly based pathology such as soft and hard disc herniations are the most common causes of cervical radiculopathy. The majority of patients are treated with an anterior cervical discectomy and fusion (ACDF). The anterior approach allows excellent exposure of the cervical spine and involves removal of the offending disc. It is muscle sparing and involves minimal blood loss. Once the discectomy is performed, the posterior longitudinal ligament can be resected, offering direct visualization of the dura and exiting nerve roots. Fashioned iliac crest autograft, bone-banked allograft, or an interbody device is placed in the decompressed interspace to impart stability and to promote bony fusion across the motion segments. The interbody graft restores intervertebral height and indirectly expands the neuroforaminal space. Advantages of the anterior approach include access to both central and lateral disc herniations, low infection and wound complication rates, and relatively minimal postoperative pain. The major disadvantages of ACDF are the risks for nonunion at the fusion site and persistent speech and swallowing difficulties due to retraction of the esophagus and laryngeal nerves.

Some patients may elect to have a cervical disc arthroplasty instead of an ACDF. The approach and manner of decompression are essentially similar to that for a fusion, except an artificial disc is placed in the interspace. The theoretical advantage of cervical disc arthroplasty (CDA) is preservation of motion at the surgical level, potentially mitigating the risk of adjacent segment disease and subsequent need for reoperation. It also eliminates the risk for pseudarthrosis. ACDF and CDA have been shown to have essentially equivalent patient-reported outcomes in shorter-term clinical trials (2–7 years); however, debate persists regarding CDA's effectiveness in decreasing adjacent segment disease and reoperation rate. Cervical adjacent segment disease is believed to occur at an annual incidence of about 3%, regardless of the surgery performed, and it is unclear if this is a consequence of fusion or due to the natural history of disc degeneration. The long-term mechanical durability and clinical outcomes data for cervical disc arthroplasty have also not yet been realized, since it's a relatively new technology.

A posterior approach involving a laminoforaminotomy can be used to address anterolateral disc herniations or foraminal stenosis. The posterior approach to the spine involves dissection through the muscular raphe in the midline of the neck. Direct access to the compressed nerve root is achieved with removal of bone from the overlying facet and lamina, without destabilizing the motion segment. Proponents of the posterior laminoforaminotomy value the direct visualization of the nerve root and avoidance of fusion and its attendant complications. Drawbacks of this procedure include inability to restore foraminal height with an interbody graft, as well as risk for recurrence as degenerative changes ensue. A high rate of clinical success is to be expected for surgical decompression of the cervical nerve roots, regardless of approach, with reported relief of arm pain and improvements in motor and sensory function appreciated by more than 80% of patients.

Cervical Myelopathy and Myeloradiculopathy

Definition and Epidemiology

Cervical spondylotic myelopathy is the most common cause of spinal cord dysfunction in adults, and its incidence is likely underreported. Cervical spondylotic myelopathy results from age-associated degenerative changes to structures about the spinal cord, including disc degeneration, ligamentous hypertrophy, and osseous changes. These anatomic changes encroach upon the spinal canal and can lead to direct compression of the cord. Congenital spinal stenosis anatomically predisposes the development of cervical myelopathy. Patients with cervical spondylotic myelopathy have a much greater risk for spinal cord injury. Primary care physicians play an important role in the management of cervical myelopathy, as early detection and prompt referral for surgical evaluation can greatly improve patient outcomes.

Clinical Presentation

The pathophysiologic effects of spinal cord compression are thought to be a combination of direct mechanical effects on the neural tissue and related alterations in vascular supply. Presenting symptoms can include gait instability, diminished manual dexterity, motor weakness, sensory loss, incontinence, and permanent functional disability. The spectrum of disease severity and variation in symptomatology are commensurate with the many different manners in which the spinal cord can be functionally compromised by compression. For example, pathology that affects the dorsal column may predominantly manifest with proprioceptive loss in the extremities. The clinical course of cervical spondylotic myelopathy is marked by periods of neurologic stability with stepwise deterioration of neurologic function.

A thorough history and physical exam helps to illicit subtle cues of spinal cord dysfunction. Patients may endorse changes in their gait, demonstrate instability on exam, and have difficulty with heel-to-toe walking more than a few steps. Patients may also report difficulty performing fine motor tasks, like buttoning a shirt or using chopsticks. The examiner can test hand dexterity with the grip and release test, where patients rapidly open and close their hands while being timed. Patients are normally able to do this about 20 times in 10 s. This test of manual dexterity can be used to survey stability of neurologic function over time. Additional evidence of spinal cord dysfunction occurs with extension of the neck causing an electrical shocklike sensation to shoot down the spine, the so-called Lhermitte's sign. This maneuver dynamically decreases the space available for the spinal cord and exacerbates symptoms.

Patients may also exhibit long tract signs, which are indicative of damage to the corticospinal tracts. The Hoffman's reflex, for example, should raise concern for cervical myelopathy when positive. To test this the examiner flicks the distal phalanx of the index or middle finger, and a positive finding is seen with flexion of the distal phalanx of the thumb. Other clinical findings of upper motor neuron dysfunction include an extensor plantar response known as the Babinski sign, where firmly stroking the lateral border of the foot results in extension of the great toe.

It is important to note that the absence of upper motor neuron signs (i.e., hyperreflexia, Hoffman sign, inverted brachioradialis reflex, clonus, and Babinski) does not preclude the diagnosis of myelopathy. The presence of long tract signs is not highly sensitive, and patients with unequivocal cervical myelopathy may in fact manifest no such signs. Up to one-fifth of patients who otherwise are myelopathic on the basis of history, correlative advanced imaging, and subjective improvement after decompression do not have long tract signs on presentation. Certain coexisting conditions can diminish the reliability of long tract signs in detecting spinal cord dysfunction. For example, in patients with myeloradiculopathy, concurrent radiculopathy can diminish the transmission of long tract signs. Diabetes, through its affect on peripheral nerves, is also thought to have a dampening effect on the transmission of neurologic reflexes. A higher index of suspicion for myelopathy should be had for patients with diabetic peripheral neuropathy. Even in the absence of long tract signs, concerning clinical symptoms combined with correlative imaging studies should guide treatment decisions.

It is advisable for primary care physicians to remain vigilant for cervical myelopathy even in patients presenting with lumbar spine symptoms, such as neurogenic claudication and radiculopathy. A red flag symptom of gait instability should immediately stoke concern for concomitant cervical myelopathy. Interestingly, it is not an uncommon presenting clinical scenario for patients with primarily low back symptomatology to have an underlying myelopathy. In fact, there is a relatively frequent coexistence of lumbar and cervical spinal stenosis. A focused lower extremity exam may not illicit positive long tract signs, since concomitant lumbar spinal stenosis may dampen CNS signal transmission. It is therefore appropriate to screen patients presenting with lumbar spinal stenosis for concomitant cervical myelopathy by thoroughly examining both the upper and lower extremities.

Differential Diagnosis and Diagnostic Testing

The differential diagnosis for cervical myelopathy includes other central nervous system disorders as well as neuropathy and the long-term effects of alcohol abuse or certain vitamin deficiencies. When cervical myelopathy is suspected, upright plain radiographs are used to assess for alignment, segmental stability, and degree of degeneration. The condition of the spinal cord and influence of surrounding structures are evaluated with an MRI or CT-myelogram in cases where MRI is contraindicated (Fig. 2.3). The patient should be referred to a spine surgeon to discuss treatment options and establish care for routine surveillance.

Fig. 2.3 Sagittal MR image demonstrating severe spinal stenosis and myelomalacia (*black arrow*) at the level of C3–C4 in a patient with cervical spondylotic myelopathy

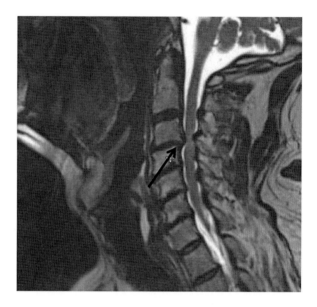

Nonoperative Management

Although surgical decompression of cervical myelopathy is the only manner in which the natural history of the disease can be altered, not all patients desire to undergo surgery. Many patients function well with mild forms of myelopathy and remain neurologically stable for years. However, there is always a risk for functional decline, which patients should reasonably be made aware of. A treatment plan is formulated between the care team and the patient after discussing the risks and benefits of surgery versus expectant management. Medical comorbidities such as diabetes, significant cardiac or renal disease, and advanced age may sway the balance of surgical risks and benefits toward nonoperative care.

There is no role for injections in patients with cervical spondylotic myelopathy. Physical therapy may improve the functional capacity of the patient, but will not alter the natural history of the disease. Anti-inflammatory medications and neuromodulators may help to alleviate radicular symptoms when simultaneously present. In general, when patients present with myelopathy, it is advised that the patient be referred to a spine specialist for consideration of surgery.

Indications for Surgery

The goal of surgery is to decompress the spinal cord and arrest further neurologic decline. The thought process surrounding decompression is that the patient is far less likely to worsen in the absence of ongoing cord compression, and this is overwhelmingly the case. Indeed, some patients experience improvement of neurologic symptoms postoperatively. Others may experience further deterioration, even after a successful decompression, but these patients are in the minority. The most common etiology for neurologic decline after an adequate decompression is the development of a new, adjacent focus of cord compression.

Patients may elect to defer surgery when there is mild evidence of spinal cord dysfunction, though this is not without some risk. It is difficult to predict which patients will have stable disease without decompression and which are at risk for further progression. These patients can be screened at regular intervals for evidence of neurologic decline. Such deterioration may be subtle, and it is advantageous for patients to be followed by the same physician over time. Evidence of decline should be indicative of the capacity for progression and once again prompt a discussion regarding surgery. Patients with more pronounced or progressive clinical findings, and/or evidence of severe cord compression, should consider surgical intervention as soon as is reasonably possible. These patients are likely to be at greater risk for further functional decline, with the possibility of a devastating spinal cord injury in the event of a traumatic event that stresses a spinal cord that is already compromised.

Operative Management and Expected Outcomes

Anterior, posterior, and combined surgical approaches may be utilized, depending on a variety of factors, including anatomic location of the compression, alignment of the spine, and consideration of distinct complications associated with each approach. Decompression is the chief goal of surgery, and selection of the approach is performed with this priority in mind. In the lordotic cervical spine, in the setting of ventral compression, a posterior laminectomy can effectively allow the cord to freely float away dorsally. The most commonly used posterior surgical technique is a laminectomy and instrumented fusion. This involves removal of the posterior lamina and segmental instrumented fusion. Advantages of this include the potential for wide decompression, stabilization to prevent subsequent post-laminectomy kyphosis, and fusion to improve pain related to spondylosis. Laminoplasty, an alternative technique, expands the diameter of the spinal canal by expanding the lamina only on one side. Laminoplasty directly decompresses posterior impinging structures and indirectly decompresses the ventral cord. Advantages of this procedure include maintained segmental distribution of axial and rotational forces and preservation of motion. This is a reasonable option in patients with poor biologic potential for bony fusion.

An anterior approach can directly address anterior pathology, such as a central disc herniation. This approach involves discectomy or corpectomy (Fig. 2.4), depending in part on the location and extent of anterior pathology. It is particularly useful when ventral compression exists in the setting of neutral or kyphotic cervical spine alignment, precluding the possibility of indirect decompression with a posterior procedure. Both anterior and posterior approaches are effective in improving patients' quality of life and have comparable outcomes. Posterior approaches have a higher rate of complications, particularly infection or wound breakdown.

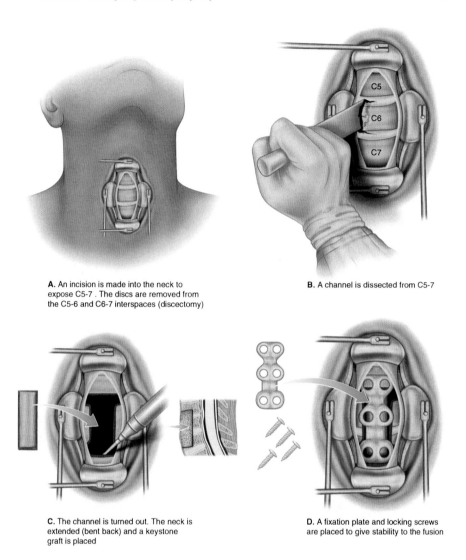

A. An incision is made into the neck to expose C5-7 . The discs are removed from the C5-6 and C6-7 interspaces (discectomy)

B. A channel is dissected from C5-7

C. The channel is turned out. The neck is extended (bent back) and a keystone graft is placed

D. A fixation plate and locking screws are placed to give stability to the fusion

Fig. 2.4 Depiction of an anterior cervical approach with corpectomy and reconstruction using a strut graft, anterior plate, and instrumentation

Ultimately, the success of the surgery is most closely linked to the adequacy of the spinal cord decompression. Surgical intervention has a better prognosis if patients with myelopathy are treated at an earlier clinical stage before severe spasticity or loss of ambulatory function occurs. Once the spinal cord undergoes irreversible chronic changes, the surgical goal is to prevent further neurologic deterioration since full recovery is often a challenge.

Table 2.1 is a synopsis of presentation, diagnostic testing, and treatment options for patients with cervical radiculopathy or myelopathy.

Table 2.1 Synopsis of presentation, diagnostic testing, and treatment options for patients with cervical radiculopathy or myelopathy

Clinical entity	Presentation	Diagnostic testing	Conservative management	Indications for surgery	Operative management
Cervical radiculopathy	– Radiating pain, with possible sensory deficits, and motor weakness in the distribution of the affected nerve root	– MRI or CT-myelogram	– Physical therapy – Anti-inflammatory medications	– Radicular symptoms refractory to conservative management – Significant motor weakness	– Anterior cervical discectomy and fusion – Cervical disc arthroplasty – Posterior laminoforaminotomy
Cervical myelopathy	– Gait instability, diminished fine motor dexterity, sensory deficits and motor weakness, hyperreflexia, bowel and/or bladder incontinence	– MRI or CT-myelogram	– Generally not advocated – Counseling about risks of disease progression – Routine surveillance of neurologic function	– Myelopathy in the setting of static or dynamic spinal cord compression	– Anterior cervical discectomy/corpectomy and fusion – Posterior cervical decompression and instrumented fusion – Posterior cervical laminoplasty

MRI magnetic resonance imaging, *CT* computed tomography

Suggested Reading

Carette S, Fehlings MG. Clinical practice. Cervical radiculopathy. N Engl J Med. 2005;353(4):392–9. https://doi.org/10.1056/NEJMcp043887.

Lebl DR, Bono CM. Update on the diagnosis and management of cervical spondylotic myelopathy. J Am Acad Orthop Surg. 2015;23(11):648–60. https://doi.org/10.5435/jaaos-d-14-00250.

Molinari WJ 3rd, Elfar JC. The double crush syndrome. J Hand Surg Am. 2013;38(4):799–801; quiz 801. https://doi.org/10.1016/j.jhsa.2012.12.038.

Rhee JM, Heflin JA, Hamasaki T, Freedman B. Prevalence of physical signs in cervical myelopathy: a prospective, controlled study. Spine (Phila Pa 1976). 2009;34(9):890–5. https://doi.org/10.1097/BRS.0b013e31819c944b.

Rhee JM, Yoon T, Riew KD. Cervical radiculopathy. J Am Acad Orthop Surg. 2007;15(8):486–94.

Part III
Lumbar Spine

Chapter 3
Lumbar Disc Herniation and Radiculopathy

Christopher M. Bono

Abbreviations

CSF   Cerebrospinal fluid
EMG   Electromyograph
MMPI   Minnesota Multiphasic Personality Inventory

Definition and Epidemiology

Lumbar disc herniations with radiculopathy are common. Most believe them to be a point along the so-called degenerative cascade, which spans from mild internal disorganization of the disc to advanced osteophyte formation, also known as spondylosis. However, disc herniations can also occur in very young individuals. Considering the body of literature devoted to disc herniations in the pediatric population, it would be hard to imagine that degenerative changes have occurred in such young patients. In the end, the situational components needed for herniation are a loss of structural integrity of the outer layer, termed the annulus fibrosus (or annulus for short), and an abrupt increase in intradiscal pressure that exceeds the threshold at which the inner portion of the disc (nucleus pulposus) is contained. This can be the result of a high-impact mechanism, such as a sports injury, or something as mundane as a sneeze. In many, if not most cases, there is no recognizable point of "injury," with symptoms developing without clear incident.

The prevalence of symptomatic herniated discs has been estimated to be about 1–3%. For a variety of postulated reasons, they are more common in persons aged 30–50 years old, with a male predilection. In this age category, the nucleus is still fairly well hydrated yet associated with an increasing prevalence of annular tears. This is coincident with a disproportionately higher prevalence of more physically demanding jobs in men. There are some anatomical location differences that have been appreciated, with younger patients more frequently

C.M. Bono (✉)
Department of Orthopaedic Surgery, Harvard Medical School, Brigham and Women's
Hospital, Boston, MA, USA
e-mail: cbono@partners.org

© Springer International Publishing AG 2018
J.N. Katz et al. (eds.), *Principles of Orthopedic Practice for Primary Care
Providers*, https://doi.org/10.1007/978-3-319-68661-5_3

presenting with lower lumbar disc herniations (L4-5, L5-S1), while upper lumbar disc herniations (L2-3, L3-L4) are more common in older individuals.

Clinical Presentation

The hallmark of clinical presentation of a lumbar disc herniation is radicular lower extremity pain. In its most classic and straightforward form, a patient's pain would closely follow the distribution of a single-lower lumbar nerve root. For example, a patient with an L5-S1 right-sided paracentral (i.e., not immediately in the midline, but slightly off to one side) herniation should complain of pain in the S1 distribution, which can extend from the buttock, down the posterior calf, and into the lateral plantar surface of the foot. In reality, patient's complaints vary considerably and do not always follow such discrete dermatomal patterns.

Patients can also complain of varying degrees of numbness and weakness, while neither is requisite for the clinical diagnosis. Again, these complaints ideally follow a specific nerve root distribution. Using the example from above, the patient might complain of push-off weakness on the right side with ambulation, a manifestation of diminished strength of plantarflexion, controlled by the S1 nerve root. Similarly, there may be a complaint of numbness along the lateral and plantar surface of the foot on the affected side.

When evaluating a patient with a suspected lumbar disc herniation, it is important to note any events leading up to the current endorsement of symptoms as well as the patient's prior musculoskeletal health status. It is not uncommon for patients to have a history of a short period of prodromal back pain immediately preceding the complaint of leg pain. It is presumed that this is the time at which the disc herniation actually occurs, an event that may cause back pain secondary to the expansion of an annular tear. Leg symptoms are not immediately noted in many cases, even in the presence of large disc herniations with substantial nerve root compression. This phenomenon is perhaps explained by the fact that acute compression of a nerve root does not result in pain. It requires enduring compression and the onset of inflammation. It is also important to note if the patient has had a long history of recurrent or chronic back pain episodes. It is critical to delineate these prior events from the current episode of radicular pain, as it is the latter that will be the focus of current treatment and will have the highest likelihood resolving.

Patients with a lumbar disc herniation and radiculopathy should be differentiated from those with spinal stenosis and neurogenic claudication. With the former, patients will have unremitting, radiating lower extremity pain. This is not relieved by sitting and is more often aggravated by it. Lying supine and sleeping can be equally troubling. In the exam room, lumbar disc herniation patients usually prefer to stand and report that walking, and even running, is more comfortable for them. In contrast, patients with lumbar stenosis and neurogenic claudication are most comfortable at rest, either sitting or lying down. They experience the most pain when they ambulate distances, feeling relief by flexing forward or sitting for a short period of time. Patients should be asked about bowel and bladder incontinence and perianal anesthesia. Though exceedingly rare, these complaints can indicate the presence of a cauda equina syndrome, which should be urgently evaluated and treated if indeed present.

The physical examination of an affected patient should consist of a detailed motor and sensory assessment of the lower extremities. The patella tendon (L3/4) and Achilles (S1) tendon reflexes should also be evaluated. Isolated, unilateral loss of one of the reflexes can be a sign of nerve root compression from a disc herniation. There are some provocative maneuvers that can also be helpful in establishing the clinical diagnosis. With the patient lying supine, a straight leg raise test can be performed by elevating the extremity with the knee extended. The test is considered positive if radicular leg pain is reproduced with 30–70° of hip flexion on the affected side. The same test can be performed on the contralateral side and, if positive, will reproduce pain on the ipsilateral lower extremity. This is a very specific, but not sensitive, physical exam finding for a lower lumbar disc herniation. Straight leg raises may also be performed with the patient seated on an exam table. Upper lumbar disc herniations may be associated with a positive femoral stretch test, which is performed with the patient supine and the examiner slowly raising the lower leg with knee flexion. Radicular pain in the thigh is considered positive.

The patient's gait should be observed during evaluation as well. While gait can be affected simply by pain, a Trendelenburg sign may also be present, noted as the hip sagging on the affected side, a result of hip abductor weakness. A foot drop may also be noted in certain scenarios. Patients often compensate for this by "high stepping" to accommodate for the lack of ability to dorsiflex the foot.

Differential Diagnosis and Suggested Diagnostic Testing

The differential diagnosis of radiating lower extremity pain is wide. It can be related to any process that causes nerve root or cauda equina compression, such as spinal stenosis, tumor, abscess, or epidural lipomatosis (an accumulation of fat inside the spinal canal). Processes such as infection or neoplasm can be associated with so-called red flag signs and constitutional symptoms (e.g., fever, night sweats, weight loss, malaise). Peripheral nerve entrapment can also present similarly. This can occur in the pelvis within the piriformis fossa, about the knee (most commonly near the fibular head where the common peroneal nerve is most vulnerable), or even in the lower leg. Nonneural causes should also be considered, such as vascular insufficiency, which can present with similar radicular-like leg pain.

In the primary care setting, obtaining plain films of the lumbar spine in a patient with a suspected lumbar disc herniation is generally of low yield. Disc herniation cannot be visualized on plain films. In addition, they are not highly sensitive for ruling out other more concerning pathology, such as tumor or infection. Plain films have a potential role in preoperative planning, as spinal alignment and other morphological variations may influence surgical decision-making. However, these can be deferred until a decision for surgery has been reached.

A non-contrast enhanced MRI is the imaging modality of choice for the detection of lumbar disc herniation (Fig. 3.1). It provides superior visualization of the soft tissues, ligaments, discs, neural elements, and spinal fluid. Furthermore, it is highly sensitive for the presence of tumor or infections. It must be appreciated, however, that the prevalence of disc herniations is not insubstantial in asymptomatic individuals. One classic study found a 20% prevalence of disc herniations in an asymptomatic population less than 60 years old. The use of contrast should be reserved for those with particular findings on a non-contrast enhanced MRI, such as the presence of a suspected neoplastic lesion. Some feel that contrast-enhanced studies are necessary in patients who have had previous lumbar surgery; however, this has been contested. CT myelography is a reasonable advanced imaging study. However, this should be reserved for patients who have a clear contraindication to MRI.

Electrodiagnostic studies, such as electromyographs (EMGs) and nerve conduction studies, are rarely needed in the routine work-up of a lumbar disc herniation. Such tests should be reserved for patients in whom the diagnosis is unclear or concomitant

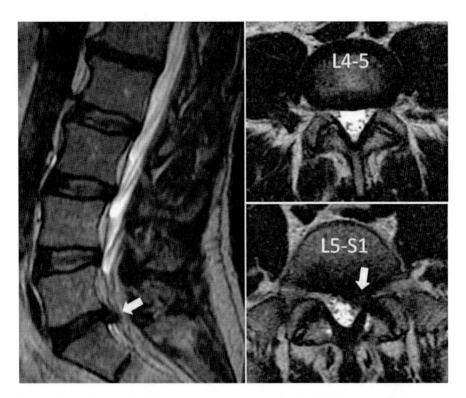

Fig. 3.1 Sagittal and axial MR images of a patient with a left-sided L5-S1 paracentral disc herniation (*white arrows*). MRI is the diagnostic modality of choice as it clearly demonstrates the distinction between neural elements, disc, and ligamentous structures

non-spinal pathology is suspected. It may also have a role delineating the most symptomatic level in a patient with multiple sites of nerve root compression.

Nonoperative Management

Nonoperative management of radiculopathy should begin with nonnarcotic analgesic medications for pain control. Nonsteroidal anti-inflammatory medications and acetaminophen should be considered first-line agents. Patients should be encouraged to be as mobile as possible. There is strong evidence that more than 3 days of bed rest can perpetuate back pain; this association can be reasonably extrapolated to patients with radicular pain as well. Oral steroids should be reserved for patients in excruciating pain that is severely limiting their ability to ambulate and function. Neuroleptic medications, such as gabapentin or pregabalin, can also be used to specifically target neuropathic pain.

Education is perhaps the most overlooked component of nonoperative care. Affected individuals should be informed of the generally favorable natural history of this condition. There is an approximate 90% chance of resolution or improvement of symptoms (to the point of avoiding surgery) within 3 months of onset following nonoperative care. Many individuals, in fact, likely have disc herniations with radicular pain, ascribed to a bout of "sciatica," that resolves within a couple of weeks without any formal nonoperative care or physician evaluation. In the absence of progressive neurological deficits or cauda equina syndrome, nonoperative care appears to be safe.

If a patient has had persistent radicular symptoms that have not improved within a couple of weeks of pharmacological management, physical therapy can be initiated. While most physical therapists will perform an initial evaluation, review imaging reports, and develop a specific treatment plan, the prescription ideally should request range of motion exercises and stretching. Core strengthening is a common component of physical therapy as well. Therapy is usually performed two to three times per week for 4–6 weeks.

There is also a role for epidural steroid injections for the treatment of lumbar disc herniations. These are usually not used as a first-line nonoperative treatment. Injections should be reserved for those patients who have not responded to pharmacological and physical therapy. Spinal injections can be performed by anesthesia pain physicians, physiatrists, interventional radiologists, or surgeons. There are a variety of specific injections that can be performed, with the injectionist deciding among them based on the type of herniation. A reasonable protocol for injections is as follows. After an initial injection is performed, it may take 1–2 weeks for the steroid to take effect. If leg pain resolves, there is little indication for another injection. If there is little or fair response to the first injection, a second may be attempted. Again, if the pain resolves, there is scant justification for a third injection. More so, if two injections failed to be beneficial, there is really no indication for a third attempt.

Indications for Surgery

Surgery can be electively performed in a patient who has failed a 6–12-week course of nonoperative care. In the author's practice, a decision about surgery is usually held until the 3-month mark from the onset of symptoms. An implied prerequisite for surgery is, of course, signs and symptoms that are concordant with imaging findings of a lumbar disc herniation. An indication for surgery earlier than 6 weeks would be if a patient has a progressive deficit or a functionally limiting deficit, such as a foot drop that is impeding ambulation. Substantial canal compromise due to the size of the herniation (Fig. 3.2), which may manifest as cauda equina syndrome, is also an indication for more urgent surgical intervention.

While there is a general sense that, if possible, patients should avoid spinal surgery as long as possible, this can potentially be detrimental to those with lumbar disc herniations. There is evidence that those undergoing surgery within 6–9 months of symptom onset have superior outcomes as compared to those who wait longer. The exact mechanism for this relationship is not well understood, though it is logical that long-standing compression and vascular compromise may increase the likelihood of permanent neuropathic pain.

Fig. 3.2 Sagittal MR image of a patient with a large disc herniation at L5-S1 causing near complete occlusion of the spinal canal. Such a scenario may manifest as cauda equina syndrome

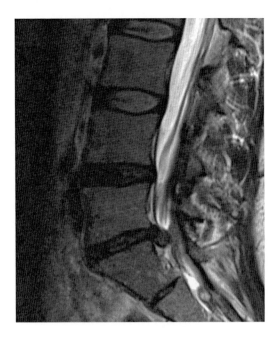

Operative Management

A lumbar discectomy can be performed using a variety of techniques. The gold standard is an open procedure, sometimes termed as microlumbar discectomy, microscopic discectomy, or simply a discectomy. By definition, a microscopic procedure is performed using an operating microscope. This does not imply that it is performed in a more minimally invasive manner or with a smaller incision. In reality, a standard open lumbar discectomy can usually be performed through a relatively small incision (4–5 cm). Tubular retractors can also be used to gain exposure and perform the surgery. It is the author's preference to perform a standard open procedure using magnifying loupes.

The patient is positioned prone after endotracheal intubation with general anesthesia on an operating Table. A small portion of the lamina above and below and part of the medial facet joint at the operative level are removed. The ligamentum flavum is then excised to allow access to the spinal canal. The descending nerve root is retracted toward the midline, which usually reveals the disc herniation (Fig. 3.3). The herniated fragment is mobilized from the surrounding soft tissues using a variety of blunt instruments. The fragment can then be removed using a grasping instrument.

Expected Outcomes

Surgical treatment of lumbar disc herniations is among the most satisfying for both surgeon and patient. In general, the chance of a successful outcome is about 80–90%. It is very important, however, to accurately characterize what "success" means to the patient prior to surgery. Based on the best available evidence, a patient can expect an 80–90% chance that leg pain (which includes buttock pain) and everyday function will substantially improve. It is clear from available data that back pain *may* improve but that it does so much less reliably than leg pain. In the authors' practice, he is reluctant to perform surgery if the primary complaint is low back pain.

Patients often present with complaints of paresthesias, numbness, and weakness. It is equally important to explain that these are not as reliably improved with surgery as pain and function. There are a number of studies that have demonstrated that measurable strength deficits often do not improve following a discectomy. Regarding numbness, it has been the author's experience that intermittent, subjective numbness has a better chance of resolving than persistent anesthesia. Discussion of these tendencies is critically important prior to surgery as patients often intuitively expect that any neurological deficits will be immediately reversed postoperatively.

It is important to recognize a number of factors that can influence surgical outcomes. It has been long thought that larger disc herniations are associated with better outcomes. More recent work has not supported this but instead has reported that the volume of herniated disc removed at surgery is more important.

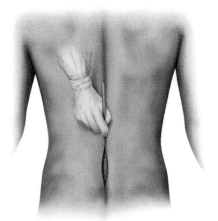

A. An incision is made over the lumbar spine from the spinous process of L4 to S1

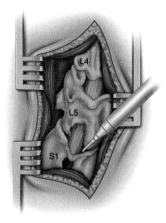

B. A left sided laminectomy is done at L5-S1 to extend the operative window

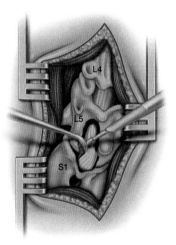

C. The posterior longitudinal ligament is removed to expose the neural elements (spinal cord and L5 root)

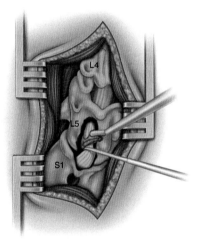

D. The neural elements are retracted medially and the herniated portion of the L5-S1 disc is removed

Fig. 3.3 After the ligamentum flavum has been removed, the descending nerve root and cauda equina are identified and retracted toward the midline. This usually reveals the annulus of the disc and the herniation. The herniated fragment is mobilized from the surrounding soft tissues and removed with a grasping instrument such as a pituitary rongeur

There is conflicting data regarding the relationship between the anatomical level or location of the herniation and surgical outcomes.

The effect of psychosocial factors on the outcomes of disc herniations cannot be overstated. Among a variety of factors assessed, one study found psychological status as measured by the Minnesota Multiphasic Personality Inventory (MMPI) to be the most predictive of surgical outcomes. Other studies have corroborated these results, with additional factors such as self-confidence and optimism to be associated with superior surgical results. Conversely, patients receiving workers' compensation are less likely to report favorable outcomes following discectomy.

There are a number of complications that can occur during or after lumbar discectomy, with infection among the most common. The risk for wound infection is influenced primarily by patient factors, including diabetes, obesity, smoking, and immunosuppression. By nature of the procedure itself, the nerve roots are being mobilized and can result in a new postoperative neurological deficit, albeit this complication is rare. Postoperative deficits can range from mild decreased sensation to a full-blown foot drop.

Dural tear and cerebrospinal fluid (CSF) leak can also occur during the procedure. If this occurs, suture repair or patching of the tear may be necessary. Postoperatively, the patient may require 1–3 days of bed rest in order to decrease the intrathecal pressure on the area of repair. Dural tears have been reported to occur in up to 4% of lumbar discectomies. Fortunately, their occurrence does not portend a poor outcome.

The risk of recurrent disc herniation varies widely and is influenced by patient age, the type of herniation, and the size of the associated annular defect. It can also be influenced by surgical technique. Recurrent herniations occur in about 5–10% of patients following a primary lumbar discectomy. Fortunately, the results of operative treatment for a recurrence are reportedly comparable to those achieved after index discectomy.

Table 3.1 presents a summary of lumbar disc herniation and radiculopathy presentation, diagnostic testing, and suggested management options.

Table 3.1 A summary of lumbar disc herniation and radiculopathy presentation, diagnostic testing, and suggested management options

Clinical entity	Presentation	Diagnostic testing	Conservative management	Indications for surgery	Operative management
Lumbar disc herniation with radiculopathy	– Unilateral, radiating leg pain – Variable degrees of mild sensory and motor deficit	– MRI to detect the site of disc herniation, level involved, and degree of compression – CT myelogram only if MRI is contraindicated	– PT: stretching, range of motion of the low back and lower extremities – Non-narcotic analgesic medications – Avoidance of extended period of bed rest	– Progressive neurological deficit or cauda equina syndrome (rare) – Persistence of substantial symptoms despite 6–12 weeks of structured nonoperative treatment	– Lumbar discectomy (also known as microdiscectomy)

Suggested Reading

Atlas SJ, Keller RB, YA W, Deyo RA, Singer DE. Long-term outcomes of surgical and nonsurgical management of sciatica secondary to a lumbar disc herniation: 10 year results from the Maine lumbar spine study. Spine (Phila Pa 1976). 2005;30(8):927–35.

Kreiner DS, Hwang SW, Easa JE, Resnick DK, Baisden JL, Bess S, Cho CH, DePalma MJ, Dougherty P 2nd, Fernand R, Ghiselli G, Hanna AS, Lamer T, Lisi AJ, Mazanec DJ, Meagher RJ, Nucci RC, Patel RD, Sembrano JN, Sharma AK, Summers JT, Taleghani CK, Tontz WL Jr, Toton JF, North American Spine Society. An evidence-based clinical guideline for the diagnosis and treatment of lumbar disc herniation with radiculopathy. Spine J. 2014;14(1):180–91.

Saal JA. Natural history and nonoperative treatment of lumbar disc herniation. Spine (Phila Pa 1976). 1996;21(24 Suppl):2S–9S.

Schoenfeld AJ, Bono CM. Does surgical timing influence functional recovery after lumbar discectomy? A systematic review. Clin Orthop Relat Res. 2015;473(6):1963–70.

Weinstein JN, Lurie JD, Tosteson TD, Tosteson AN, Blood EA, Abdu WA, Herkowitz H, Hilibrand A, Albert T, Fischgrund J. Surgical versus nonoperative treatment for lumbar disc herniation: four-year results for the spine patient outcomes research trial (SPORT). Spine (Phila Pa 1976). 2008;33(25):2789–800.

Chapter 4
Degenerative Lumbar Spinal Stenosis and Spondylolisthesis

Daniel G. Tobert and Mitchel B. Harris

Abbreviations

CT	Computed tomography
DLS	Degenerative spondylolisthesis
EMG	Electromyography
ESI	Epidural steroid injections
LSS	Lumbar spinal stenosis
MRI	Magnetic resonance imaging
NASS	North American Spine Society
NCS	Nerve conduction studies
NSAIDs	Nonsteroidal anti-inflammatory drugs
PT	Physical therapy
PVD	Peripheral vascular disease
SPORT	Spine Patient Outcomes Research Trial

Introduction

Degenerative changes in the lumbar spine primarily manifest as low back pain; less commonly the clinical presentation is claudicant or radicular in nature. Lumbar spinal stenosis (LSS) and degenerative lumbar spondylolisthesis (DLS) are two prevalent degenerative conditions that can range from mild axial pain to debilitating symptoms with signs of neurologic compromise.

The term *stenosis* derives from the Latin prefix "steno," meaning "narrowing." The term *spondylolisthesis* derives from the Latin "spondylo," meaning "spine," and "listhesis," meaning "slip." Both terms refer to radiographic observations and do not necessarily correlate with patient symptoms. As such, decisions on clinical care are

D.G. Tobert • M.B. Harris (✉)
Department of Orthopaedic Surgery, Brigham and Women's Hospital, Harvard Medical School, Boston, MA 02115, USA
e-mail: dtobert@partners.org; mbharris@partners.org

© Springer International Publishing AG 2018   47
J.N. Katz et al. (eds.), *Principles of Orthopedic Practice for Primary Care Providers*, https://doi.org/10.1007/978-3-319-68661-5_4

made based on the nature and severity of an individual's complaints. The purpose of this chapter is to further clarify the varied clinical presentation of these conditions and detail the diagnostic workup, treatment options, and expected outcomes for degenerative lumbar spinal stenosis and spondylolisthesis.

Lumbar Spinal Stenosis

Definition and Epidemiology

The prevalence of LSS has been reported in the range of 5–10% of the population, regardless of age. However, up to 40% of patients over the age of 60 meet the radiographic criteria for LSS. Fortunately, the prevalence of symptomatic LSS is lower than that observed radiographically, with between 7 and 10% of patients over 65 experiencing radiculopathy or neurogenic claudication. LSS presents equally in males and females. It should be noted that a subset of patients develop LSS earlier in life based on congenitally narrowed spinal canals. In addition, patients with achondroplasia or osteopetrosis may develop symptomatic LSS in the third or fourth decade of life.

Clinical Presentation

The manifesting symptom of LSS is leg pain, and the type of leg pain depends not only on the level of stenosis (e.g., L4–L5) but also the location within the spinal canal (e.g., central vs. lateral recess or foraminal). If the thecal sac is compressed centrally, *neurogenic claudication* often results. This condition is described by patients as a dull ache or burning sensation that originates in the low back or gluteal region and travels down the lower extremities without following a specific nerve root distribution. Pain radiating distal to the knee is not required for the diagnosis, as patients can present with pain solely in the gluteal region. This sensation is typically worse when walking or with activities involving extension of the lumbar spine, such as sitting or standing upright for a prolonged period of time. Anatomical studies have demonstrated further narrowing of the lumbar spinal canal in extension, increasing the severity of compression on an already compromised thecal sac. Flexion in the lumbar region results in an expansion of the contours of the spinal canal. This accounts for observations that symptoms are often partially alleviated when leaning forward or pushing a grocery cart.

Aside from neurogenic claudication, LSS can result in lumbar radiculopathy. This symptom arises from compression of a nerve root as it exits the thecal sac. Unlike neurogenic claudication, patients with nerve root compression describe leg pain and paresthesias in a specific nerve root distribution. The L5 nerve root is most commonly affected in the setting of LSS. Classic symptoms manifest as pain radiating down the outside aspect of the thigh, wrapping around the front of the leg and ending in the webspace of the first and second toes, with associated paresthesias.

Physical examination findings are not consistent in LSS, and typically patients are neurologically intact. Provocative nerve root tension signs, such as the straight leg raise test, are frequently negative in LSS. Careful extension of the lumbar spine with examiner assistance or asking to the patient to stand for a period of time during the exam may provoke neurogenic claudication symptoms. In large population studies, frank motor weakness is present only 25% of the time, and sensory changes are seen in approximately 20–50% of patients. Decreased reflexes in the patella and Achilles tendon can also be seen in LSS and may be asymmetric. Any presence of an upper motor neuron sign, such as hyperreflexia, dense lower extremity paralysis, sustained ankle clonus, or an upgoing great toe excursion during the Babinski maneuver, should alert the clinician to coexistent pathology elsewhere in the spine (e.g., cervical or thoracic regions) or involving the brain.

Differential Diagnosis and Suggested Clinical Testing

The demographic predisposed to LSS is also at risk of other degenerative musculoskeletal conditions including peripheral joint arthritis, peripheral vascular disease, and neuropathy. Hip arthritis most commonly presents with groin pain exacerbated by weight-bearing or movements involving the hip. On physical examination, patients will exhibit a painful loss of hip flexion and internal rotation. If there is concern for hip joint pathology, a standing AP view of the pelvis should be obtained to assess that area. Often, radiographic evidence of degenerative pathology in both the lumbar spine and hip is present. This entity, termed the "hip-spine syndrome," is increasingly being recognized as a relatively common condition in the aging population. Musculoskeletal specialists often use diagnostic injections to help characterize the contributions of each area to a patient's pain.

Peripheral vascular disease (PVD) can result in *vascular claudication*, and symptoms can overlap significantly with neurogenic claudication. Clues that aid the clinician during history and physical examination are summarized in Table 4.1. Patients with PVD will generally describe a set distance or amount of exertion before symptoms develop, regardless of position. Typically, the pain begins distally near the ankle and moves proximally during vascular claudication. In addition, predisposing factors for PVD are well known, including diabetes mellitus, smoking, and hyperlipidemia. Physical exam findings for patients with PVD include diminished distal pulses, hairless extremities, lipodermatosclerosis, or frank ulceration. Concern for PVD should prompt measurement of ankle-brachial indices and noninvasive arterial/venous flow studies.

Table 4.1 History and physical exam findings that help differentiate between neurogenic claudication, radiculopathy, and vascular claudication

	Neurogenic claudication	Radiculopathy	Vascular claudication
Location	Proximal to distal, non-dermatomal	Proximal to distal, dermatomal	Distal to proximal, non-dermatomal
Quality	Dull, achy	Sharp	Dull, achy
Severity	Variable	Variable	Variable
Timing	Related to posture, can be constant	Generally constant but can be related to posture	Only with activity unless end stage
Aggravating factors	Standing, sitting, walking upright	Certain movements or extension reliably worsen	Walking uphill, increased physical exertion
Alleviating factors	Leaning forward, walking uphill	Certain movements and flexion improve	Cessation of activity unrelated to position
Physical exam	Palpable pulses, no distal skin changes	Palpable pulses, no distal skin changes	Hairless, shiny legs, diminished or absent pulses

Diabetic neuropathy also results in symptoms that can mimic LSS. However, diabetic neuropathy is not activity related and usually arises in a "stocking and glove" distribution. Less common mimickers of LSS include multiple sclerosis, transverse myelitis, or compressive lesions of the lumbosacral plexus.

When LSS is suspected after history and physical examination, imaging is required to confirm the diagnosis and evaluate the extent of disease. Plain films of the lumbar spine should be obtained with upright AP, lateral, and flexion/ extension views. These views often show diffuse degenerative changes but are helpful insofar as they portray the sagittal and coronal alignment of the lumbar spine while under physiologic loading. Flexion and extension views aid in the evaluation of spondylolisthesis. Magnetic resonance imaging (MRI) is the most useful modality when evaluating for LSS. The images obtained from MRI are able to delineate relationships between osseous, soft tissue, and neural structures of the lumbar spine. Therefore, MRI helps define the degree of stenosis (narrowing) and the specific neural structures involved (Figs. 4.1 and 4.2). This information, in combination with a history and physical exam, can definitively establish the diagnosis of LSS.

If MRI is contraindicated because of pacemaker devices or other ferromagnetic implants, computed tomography (CT) with myelography can be used. The soft tissue resolution of CT with myelography is much lower in comparison to MRI, and the study is invasive. Nonetheless, a CT myelogram can determine the level(s) of stenosis and differentiate soft tissue pathology that is anterior, posterior, or lateral to the thecal sac. Electromyography (EMG) and nerve conductions studies (NCS) are not a standard part of the LSS workup and should not be ordered unless evaluation of a secondary diagnosis is warranted.

Fig. 4.1 Sagittal MRI image demonstrating loss of disk space height, disk protrusions, and buckling of the ligamentum flavum at L3–4 and L4–5 in the setting of two-level spondylolisthesis (*red circle*)

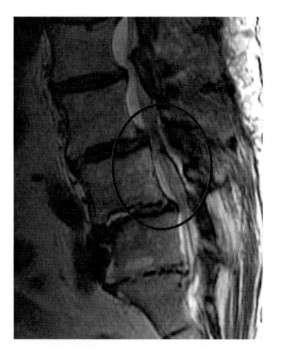

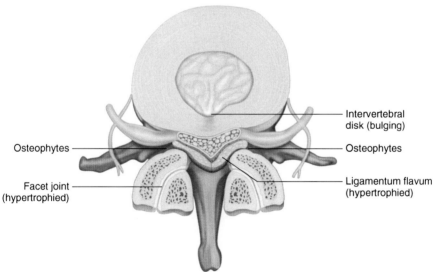

Fig. 4.2 Pictorial demonstrating stenosis resulting from a combination of central disk bulging, facet joint osteophytes, and ligamentum flavum hypertrophy

Nonoperative Management

The natural history of LSS has not been clearly defined, but existing research can help guide the clinician when counseling patients about treatment strategies. A well-done natural history study has demonstrated that 70% of patients with LSS have similar symptoms after an average follow-up of 4 years, with 15% worsening clinically and another 15% reporting symptomatic improvement.   Oral medications can be helpful in the management of LSS. Nonsteroidal anti-inflammatory drugs (NSAIDs) can provide partial symptom relief but have well-known renal, gastrointestinal, and cardiovascular side effects with prolonged use. Opioid medications should be avoided due to the risk of dependence, gastrointestinal effects, and cognitive alterations.

Physical therapy (PT) focused on core strengthening and range of motion should be tried as an initial therapy if not otherwise contraindicated by other medical conditions. Patients should be counseled to attempt at least 6 weeks of therapy with daily completion of a home exercise program before reassessing symptoms. In a randomized controlled trial comparing PT to surgical treatment in patients with LSS, nearly half of the patients who were treated with PT alone noted some degree of improvement at 2-year follow-up.

Epidural steroid injections (ESI) under fluoroscopic guidance are commonly used to treat symptoms from LSS. The premise behind an accurately placed ESI is that a reduction of local inflammatory mediators will help improve pain. However, a randomized controlled trial of 400 patients with moderate to severe symptomatic LSS found ESI had no benefit at 6-week follow-up. ESI may be more beneficial for patients with LSS who present with radicular symptoms as opposed to those manifesting neurogenic claudication. Physicians treating patients with LSS and considering ESI should take into account the patient's predominant complaint, as well as their candidacy for other nonoperative and surgical interventions, before proceeding with a referral for injections.

Indications for Surgical Management

An absolute indication for surgical management is a progressing neurologic deficit or bowel and bladder dysfunction. Fortunately, this scenario is exceedingly rare in LSS, presenting in less than 1% of patients. In most instances, surgical management is typically recommended following a patient's failure to satisfactorily derive benefit from a nonoperative treatment regimen.

A shared decision-making approach between patient and provider should be used when discussing surgical management. The clinician should understand the patient's level of function prior to the onset of LSS in contrast to their level of function at the time of presentation. Walking distance is a good metric for assessing functional status. A patient who would otherwise be able to walk long distances but is limited to one or two city blocks because of LSS symptoms experiences significant quality of life impairment. Ultimately, however, it is the patient who must conclude that their quality of life has deteriorated to the point where surgical treatment should be considered.

A discussion of surgery begins by assessing the patient's expectation for treatment. This information helps guide the discussion of surgical management and will often prevent a less favorable patient-reported outcome. Careful scrutiny of the medical history should be performed to help manage perioperative risk. For example, patients with significant cardiovascular comorbidities not evaluated within a year should be referred to a cardiologist for evaluation and perioperative risk assessment. If a patient is anticoagulated, a clear plan for cessation and resumption of anticoagulant therapies should be devised with the patient's other physicians. While this care coordination can be cumbersome in the increasingly fragmented medical care system, it is essential to prevent surgical complications.

Operative Management

Operative treatment of LSS is increasingly common. Between 1994 and 2006, surgery performed for LSS increased by over 900%. Technological advances have provided a multitude of options for the spine surgeon. Nonetheless, the succinct goal of operative treatment is decompression of the neural elements that are believed to be the cause of the claudicant or radicular symptoms. This is categorically accomplished by removal of the offending surrounding structures while maintaining spinal stability.

Depending on the extent of stenosis, a *laminotomy* or *laminectomy* can be performed, which entails removal of a portion or the entire lamina at a given level.

A laminectomy is performed in conjunction with fusion, or *arthrodesis*, if there is concern for concomitant instability. Instability can exist preoperatively or as a result of surgical decompression. Preoperative instability is assessed with flexion/extension radiographs but can often be inferred on MRI or CT imaging. Typically, if more than 50% of the facet joints are removed during decompression, a surgeon will perform a fusion at the time of surgery.

Many patients inquire about the use of micro-endoscopic techniques for lumbar spine surgery. This is usually performed when single-level stenosis is present lateral to the thecal sac, or the *lateral recess* of the spinal canal. The advantages of this technique are a less extensive soft tissue dissection and a smaller surgical scar. However, this method risks incomplete decompression, and some studies have shown a higher rate of dural tear. At the time of this writing, decompression with open laminectomy or laminotomy remains the gold standard for operative management of LSS.

Expected Outcomes

Achieving a successful outcome following treatment of LSS begins with a transparent discussion between the patient and clinician about available treatment options and the patient's expectations. Numerous studies have reported patient satisfaction rates in the range of 80% following decompression for LSS. Other research has shown that the patients least satisfied with surgical treatment are those that have back pain as their predominant symptom. This highlights the crucial role of listening to the patient's history when evaluating a patient for LSS. Other factors that portend a less favorable surgical outcome are increased medical comorbidities and increased baseline functional disability. Patients with diabetes, obesity, and rheumatoid arthritis are at increased risk of a surgical site infection postoperatively.

Degenerative Spondylolisthesis

Definition and Epidemiology

Broadly, spondylolisthesis refers to translation of a vertebral body in relation to adjacent vertebral structures. Spondylolisthesis can be further distinguished by whether a developmental anomaly is present, the neural arch is intact (i.e., the posterior osseous structures are in continuity with the anterior vertebral body), or if spondylolisthesis occurs at a level adjacent to a fused segment. This section focuses on degenerative spondylolisthesis (DLS), which refers to translation with an intact neural arch in the setting of predisposing arthritic changes.

L4–L5 is the most common level where DLS occurs, and the patient is typically in the fifth decade of life or later. DLS is present four times more often in females than in males. This skew in prevalence is thought to be a result of increased ligamentous laxity observed in females secondary to hormonal differences, but definitive causality has not been established. In addition, genetic factors are thought to play a role in the development of DLS, and the condition may be more prevalent in African-American women. A population study found radiographic evidence of DLS in approximately 8% of females and 3% of males, and these numbers vary slightly depending on the ethnicity studied.

Clinical Presentation

The most common presenting complaint in the setting of DLS is neurogenic claudication that results from concomitant spinal stenosis at the level of the listhesis. As the cephalad vertebral body translates anteriorly, the space available for the thecal sac becomes dynamically stenotic. Patients describe a limit to their ability to maintain a standing position or walking before needing to lean forward or sit down. A patient's symptoms may be described as less severe when riding a bike or pushing a grocery cart, which is attributed to flexion of the lumbar spine during these activities and decreased compression on the thecal sac.

Less commonly in DLS, patients report radicular symptoms or purely axial back pain. The most common level for radiculopathy to develop in DLS is at L5. A concomitant motor weakness of great toe extension and ankle dorsiflexion can occur if the L5 nerve root is involved but is not observed in the majority of cases.

Differential Diagnosis and Suggested Clinical Testing

Similar to the differential diagnoses for LSS, degenerative changes in the hip and knee must be considered in the event of DLS. Osteoarthritis of the hip can refer pain to the medial aspect of the knee through the anterior branch of the obturator nerve, and a patient's description of this can mimic radicular pain. Degenerative hip pain can be exacerbated immediately on standing and with internal rotation of the femur, and a weight-bearing plain film of the pelvis is recommended to look for the presence of degenerative hip pathology.

Peripheral vascular disease should always be considered in a patient with activity-related leg pain. As noted in Table 4.2, the factors that distinguish vascular claudication from neurogenic claudication are a fixed physical activity limit that does not vary with position, improvement of symptoms by standing upright, diminished or absent distal lower extremity pulses, and skin changes from chronic hypoperfusion.

There is often radiographic evidence of DLS as a patient is being worked up for a complaint of low back, leg, gluteal, or hip pain. The challenge for the clinician is to distinguish DLS as the primary etiology of a patient's symptoms or merely a secondary radiographic finding. The most useful radiographic study in the evaluation of DLS is a weight-bearing lateral lumbar plain film. The weight-bearing film is important because it evaluates the alignment of the lumbar spine during physiologic loading, and spondylolisthesis can be missed if a lateral radiograph is taken in the supine position and the translated vertebral body reduces to its anatomic position. Flexion/extension views are useful if the initial upright lateral film is equivocal or to evaluate for a mobile spondylolisthesis.

Because the symptoms of LSS and DLS overlap almost completely, a lumbar spine MRI helps evaluate for stenosis in the setting of DLS. However, similar to plain films taken in the supine position, the lack of anterior translation on MRI does not rule out DLS. Subtle clues on MRI can alert the clinician to the presence of spondylolisthesis. On the axial sequences, a facet joint effusion greater than 1.5 mm is suggestive of DLS and should prompt weight-bearing plain films if they have not been already obtained.

Table 4.2 A summary of degenerative lumbar spinal stenosis and spondylolisthesis with a synopsis of presentation, diagnostic testing, and suggested management options

Clinical Entity	Presentation	Diagnostic testing	Conservative management	Indications for surgery	Operative management
Lumbar spinal stenosis	– Neurogenic claudication – Radiculopathy	– MRI/CT—myelogram if MRI contraindicated	– PT – Non-opioid oral medications – Lifestyle modification	– Rapidly progressive neurologic deficit – Failure of nonoperative regimen	– Laminotomy – Laminectomy – Laminectomy with fusion
Degenerative spondylolisthesis	– Neurogenic claudication – Radiculopathy	– Upright lateral lumbar plain film – MRI to evaluate extent of stenosis	– PT – Non-opioid oral medications – Lifestyle modifications	– Rapidly progressive neurologic deficit – Failure of nonoperative regimen	– Laminectomy without fusion (elderly, frail) – Laminectomy with fusion

Nonoperative Management

All patients with DLS should receive nonoperative therapies as first-line treatment. The majority of patients will not require operative management in the absence of a progressive neurologic deficit. Natural history studies regarding DLS are limited. One study followed a group of 40 patients with DLS for an average of approximately 8 years, and only 10% developed worsening symptoms during this time period. Interestingly, none of the patients whose symptoms worsened developed radiographic progression of the spondylolisthesis. There is not a correlation between radiographic severity of DLS and clinical symptoms.

As with LSS, nonoperative treatment modalities include physical therapy and non-opioid oral medications. The North American Spine Society (NASS) published an updated evidence-based clinical guideline in 2014 on the treatment of DLS and concluded there is insufficient evidence to make a recommendation for or against injections, although this modality is frequently employed, especially in those patients adamantly against consideration of surgery.

Indications for Surgical Management

Absent of a progressive neurologic deficit attributable to DLS, the indications for surgical management are based on the severity of a patient's symptoms and the extent of their response to conservative care. The Spine Patient Outcomes Research Trial (SPORT) prospectively randomized over 600 patients with DLS to nonoperative or operative treatment. As a result of substantial crossover between the two cohorts, the publication of this trial included both intention-to-treat and as-treated analyses. Using as-treated analysis, a statistically significant improvement in pain and function was found at 4-year follow-up in the operative group.

The opportunity for symptom alleviation and functional improvement with surgical treatment must be weighed against the risks. Typically, operative treatment can be considered if symptoms related to DLS have led to a loss of independence in daily activities. Likewise, if symptoms have led to an unacceptable degradation in the quality of life for a patient, then surgical treatment can be offered.

Operative Management

The typical surgical treatment for symptomatic DLS is decompression of the stenotic areas and arthrodesis (Fig. 4.3). As described above, a laminectomy is typically performed to decompress the thecal sac dorsally. There are retrospective studies in the literature that maintain positive results can be achieved following decompression alone (without arthrodesis) in the setting of low-grade

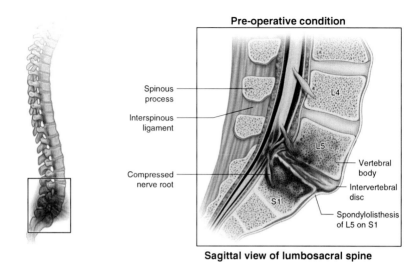

Pre-operative condition

Spinous process

Interspinous ligament

Compressed nerve root

L4

L5

Vertebral body

Intervertebral disc

S1

Spondylolisthesis of L5 on S1

Sagittal view of lumbosacral spine

Post-operative fixation

Post-operative fixation

Vertebral body

Intervertebral disc

Nerve root

L4

L5

S1

Rod

Pedicle screw

Bone graft

L4

S2

Posterior view of lumbosacral spine

Fig. 4.3 Schematic demonstrating a lumbar spondylolisthesis treated with an instrumented fusion-based procedure. Screws and connector rods are used to stabilize the fusion site and allow for osseous integration

spondylolisthesis. For an elderly patient with multiple comorbidities and low functional activity, decompression alone may be a viable option.

However, higher-quality data demonstrates superior and more durable results which can be achieved when arthrodesis is performed in addition to decompression in the setting of DLS. This is reflected in the NASS clinical guideline for DLS, where a stronger recommendation is made for both decompression and arthrodesis as compared to decompression alone. Arthrodesis is often performed with instrumentation based on data suggesting it can improve fusion rates. However, there is no evidence to support a contention that the use of instrumentation improves clinical outcomes. Given the lack of objective high-quality data, the decision for instrumentation is made by the treating surgeon based on their clinical experience, patient factors, and surgical goals.

Expected Outcomes

The natural history of symptomatic DLS favors nonsurgical management, and of those who undergo operative treatment, the majority can expect a positive outcome. The SPORT reported that 86% of patients were satisfied with the results of surgical intervention.

Numerous studies have evaluated factors that influence outcomes in the surgical treatment of DLS, but few provide high-quality data. There are suggestions in the literature that patients who achieve fusion, regardless of instrumentation, experience superior clinical outcomes. As such, factors that predispose a patient to pseudarthrosis after an attempted fusion, such as smoking and chronic steroid use, may influence the ultimate surgical result. The duration of symptoms prior to surgical treatment does not appear to influence outcomes. Obesity as defined by a body mass index over 30 kg/m^2 is associated with an increased surgical site infection rate and need for reoperation.

Suggested Reading

Friedly JL, Comstock BA, Turner JA, et al. A randomized trial of epidural glucocorticoid injections for spinal stenosis. N Engl J Med. 2014;371(1):11–21.

Katz JN, Stucki G, Lipson SJ, Fossel AH, Grobler LJ, Weinstein JN. Predictors of surgical outcome in degenerative lumbar spinal stenosis. Spine. 1999;24(21):2229–33.

Kreiner DS, Shaffer WO, Baisden JL, et al. An evidence-based clinical guideline for the diagnosis and treatment of degenerative lumbar spinal stenosis (update). Spine J. 2013;13(7):734–43.

Matsunaga S, Ijiri K, Hayashi K. Nonsurgically managed patients with degenerative spondylolisthesis: a 10- to 18-year follow-up study. J Neurosurg. 2000;93:194–8.

Matz PG, Meagher RJ, Lamer T, et al. Guideline summary review: an evidence-based clinical guideline for the diagnosis and treatment of degenerative lumbar spondylolisthesis. Spine J. 2016;16(3):439–48.

Miyamoto H, Sumi M, Uno K, Tadokoro K, Mizuno K. Clinical outcome of nonoperative treatment for lumbar spinal stenosis, and predictive factors relating to prognosis, in a 5-year minimum follow-up. J Spinal Disord Tech. 2008;21(8):563–8.

Weinstein JN, Lurie JD, Tosteson TD, et al. Surgical compared with nonoperative treatment for lumbar degenerative spondylolisthesis. Four-year results in the spine patient outcomes research trial (SPORT) randomized and observational cohorts. J Bone Joint Surg Am. 2009;91(6):1295–304.

Part IV
Osteoporosis

Chapter 5
Osteoporosis, Vertebral Compression Fractures, and Cement Augmentation Procedures

Marco L. Ferrone and Andrew J. Schoenfeld

Osteoporosis

Definition and Epidemiology

Osteoporosis lies at the far end of the bone mineral density spectrum, with osteopenia being a more mild manifestation. Osteoporosis is defined as loss of bone mass and disruption of internal architecture, which can lead to fragility fractures. Osteoporosis may also be present in the absence of fractures. As the population ages, the rate of osteoporosis is predicted to increase in the next 50 years by a factor of three. At present, it is estimated that osteoporosis affects ten million individuals in the United States, 80% of whom are women, with another 18 million diagnosed with osteopenia.

Osteoporosis variably affects the global population and is less prevalent in the developing world and far more common in Europe. In the United States, known risk factors include female gender; Caucasian or Asian race; a family history of osteoporosis; consumption of caffeine, nicotine, and alcohol; low body weight; deficiencies of dietary calcium and vitamin D; insufficient physical activity; and advancing age. Obesity, or higher BMI, has been shown to be protective against the development of osteoporosis.

M.L. Ferrone
Department of Orthopaedic Surgery, Brigham and Women's Hospital/Dana Farber Cancer Institute, Harvard Medical School, 75 Francis Street, Boston, MA 02115, USA
e-mail: mferrone@partners.org

A.J. Schoenfeld (✉)
Department of Orthopedic Surgery, Brigham and Women's Hospital, Harvard Medical School, Boston, MA, USA
e-mail: ajschoen@neomed.edu

© Springer International Publishing AG 2018   63
J.N. Katz et al. (eds.), *Principles of Orthopedic Practice for Primary Care Providers*, https://doi.org/10.1007/978-3-319-68661-5_5

Clinical Presentation

Osteopenia and osteoporosis are clinically silent until fractures develop. This fact speaks to the critical necessity for testing individuals who may otherwise be at risk. Patients who present with a fragility fracture should be evaluated for osteoporosis during, or after, treatment of the injury.

Differential Diagnosis

Osteoporosis is characterized as primary and secondary. Primary osteoporosis can occur in both genders but is most typical of postmenopausal women. Secondary osteoporosis is caused by medications and other medical conditions or diseases, as seen in patients using glucocorticoids and with hypogonadism or celiac disease.

Although osteoporosis is most commonly the result of bone loss, it can also be the result of a failure to achieve optimal bone mass as a young adult. In this setting, osteoporosis is not due to accelerated bone loss but rather suboptimal development, which can be impaired by malnutrition, malabsorption, eating disorders, chronic disease, or severe inactivity.

Diagnostic Testing

Screening laboratory tests are carried out in all patients being evaluated for primary osteoporosis and should include a basic metabolic panel, complete blood cell count, liver function tests, thyroid function tests, gonadal hormone levels, and serum 25-hydroxyvitamin D level. Vitamin D deficiency is one of the most common causes of reduced bone mineral density, especially in men. Laboratory tests for secondary osteoporosis should be directed at the suspected underlying cause of the condition.

While plain radiographs and advanced imaging studies such as computed tomography (CT) are often used in the workup of patients with osteoporosis, radiolucency associated with the condition will not readily be present until the loss of more than 30% of bone mineral density. As a result, these imaging modalities are not reliable screening tools for osteoporosis in the absence of suspected fracture.

Dual-energy X-ray absorptiometry (DEXA) is the most widely validated method of measuring bone mineral density (BMD). DEXA scans measure BMD within the lumbar spine and proximal femur. DEXA scores are reported as a T-score, with the value in standard deviations (SD) as compared to a healthy young adult white woman, and a Z-score, where the value is given in SD as compared to age-, race-, and sex-matched controls. T-scores of −1.0 or greater are considered normal. Those in the range of −1.0 to −2.5 are reflective of osteopenia. Patients with scores that are lower than −2.5 are considered to have frank osteoporosis. An osteopenic score in the presence of a fragility fracture is also considered reflective of osteoporosis.

Nonoperative Management

Osteoporosis in and of itself is not a surgical condition and can be treated with a variety of medical interventions ranging from calcium and vitamin D supplementation to disease-modulating agents. The opportunity to address all modifiable risk factors should also be recognized, including smoking, alcohol, exercise, living situation, use of walking aides, and visual disturbances.

While correcting vitamin D deficiency and calcium intake are the most common interventions and those with the lowest side-effect profile, a number of medications to preserve bone stock should also be considered. Bisphosphonate medications are typically considered a first-line treatment for patients with osteoporosis. There are two classes of bisphosphonates, based on whether the medication contains nitrogen. The nitrogen-containing bisphosphonates (alendronate, pamidronate, ibandronate, risedronate) inhibit farnesyl pyrophosphate synthetase, the enzyme required for osteoclasts to resorb bone. The non-nitrogen-containing bisphosphonates (clodronate, etidronate, tiludronate) precipitate the apoptosis of osteoclasts by creating a toxic analog of adenosine triphosphate. Bisphosphonates have been shown to reduce the risk of fragility fractures by approximately 50% following 1 year of use. Side effects from the oral formulations include esophageal erosions and stomach inflammation, while intravenous formulations can cause flu-like symptoms. All bisphosphonates carry a risk of osteonecrosis of the jaw, as well as atypical fractures with long-term use. The most characteristic manifestation of these atypical fractures mainly present in the subtrochanteric region of the femur.

Calcitonin is another medication that can be used in the treatment of osteoporosis. This medication is administered intranasally and binds to osteoclasts, thus inhibiting bone resorption. It is not generally considered first-line therapy but may be used in patients who cannot tolerate bisphosphonates. While BMD has been shown to increase with the use of calcitonin, specific studies have reported these to be only modest for the most part. Common side effects are related to the means of intranasal administration, including topical irritation, rhinitis, and bleeding. There is some concern regarding a link between calcitonin use and the risk of malignancy, but evidence for this is inconclusive at present.

Denosumab is a monoclonal antibody administered monthly as a subcutaneous injection. Denosumab works through the biochemical pathway that facilitates the differentiation of osteoclasts. Denosumab has been shown to increase BMD in postmenopausal women and leads to concomitant reductions in fragility fractures. Denosumab is typically well tolerated by most patients but carries similar risks of osteonecrosis of the jaw as the bisphosphonates. The main obstacle to use of denosumab tends to be its high cost and insurance approval.

Teriparatide is a recombinant version of parathyroid hormone, administered subcutaneously daily, and is the only known anabolic agent used to treat osteoporosis. It has been approved for use in the United States since 2002 and has been found to increase BMD by 8% and reduce the risk of fragility fractures after 1 year of use. Overall, teriparatide leads to greater increases in BMD than the other anti-osteoporotic medications. Obstacles to use include cost, the requirement for daily injection, and concerns for osteosarcoma. Due to this warning, teriparatide is contraindicated in patients with a history of some cancers and Paget's disease. Other side effects are typically well tolerated, including mild nausea, dizziness, and headaches.

Expected Outcomes

Patients who are found to be osteoporotic or develop fragility fractures should be considered for some type of medication to decrease the risk of future fracture. Sizable reductions in fracture risk can be achieved even after only a short period of appropriate medication use. If a patient fails to respond satisfactorily to first-line medications based on DEXA or develops another fragility fracture while on appropriate medications, consideration should be given to the use of denosumab or teriparatide.

Vertebral Compression Fractures

Definition and Epidemiology

It is estimated that worldwide, approximately nine million fractures occur as a direct result of osteoporosis. The most common locations of these fragility fractures include the hip, distal radius, and vertebral body in the thoracic and lumbar spine. The lifetime risk of an osteoporotic fracture is between 30 and 40% in the developed world for women and about 10–15% for men. Osteoporotic fractures account for significant disability-adjusted life years (DALYs) lost. For perspective, when considering DALYs lost, osteoporotic fractures are more impactful than most cancers, rheumatoid arthritis, and hypertension.

Approximately 1.5 million vertebral compression fractures (VCF) occur annually in the United States. The yearly incidence is 10.7 per 1000 women and 5.7 per 1000 men. The estimated annual cost of treating these injuries is $746 million. The most influential risk factor for a VCF is preexisting osteoporosis, but other issues contribute as well. These include conditions that increase the likelihood of a patient's fall, such as poor eyesight, dementia, and frailty.

Clinical Presentation

VCFs occur as a result of a flexion compression force. The clinical presentation is most often related to a fall, and patients typically complain of axial back pain with mechanical and positional components. These injuries present as anterior wedging with preservation of the posterior wall of the vertebral body and without

Fig. 5.1 Sagittal reconstruction MRI image demonstrating an acute compression fracture at T11 (*red arrow*) in an elderly patient with prior compression fractures at T9 and T12. The fracture at T9 was previously treated with a cement augmentation procedure

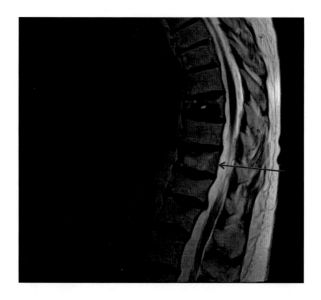

retropulsion into the spinal canal. For these reasons, neurologic function is generally preserved. The injury may be localized to a single level or multiple levels can fracture simultaneously. In severe cases, patients may present with acute fractures in the setting of multiple old compression injuries or fractures in various stages of healing (Fig. 5.1). In other settings, individuals may develop a new compression fracture within a previously injured vertebral body (a so-called acute on chronic compression fracture). These types of injuries may be more difficult to detect and necessitate advanced imaging modalities such as CT or magnetic resonance imaging (MRI).

Presenting complaints are generally consistent with axial back at the injured level and reproducible tenderness to palpation on physical exam. Over time, multiple VCF may be acquired, leading to kyphotic posture, loss of height, and chronic back pain.

Differential Diagnosis

The differential diagnosis for VCFs may include advanced degenerative changes or spinal deformity, elder abuse, infection, and malignancy.

Diagnostic Testing

Plain radiographs, including high-quality anteroposterior and lateral views, often can demonstrate not only the fracture but also give a general sense of the bone quality. CT scans can show more detail and bony architecture, but both CT and plain films are unreliable when it comes to determining the acuity of the VCF. MRI is most helpful in this regard and can also provide useful information on the status of the neural elements and integrity of the spinal canal. MRI may be used to detect the presence of new acute injury within a previously existing compression deformity. In the setting where multiple vertebral bodies are fractured and one is being considered for an intervention, determining the acuity of the symptomatic level can be critical for appropriate care. CT and MR imaging are also helpful when ruling out underlying malignancy or infection.

Nuclear medicine scans can be useful in determining the acuity of a fracture and in ruling out underlying malignancy. The specificity can be vastly improved with use of single-photon emission computed tomography (SPECT) technology. Nuclear medicine studies are not considered part of the standard evaluation of patients who are otherwise not at risk for a malignant process and where CT or MRI studies are conclusive regarding a diagnosis. Establishing an underlying diagnosis of osteoporosis in the setting of previously identified VCF can be achieved using DEXA imaging, as outlined above.

Nonoperative Management

Nonoperative treatment is the preferred course of care for most VCFs. Immediate treatment centers around analgesia and activity modification. Immobility and bed rest should be minimized as they predispose patients to the development of urinary tract infections, bedsores, deep venous thrombosis, pneumonia, and deconditioning. When considering analgesics, care must be taken to balance the need for pain control with the risk of delirium, impaired sensorium and further falls. Nonsteroidal medications should be the first line of treatment unless they are contraindicated. A short course of narcotic medications can be considered in those who fail management with nonsteroidals. If appropriate, bisphosphonates and calcitonin that are begun in the acute post-injury period have been found to have an analgesic effect.

Bracing can be considered as an adjunct for pain control. The use of a brace may provide some stability to the fractured segment and off-load painful paraspinal musculature. The use of a brace has not been shown to prevent the development of kyphosis or accelerate the healing process. If utilized, bracing is typically trialed for a period of 4–6 weeks or until the patient does not have substantial fracture related pain while not wearing the brace. The patient should be gradually weaned from the brace as they slowly return to full activities. In this time period, physical therapy can also serve as a useful adjunct to maintain mobility, improve core strength, and provide additional pain relief modalities.

Indications for Operative Management

Operative intervention is used sparingly for VCFs. Open surgical procedures are reserved for cases of neurologic compromise, frank instability in the setting of a VCF, or severe deformity. Poor bone quality which contributed to the development of the VCFs is a complicating factor for open spinal reconstruction with instrumentation. There is, however, a more widely accepted role for cement augmentation (Fig. 5.2), which is typically performed percutaneously with image guidance. Patients with radiographically confirmed acute compression fractures (generally within 90 days of symptom onset) may be considered for a cement augmentation procedure if they have severe pain that has proven refractory to conservative measures, including the use of a back brace or in patients for who bracing is contraindicated.

Vertebroplasty

Vertebroplasty was originally developed in 1984 for the treatment of painful spinal hemangiomas and spinal fractures secondary to malignancy. The technique uses bone cement, (polymethylmethacrylate (PMMA)), which is injected through the cannulae into the vertebral body defect. Image guidance is used to place the cannulae within the fractured vertebral body, as well as to monitor for cement extrusion. The imaging used can be fluoroscopic or CT guided. The cement interdigitates with the trabeculae of the bone and is allowed to cure, thus stabilizing the fracture.

Fig. 5.2 Lateral plain film radiograph of a patient with a compression fracture at L1 that was treated using a cement augmentation procedure

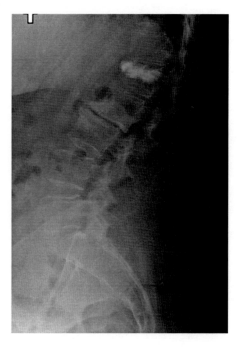

Kyphoplasty

Kyphoplasty, a variation of the vertebroplasty procedure using inflatable bone tamps, was developed in 1996. The concept is similar to vertebroplasty, as both rely on percutaneous working cannulae placed into the fracture site. Kyphoplasty, however, relies on the use of a balloon that is inflated creating a void into which the cement is placed under low pressure (Fig. 5.3).

Both procedures have very similar safety profiles, and many of the perceived advantages of kyphoplasty, including restoration of vertebral body height and correction of focal kyphosis at the fracture site, have not been reliably demonstrated in larger studies. Kyphoplasty is the more expensive procedure (as much as ten times

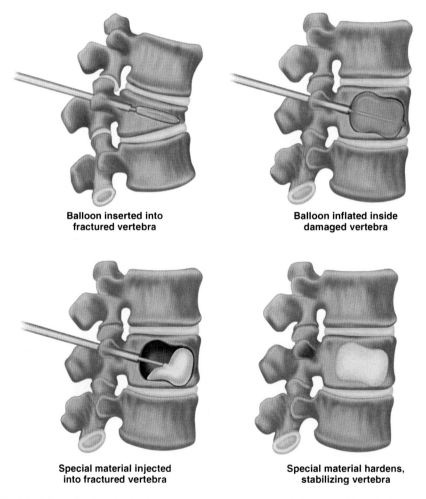

Balloon inserted into
fractured vertebra

Balloon inflated inside
damaged vertebra

Special material injected
into fractured vertebra

Special material hardens,
stabilizing vertebra

Fig. 5.3 Schematic of the kyphoplasty procedure. A balloon tamp is introduced into the fractured vertebral body and inflated. The balloon is then removed, and the resultant cavity is back filled with bone cement, inserted under low pressure

the cost of vertebroplasty) but also the only one of the two to have level I evidence supporting its use. Risks are mainly from cement extravasation and include neurologic compromise as well as cement or fat emboli traveling to the lungs. Historically, vertebroplasty was performed by interventional radiologists in imaging suites using local anesthetics, while kyphoplasty was performed by spine surgeons in operating rooms under general anesthesia.

Expected Outcomes

Cement augmentation has a role in patients with intractable pain. Good to excellent results, measured by degree of pain relief, can be expected in the range of 75–100% for both vertebroplasty and kyphoplasty, as well as nonoperative management. Cement augmentation procedures have not been shown to expedite the rehabilitation process, decrease the likelihood of kyphosis, or reduce the potential for future fractures. Regardless of the choice of management, most patients are able to return to pre-injury levels of function by 12 weeks following fracture. Patients with such injuries are at elevated risk for future fractures, and the most effective means of minimizing the potential for subsequent VCFs is through the use of appropriate osteoporosis medication and maintenance of physical activity. Even after healing a VCF, patients are more likely to have residual issues with back pain. Patients also may develop post-fracture sequelae, including chronic pain and/or post-traumatic kyphosis (PTK) at the fracture site (Fig. 5.4). VCFs at the thoracolumbar junction

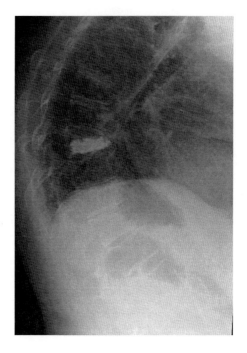

Fig. 5.4 Lateral plain film radiograph of a patient who developed post-traumatic kyphosis subsequent to a compression fracture at the thoracolumbar junction. The post-traumatic deformity developed, despite the patient having been treated with a cement augmentation procedure

Table 5.1 Summary of osteoporosis and VCFs with a synopsis of presentation, diagnostic testing, and suggested management options

Clinical entity	Presentation	Diagnostic testing	Conservative management	Surgical indications and operative management
Osteoporosis	– Clinically silent unless screened for – May be diagnosed following a sentinel fragility fracture (e.g., hip, wrist, or spine)	– DEXA	– Bisphosphonates, calcitonin, denosumab, teriparatide – PT to improve core strengthening, joint mobility and function - "Fall proofing" living space	Not applicable
Vertebral compression fracture	– Focal pain within the thoracic or lumbar spine	– Plain film radiographs – CT – MRI—determine fracture acuity	– Rest, NSAIDs – PT – Bracing	– Cement augmentation if pain is refractory to conservative care – Open reconstruction in the event of neurologic compromise, instability, or post-traumatic kyphosis

DEXA dual-energy X-ray absorptiometry, *PT* physical therapy, *CT* computed tomography, *MRI* magnetic resonance imaging, *NSAIDs* nonsteroidal anti-inflammatory drugs

have the highest likelihood of progressing to PTK. PTK can be very disabling, and some individuals may require open spinal osteotomy and instrumented reconstruction to correct a severe kyphosis.

Table 5.1 is a summary of osteoporosis and VCFs with a synopsis of presentation, diagnostic testing, and suggested management options.

Suggested Reading

Kallmes DF, Comstock BA, Hegerty PJ, et al. A randomized trial of vertebroplasty for osteoporotic spinal fractures. N Engl J Med. 2009;361:569–79.

Kim HJ, Yi JM, Cho HG, et al. Comparative study of treatment outcomes of osteoporotic compression fractures without neurologic injury using a rigid brace, a soft brace, and no brace. J Bone Joint Surg Am. 2014;96(23):1959–66.

Wardlaw D, Cummings SR, Van Meirhaeghe J, et al. Efficacy and safety of balloon kyphoplasty compared with non-surgical care for vertebral compression fracture (FREE): a randomised controlled trial. Lancet. 2009;373:1016–24.

Part V
Hip

Chapter 6
Hip Soft Tissue Injuries

Eziamaka C. Obunadike and Cheri A. Blauwet

Abbreviations

AP	Anteroposterior
FABER	Flexion, abduction, and external rotation
GTPS	Greater trochanteric pain syndrome
MRI	Magnetic resonance imaging
NSAIDs	Nonsteroidal anti-inflammatory drugs
P	Physical therapy
U/S	Ultrasound

Introduction

Soft tissue injuries involving extra-articular regions of the hip have the potential to cause significant functional morbidity and reduction in quality of life. Additionally, given the complexity of anatomy in the hip and lumbopelvic region, these entities may be difficult to differentiate and diagnose due to commonly overlapping pain patterns. Here we describe the most common soft tissue disorders involving the hip, categorizing each diagnosis as those that present as anterior, lateral, and posterior hip pain in order to best aid clinicians in considering a differential and expeditiously initiating the correct diagnosis and treatment approach. It is important to note that

E.C. Obunadike • C.A. Blauwet (✉)
Department of Physical Medicine and Rehabilitation, Spaulding Rehabilitation Hospital/
Brigham and Women's Hospital, Harvard Medical School,
300, 1st Avenue, Boston, MA 02129, USA
e-mail: eobunadike@partners.org; cblauwet@bwh.harvard.edu

© Springer International Publishing AG 2018   75
J.N. Katz et al. (eds.), *Principles of Orthopedic Practice for Primary Care Providers*, https://doi.org/10.1007/978-3-319-68661-5_6

the majority of hip soft tissue injuries can improve, or resolve, with appropriate rehabilitation and nonoperative treatment strategies.

Anterior Hip/Groin Disorders

Osteitis Pubis

Definition and Epidemiology

Osteitis pubis is a noninfectious inflammatory process involving the symphysis pubis, a nonsynovial, nonvascular joint composed of fibrocartilage. Primary osteitis pubis is caused by repetitive microtrauma alone or in conjunction with opposing shearing forces across the pubic symphysis, especially with repetitive movements associated with sports that involve kicking (e.g., soccer) or repetitive hip abduction/adduction activities. Many cases of osteitis pubis are secondary, however, and can occur during or after pregnancy or as a sequela of infection or trauma.

Clinical Presentation

Osteitis pubis typically presents as midline groin pain with or without radiation to the medial or anterior thigh or abdomen. Primary osteitis may be aggravated with activity and relieved by rest. Similar to other causes of hip or pelvic pain, osteitis pubis can be accompanied by a waddling gait or limp. On physical examination, patients will have point tenderness to palpation directly over the symphysis pubis. Pain may also be elicited with passive hip internal rotation and/or active hip adduction.

Differential Diagnosis

Other causes of groin pain that can present similarly to osteitis pubis include inguinal hernia, pubic rami stress fracture, intra-articular hip disease, genitourinary disease, osteomyelitis, and athletic pubalgia.

Diagnostic Testing

The diagnosis of osteitis pubis is often determined by history and physical examination alone. Gradual onset of midline anterior pelvic pain, along with pubic symphysis tenderness or pain with resisted adductor testing, is characteristic of osteitis pubis.

Plain radiographs are often obtained when the etiology of pain is unclear or if symptoms persist despite conservative treatment. The preferred image is an anteroposterior (AP) pelvis film. Positive findings are usually not apparent until at least 4 weeks after the onset of symptoms and include subchondral erosive change, joint irregularity, and sclerosis. Of note, these findings may also be present among asymptomatic individuals. If pelvic instability is suspected (e.g., difficulty walking, waddling gait), flamingo stress views should be obtained which can reveal vertical pelvic instability (>2 mm of vertical displacement). Ultrasound may also be used to rule out inguinal hernia as well as to visualize dynamic widening at the pubic symphysis.

If the diagnosis is still in question after examination and plain film imaging, an MRI can be obtained and may reveal high signal intensity within the pubic symphysis or periarticular subchondral edema. With chronic disease, subchondral sclerosis and osteophytes may be seen. Radionuclide scanning (e.g., bone scan) should be reserved for patients in whom MRI and/or ultrasound are equivocal.

Nonoperative Management

Management is initially conservative, consisting of relative rest from provocative activities, ice, nonsteroidal anti-inflammatory drugs (NSAIDs), and physical therapy. Core and lumbopelvic strengthening, adductor stretching, and balance control are key components of the rehabilitation program. In cases of concomitant pelvic floor dysfunction, pelvic floor therapy may also be considered. In recalcitrant cases, pubic symphyseal corticosteroid injection or an oral prednisone taper may be trialed.

Indications for Operative Management

Depending on the degree of instability and dysfunction, various surgical procedures have been described, ranging from simple debridement to symphyseal joint fusion. The majority of surgical interventions are considered salvage procedures with limited proven efficacy and are solely reserved for the most recalcitrant cases.

Expected Outcomes

Recovery is generally expected with conservative treatment. Several weeks to months may elapse, however, before symptoms completely resolve. Sports participation is permissible as long as symptoms are tolerable and there is no evidence of instability.

Athletic Pubalgia

Definition and Epidemiology

Athletic pubalgia is a clinical syndrome of groin pain without demonstrable inguinal hernia and is usually encountered in high-level athletes. It is more common in men than women. It is also more common with sports and exercises that require repetitive cutting such as ice hockey, soccer, football, and rugby.

Athletic pubalgia results from repetitive trauma and/or loading of the pelvic stabilizers, commonly involving the confluence of the rectus abdominis insertion and origin of the adductor longus on the pubic tubercle (Fig. 6.1). Muscle imbalance between strong proximal thigh muscles and relatively weaker lower abdominal muscles is thought to play a pivotal role in the development of this overuse injury. Athletic pubalgia is an overarching term describing a range of pathology in this region, often including distal rectus abdominis strain, partial tear or avulsion, adductor longus tendinopathy, enthesopathy, or partial tear, or a combination of these entities.

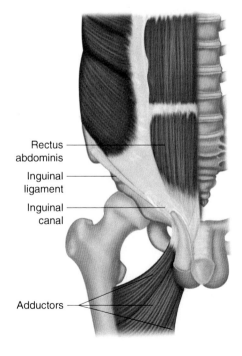

Fig. 6.1 The pertinent anatomy involved in cases of athletic pubalgia. Pathology typically occurs in the region of the rectus abdominis and proximal adductor longus aponeurosis. Although the inguinal canal is located just adjacent to this, athletic pubalgia is a musculoskeletal condition that typically occurs in the absence of a true inguinal hernia

Rectus abdominis

Inguinal ligament

Inguinal canal

Adductors

Clinical Presentation

Symptoms of athletic pubalgia typically develop in an insidious fashion without sudden or traumatic pain. Groin pain just lateral to midline is the predominant symptom. Pain may radiate toward the inner thigh, perineum, and rectus musculature and to the testicles in approximately 30% of men due to entrapment of the ilioinguinal, iliohypogastric, or genitofemoral nerves. Patients may become symptomatic with sports activity, coughing, or Valsalva maneuvers.

In contrast to cases of true inguinal hernia, physical examination of the groin typically fails to detect a bulge or the sensation of an impulse with coughing or straining. There may be tenderness to palpation of the pubic tubercle just lateral to midline over the rectus/adductor aponeurosis. With acute injuries, there may be associated swelling. Patients should be tested for pain with resisted hip flexion and hip adduction, as well as for pain following abdominal muscle contraction.

Differential Diagnosis

The differential diagnosis for athletic pubalgia is similar to that of osteitis pubis, as noted above. Additionally, it important to note that athletic pubalgia may coexist with intra-articular hip pathology in athletes, such as femoroacetabular impingement or labral tear.

Diagnostic Testing

The diagnosis of athletic pubalgia is largely clinical. Plain radiographs may be helpful for differentiating between a true osteitis pubis (with radiographic findings as noted above) versus isolated soft tissue injury, as seen in athletic pubalgia. MRI can be helpful in the diagnosis of athletic pubalgia; however, findings are often quite subtle and require a specific athletic pubalgia protocol to improve sensitivity. In positive cases, findings may include increased signal intensity on T2-weighted imaging involving the anteroinferior aspect of the pubic symphysis (also known as a "secondary cleft sign"). Other findings may include osteitis pubis, tenoperiosteal disruption or frank tear of the adductor aponeurosis, and marrow edema at the pubic tubercle.

Ultrasound offers the best method for diagnosing abnormalities within the superficial inguinal canal including visualization of occult hernias. Ultrasound is also useful in evaluation of pathology at the rectus abdominis/adductor aponeurosis.

Nonoperative Management

Generally, the acute management of groin pain suspected to be athletic pubalgia consists of conservative care, rest from offending activities, ice, trial of anti-inflammatory medications, and physical therapy. Gradual restoration of flexibility and core strengthening and stability is integral to functional recovery. In recalcitrant cases unresponsive to conservative management, diagnostic/therapeutic injections (typically guided by ultrasound imaging) can be helpful.

Indications for Operative Management

When pain continues despite appropriate conservative care and the athlete cannot return to their previous activity, surgery may be considered. Surgical treatment of athletic pubalgia consists of both open and laparoscopic approaches and depends upon the underlying etiology. True hernias are repaired with or without the use of mesh. Other surgical procedures include repair of the adductor/rectus abdominis aponeurotic plate, adductor longus tenotomy or release, and decompression of the genital branch of the genitofemoral nerve.

Expected Outcomes

Prognosis is highly favorable, although some may experience recalcitrant symptoms. If the symptoms are not severe, continued sports participation may be allowed. Surgical repair, when indicated, has been shown to be successful in a majority of cases. Generally, the athlete is allowed to return to play in 2–6 weeks with a laparoscopic repair and 1–6 months following open repair.

Acute Adductor Strains

Definition and Epidemiology

Adductor strains are a common cause of acute groin pain, particularly in athletes and active individuals. These injuries often occur in association with sports that involve kicking or rapid changes of direction with pivoting, such as ice hockey, tennis, basketball, and squash, wherein the adductor group sustains repetitive and rapid eccentric contraction.

Adductor injuries are classified according to anatomy and severity. The adductor longus is most commonly involved, secondary to its relative length, greater tendon to muscle ratio, and weaker attachment at the pubic crest. Grade 1 injuries involve a low-grade tear of a small number of muscle and/or tendon fibers, causing pain but minimal loss of strength or motion. Grade 2 injuries constitute high-grade partial tears, causing pain, swelling, and decreased motion and strength, but not complete loss of function. Grade 3 injuries involve complete disruption of the muscle-tendon unit with loss of muscle function.

Clinical Presentation

The patient should be asked to describe the onset of pain (acute or chronic), its severity, and any radiating features. Features may include tenderness to palpation of the injured myotendinous region, bruising, and, in the case of grade 3 injuries, a palpable defect. Pain is reproduced with resisted adduction, often with associated loss of muscle power.

Differential Diagnosis

Alternative diagnoses to be considered include athletic pubalgia, osteitis pubis, ilioinguinal/obturator nerve entrapment, stress fractures of the pelvis and femoral neck, intrinsic hip pathology (femoroacetabular impingement, labral tear, chondral lesion, osteoarthritis), and referred pain from the lumbar spine. Many of these pathologies may refer pain to the adductor region; however, palpation and provocative testing of the adductors are less likely to reproduce symptoms.

Diagnostic Testing

In many cases, the diagnosis of adductor strain is straightforward and based solely on history and physical examination. In such cases, diagnostic imaging is not necessary. When diagnosis is less clear or there are findings concerning for a grade 3 injury, imaging studies are obtained. Pelvis and hip radiographs can be used to exclude other conditions such as osteitis pubis or femoroacetabular impingement. Anteroposterior (AP) views of the pelvis are recommended at a minimum. Musculoskeletal ultrasound can further visualize the adductor myotendinous structure, bony attachment sites, and associated nerves. Ultrasound is useful for determining the exact location and extent of injury as well as for monitoring recovery.

Obtaining an MRI is generally not necessary for evaluating most adductor injuries, especially with the high sensitivity and low cost of ultrasound. Indications for MRI include suspected tendon avulsion, complex injuries involving more than one structure, injuries that fail to improve despite compliance with an appropriate rehabilitation program, and patients with chronic or recurrent groin pain in which diagnosis remains in question.

Nonoperative Management

Although the recommended treatment course for adductor strain is dictated by the severity of symptoms, this generally consists of a period of protected weight bearing and rest from provocative activities. In the acute phase, ice and compression may be utilized as needed to reduce associated hemorrhage and edema. Complete immobilization should be avoided as this promotes muscle stiffness and scarring. The use of anti-inflammatory analgesic medications is controversial but is typically helpful in the acute phase. It is also appropriate to begin early mobilization with physical therapy. Rehabilitation should be focused on balancing muscle length and strength. Isometric exercises are utilized initially for pain management, progressing to eccentric exercises to strengthen the myotendinous region and facilitate tissue healing. Core and lumbopelvic strengthening involving the hip abductors, lateral hip rotators, and hamstrings should also be performed. The patient may resume activity when both range of motion and muscle strength are fully restored.

Indications for Operative Management

There is no high-level evidence that surgical repair of grade 3 adductor strains yields superior outcomes to nonsurgical management. Surgery is typically reserved for complete avulsions at the adductor longus origin. Open repair with suture anchors is the surgical treatment of choice.

Expected Outcomes

Prognosis varies depending upon the extent of injury and patient activity. In general, grade 1 adductor strains require between 10 and 21 days before the patient can return to sports. Grade 2 injuries require 4–6 weeks, and grade 3 tears or avulsions may require 2–3 months before complete recovery.

Iliopsoas Muscle-Tendon Complex Disorders

Definition and Epidemiology

The iliopsoas muscle-tendon complex is directly anterior to the hip joint and consists of three muscles—psoas major, psoas minor, and iliacus. Iliopsoas pathology is often overlooked as a cause of hip pain but includes a number of clinically significant syndromes including iliopsoas tendinitis or tendinopathy, iliopsoas bursitis, and internal snapping hip syndrome (coxa saltans).

Iliopsoas tendinitis and/or tendinopathy affects young adults more commonly, with a slight female predominance. Acute injuries typically involve an eccentric contraction of the iliopsoas muscle but also may be due to direct trauma. Overuse injury is more likely to lead to iliopsoas tendinopathy and may occur in activities involving repeated hip flexion or external rotation of the thigh, including dancing, rowing, running (particularly uphill), track and field, soccer, and gymnastics.

Internal snapping hip is most commonly caused by the iliopsoas tendon sliding over the femoral head, the iliopectineal eminence, or internally over the iliacus muscle when the hip is ranged from flexion/external rotation to extension/internal rotation, resulting in a palpable and often audible snap in the region of the groin.

Clinical Presentation

Patients often present with complaints of an insidious onset of anterior hip or groin pain. Initially, the patient may note pain with specific sports-related activities that require forceful hip flexion or adduction, such as jogging, running, or kicking. Pain with simple activities such as putting on socks and shoes, rising from a seated position, and walking upstairs or inclines may also be reported. Runners often describe anterior groin pain when trying to lengthen their stride during speed training or with uphill running.

On physical examination, there may be tenderness to palpation along the course of the iliopsoas myotendinous junction just anterior to the hip joint. With the patient supine and with their heels raised off the table to approximately 15°, tenderness can be assessed by palpating the psoas muscle below the lateral inguinal ligament at the femoral triangle. Pain is exacerbated by iliopsoas activation. Hip range of motion may also be painful as will a flexion, abduction, and external rotation (FABER) test. Secondary dysfunction of the hip flexor muscle-tendon complex due to an underlying intra-articular disorder commonly occurs.

Differential Diagnosis

Other causes of anterior hip or groin pain include intra-articular pathology (e.g., labral tear, osteoarthritis), rectus femoris injury, adductor injury, athletic pubalgia, osteitis pubis, and occult hernia.

Diagnostic Testing

Plain radiographs of the pelvis and hip are initially helpful in evaluating for underlying intra-articular hip pathology or other osseous abnormalities. Ultrasonography has been used more frequently as a noninvasive diagnostic adjunct in the diagnosis of iliopsoas muscle-tendon injuries. Demonstration of a thickened or irregular iliopsoas tendon with or without distension of the iliopsoas bursa is a typical associated finding. In cases of internal snapping hip, dynamic ultrasound can assess for visible and palpable snapping of the iliopsoas tendon. As the iliopsoas bursa is frequently contiguous with the hip joint, the presence of bursitis may be indicative of underlying intra-articular pathology.

In refractory cases, MRI can prove useful by allowing for concomitant evaluation of the iliopsoas complex as well as the hip joint itself. Given overlapping clinical presentations, advanced imaging may be helpful in determining the more significant pain generator. In cases of iliopsoas tendinitis or tendinopathy,

T2-weighted images may demonstrate increased signal intensity either in a peritendinous distribution (tendinitis) or within the tendon itself (tendinopathy). In cases of acute myotendinous injury, both T1- and T2-weighted images may depict a region of high signal intensity.

Nonoperative Management

Iliopsoas injuries are typically managed conservatively. Rehabilitation should involve progressive iliopsoas loading complemented by core and lumbopelvic stabilization. Soft tissue mobilization and hip flexor stretching to restore the muscle-tendon unit to its full length should also be emphasized to promote biomechanical optimization. Joint mobilization of the hip and lumbosacral region may be considered. For recalcitrant cases, judicious use of ultrasound-guided corticosteroid injection to the iliopsoas tendon sheath and/or iliopsoas bursa may be of both therapeutic and diagnostic value.

Indications for Operative Management

In refractory cases, endoscopic release or lengthening of the iliopsoas tendon may be performed.

Expected Outcomes

Prognosis for recovery of iliopsoas muscle-tendon complex disorders is excellent. The presence of tendinopathy may prolong recovery; however, even this condition generally responds to conservative care. For cases requiring surgery, return to sports can be anticipated in 3–4 months postoperatively.

Lateral Hip Disorders

Greater Trochanteric Pain Syndrome

Definition and Epidemiology

Greater trochanteric pain syndrome (GTPS) is a clinical entity involving several conditions such as tendinopathy of the gluteus medius and minimus at their insertion on the greater trochanter, with variable involvement of the regional bursae. The gluteus medius and minimus muscles play a primary role in hip abduction and pelvic stabilization in walking, running, and single-leg stance. Mechanically induced tissue failure is a key feature of GTPS. Similar to rotator cuff tendon pathology in the shoulder, involvement of the gluteus minimus and medius can range from peritendinitis to full-thickness tears. Typically, there are three main bursae in the trochanteric region: subgluteus medius, subgluteus minimus, and subgluteus maximus bursae (Fig. 6.2). The subgluteus maximus bursa is often implicated as the source of pain in greater trochanteric bursitis, which often accompanies the tendon pathology described above.

GTPS is common, with female-to-male incidence of approximately 4:1. Age at presentation is most common in the fourth through sixth decades of life. Risk factors include female gender, obesity, knee pain, iliotibial band tenderness, and low back pain. Other conditions associated with GTPS include external snapping hip; scoliosis; leg-length discrepancy; intra-articular conditions of the hip, knee, and foot; and painful foot disorders such as plantar fasciitis.

Clinical Presentation

The key complaint in patients with GTPS is dull pain in the lateral hip and point tenderness over the greater trochanter. Pain may increase with running, ambulation, prolonged standing, climbing stairs, and direct pressure when lying on the painful side. A useful clinical question asks patients to "point where the pain is." Patients with GTPS point to the lateral hip, whereas those with intra-articular hip disease generally point to the groin and the anteromedial thigh.

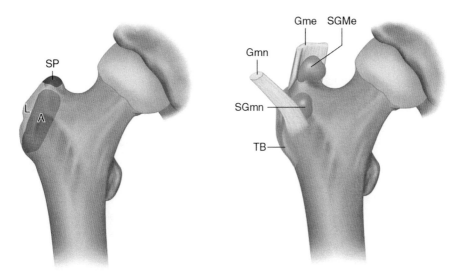

Fig. 6.2 The pertinent anatomy involved in cases of greater trochanteric pain syndrome. Note the complex anatomy of the greater trochanteric region of the lateral hip. The figure on the left depicts the anterior, lateral, and superoposterior facets of the greater trochanter. The figure on the right depicts the insertion of the gluteus minimus on the anterior facet and gluteus medius on the lateral and superoposterior facet of the greater trochanter, with the associated subgluteus minimus, subgluteus medius, and greater trochanteric bursa. With permission from *Radsource—ProtonPACS.* http://radsource.us/gluteus-minimus-tear-trochanteric-bursitis/

Fig. 6.3 Patient with
findings of mild
Trendelenburg
(contralateral pelvic tilt)
upon left single-leg squat.
This finding is common in
cases of hip abductor
(gluteus medius) weakness
or tear

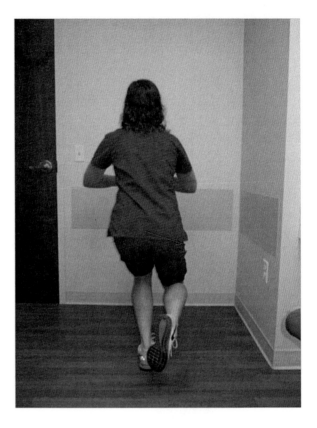

On physical examination, patient should be tested for pain with single-leg stance, single-leg squat, and isolated hip resisted abduction from a side-lying position. Patients with more severe symptoms will also have weakness with a positive Trendelenburg sign with single-leg squat (Fig. 6.3). Tenderness to palpation of the greater trochanteric prominence is the key physical examination finding of GTPS.

Differential Diagnosis

A variety of other conditions can result in lateral hip pain and include intra-articular hip disorders, sacroiliac joint disease, referred pain from lumbar spine disorders, external snapping hip syndrome, and piriformis syndrome.

Diagnostic Testing

Initial imaging should include plain radiographs to assess for bony involvement (e.g., hip degenerative changes) that may be an underlying exacerbant of symptoms. In chronic cases of GTPS secondary to gluteus minimus or gluteus medius

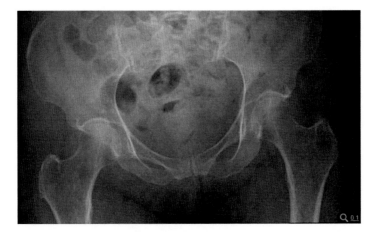

Fig. 6.4 Radiographic findings consistent with bilateral chronic gluteus minimus/medius tendinopathy with associated enthesopathy at the greater trochanter

tendinopathy, one may see enthesopathy and/or calcifications adjacent to the greater trochanter (Fig. 6.4). MRI or ultrasound can be used to detect soft tissue pathology such as bursitis, tendinopathy, enthesopathy, and partial- or full-thickness tendon tears. MRI can additionally be helpful in the evaluation of intra-articular hip disorders or bone stress injury involving the pelvis or femoral neck.

Nonoperative Management

GTPS is a self-limited condition in the majority of patients. Therefore, the goal of treatment is to relieve symptoms and prevent functional impairment. Supportive management includes activity modification, massage, stretching and tissue lengthening of the IT band, and strengthening exercises for the hip abductors, core, and lumbopelvic stabilizers. For patients whose symptoms do not improve, a single steroid injection to the bursa (if identified) or peritendinous region of the gluteus minimus or medius can be trialed. It is recommended that this be performed under image guidance (typically ultrasound) in order to avoid intra-tendinous injection of steroid, which can result in further tendon degeneration and worsen symptoms.

Indications for Operative Management

Surgery can be considered for patients with severe pain and functional impairment after 12 months of conservative management or those who have full-thickness tears of the gluteus medius or minimus resulting in lumbopelvic instability and severe Trendelenburg gait. If the gluteus medius tendon has a full-thickness tear, it can be repaired, most commonly via an endoscopic approach with debridement of degenerative tissue, curettage of the bone surface, reattachment of the tendon using bone anchors, and direct repair of the tendon.

Expected Outcomes

GTPS, as stated earlier, is largely a self-limited condition with the majority of patients reporting 100% relief of symptoms with watchful waiting or completion of a high-quality rehabilitation program. Surgical intervention is rarely necessary. However, when performed, it has been found to be successful in recalcitrant cases of GTPS.

Hip Pointer (Iliac Crest Contusion)

Definition and Epidemiology

A hip pointer is a contusion to the iliac crest, often resulting from a direct blow sustained during sports activity or other trauma such as falls. This condition most often occurs in football, soccer, and ice hockey players.

Clinical Presentation

The patient will report a history of trauma with acute onset of pain. They may have severe pain directly over the iliac crest that worsens with movements that involve activation of the deep core and abdominal musculature such as with coughing, sneezing, or running. The condition may cause severe disability for a brief period of time, with associated swelling or ecchymosis. On physical examination, the patient should be assessed for associated regional muscle spasm.

Differential Diagnosis

Other possible etiologies include iliac crest fracture or apophysitis, abdominal wall injury, or acute strain of the muscles overlying the iliac crest, namely, the gluteus medius, the gluteus minimus, and the tensor fasciae latae. Other non-musculoskeletal causes of abdominal pain or flank pain, such as renal calculi, should be considered.

Diagnostic Testing

An anteroposterior radiograph of the pelvis is helpful to evaluate for fracture or other bony abnormality. In more severe cases, ultrasound may be utilized to evaluate for a focal muscle defect, and MRI can be helpful in the assessment of either bony or soft tissue edema.

Nonoperative Management

Initial treatment should attempt to minimize swelling or hematoma formation with the application of ice and compression. In the acute phase, the affected lower extremity should be partially immobilized with crutches and protected weight bearing. As symptoms improve, a gentle and gradual physical therapy program should be implemented, initially focusing on range of motion followed by isometric strengthening. Ultimately the patient can be progressed to aggressive multidirectional strengthening and neuromuscular rehabilitation.

Expected Outcomes

Prognosis is generally excellent, with return to full activity dictated by sufficient resolution of pain. In the case of athletes returning to play, repeated injury can be avoided via the application of protective padding to the region of the iliac crest.

Posterior Hip and Proximal Hamstring Disorders

Proximal Hamstring Strain

Definition and Epidemiology

Hamstring muscle injuries occur frequently among recreational and elite athletes. As a hip extensor and knee flexor, hamstring injuries can occur at any level in the hamstring but most commonly occur at the myotendinous junction, a 10–12 cm transition zone in which myofibrils merge with tendon in the posterior thigh. Proximal injuries, including tendon avulsion, are more common than distal injuries regardless of the muscle involved. Avulsion fractures of the ischium involving the hamstring muscle origin rarely occur in adults but may occur in skeletally immature athletes.

From a functional standpoint, the hamstring is the key player in lower limb deceleration during walking and running. In these cases, the hamstring contracts eccentrically to decelerate the leg during the end of the swing phase, when the lower extremity is fully extended in front of the athlete's body. Thus, hamstring strain often occurs during high-speed running or with kicking movements such as in soccer. Sprinters tend to injure the long head of the biceps femoris, including the intramuscular tendon and adjacent muscle fibers proximally. Hamstring strains may also occur during stretching movements with the hip in full flexion and the knee in full extension, forcing the hamstring beyond its elastic capacities. This type of injury is often seen in dancers and gymnasts and typically involves the semimembranosus muscle and its proximal tendon.

Clinical Presentation

Most individuals with proximal hamstring strain injury present acutely, complaining of a sudden onset of stabbing posterior thigh pain while performing a high-risk activity. In more severe acute injuries, there is often a feeling of a "pop." On physical examination, a palpable defect indicates a more severe injury. Focal tenderness, swelling, and bruising are common. Pain may be provoked with knee flexion or hip extension, either actively against resistance or with passive stretching.

Differential Diagnosis

In most cases, the mechanism of injury and localization of symptoms makes the diagnosis of acute hamstring strain straightforward. However, in patients with longstanding pain, recurrent symptoms, or an unclear etiology, definitive diagnosis can be more difficult. The differential for proximal posterior thigh pain includes chronic hamstring tendinopathy, lumbosacral radiculitis, sacroiliac joint dysfunction, piriformis syndrome, and posterior thigh compartment syndrome.

Diagnostic Testing

In acute cases, plain radiographs can assist with the identification of severe hamstring injury involving bony avulsion of the ischial tuberosity. In most cases, however, musculoskeletal ultrasonography and MRI are the best methods for assessing acute hamstring strain injuries. Both provide detailed information about the location and extent of injury. Ultrasound allows for dynamic assessment, providing information about tendon and muscle integrity at varying degrees of resisted contraction. Ultrasound has greater sensitivity during the acute phase of injury when inflammatory fluid or hematoma is found in the soft tissue, but sensitivity declines when scanning is delayed. MRI is more reliable than ultrasound at depicting hamstring tendon and osseous avulsion injuries and injuries at the deeper musculotendinous junction. MRI sensitivity does not wane over time and allows accurate assessment of the degree of tendon retraction and morphology if surgical intervention is required. When severe hamstring injuries (e.g., proximal hamstring avulsion) are suspected, MRI remains the imaging modality of choice.

Nonoperative Management

Most hamstring injuries, including high grade strain at the myotendinous junction, can be treated conservatively with protected weight bearing followed by a hamstring stretching and strengthening program. Initial acute management consists of rest, ice, and elevation to limit the extent of localized inflammation. Over-the-counter analgesics are generally adequate for pain relief. While concern has been raised that NSAID therapy for muscle injury may delay healing and lead to impaired function, there is no clinical evidence to suggest that short-term use of nonsteroidal anti-inflammatory medications in the treatment of hamstring injury has significant deleterious effects.

As acute symptoms resolve, gentle stretching followed by conditioning is implemented. Strengthening begins with isometric exercises with ultimate progression to eccentric isokinetic strength exercises as symptoms allow. Eccentric strength training is key for any rehabilitation program as it reduces the risk of reinjury. Return to play is only recommended when strength is at least 90% of the normal contralateral side.

Indications for Operative Management

For complete proximal avulsion ruptures of the tendinous origin from the ischium, early surgical repair is typically advocated as such an approach leads to more favorable outcomes. Surgical repair involves reattachment of the ruptured tendons to the ischial tuberosity with the use of suture anchors.

Expected Outcomes

Recovery is generally favorable with return to sports dictated by the athlete's functional performance. General guidelines include full pain-free range of motion and at least 90% of normal strength before returning to play. Recurrent injuries tend to be more severe and recovery takes longer as a result. Reflective of the highly variable nature of proximal hamstring injuries, mild strains may result in minimal lost playing time, whereas more severe injuries may take several months to fully recover.

Proximal Hamstring Tendinopathy

Definition and Epidemiology

Distinct from a hamstring strain, proximal tendinopathy often involves a slow, progressive onset of tendon thickening and disorganization near the hamstring insertion on the ischial tuberosity, often with concomitant enthesopathy or degenerative tears. In some cases, ischial bursitis may also be present.

Clinical Presentation

Patients typically report deep buttock pain near the ischial tuberosity that is aggravated when accelerating or running uphill or with direct pressure on the ischial tuberosity, as with prolonged sitting. On physical examination, there is tenderness to palpation directly over the ischial tuberosity. Pain provocation tests include the modified bent-knee stretch test, single-leg bridge, and resisted hip extension with the patient in a prone position.

Differential Diagnosis

Differential diagnosis includes lumbosacral radiculitis, ischiofemoral impingement, piriformis syndrome, intra-articular hip pathology with radiation to the buttock, and sacroiliac dysfunction.

Diagnostic Testing

Diagnostic testing is similar to that noted above in the section on proximal hamstring strain. In cases of proximal hamstring tendinopathy, ultrasound is likely to reveal thickening and disorganization of the proximal hamstring tendinous insertion, often with associated enthesopathy or small intra-tendinous calcifications. Additionally, in chronic cases, plan radiographs may also be helpful to identify enthesopathy or intra-tendinous calcifications at the ischial tuberosity.

Nonoperative Management

Early treatment should include core and lumbopelvic stabilization with particular focus on gluteal muscle activation. Progressive strengthening of the hamstrings with eccentric exercises should be implemented once the tendon is less reactive. In refractory cases, ultrasound-guided needle tenotomy with or without use of platelet-rich plasma can be attempted in order to incite a pro-inflammatory response and stimulate tendon healing. Additionally, a one-time corticosteroid injection under ultrasound guidance, targeting the peritendinous soft tissue, may be helpful in reducing pain and facilitate full participation in a progressive loading program.

Indications for Operative Management

Referral for surgery is indicated when pain persists despite prolonged conservative management or in cases of advanced tendinopathy that have progressed to high-grade partial- or full-thickness tears. Operative management consists of open tendon debridement and primary repair.

Ischiofemoral Impingement

Definition and Epidemiology

Ischiofemoral impingement syndrome is defined by posterior hip pain related to impingement of soft tissues between the ischial tuberosity and lesser trochanter of the femur, primarily involving the quadratus femoris muscle. Narrowing of the ischiofemoral space may be positional, congenital, or acquired, such as in cases of prior hip arthroplasty, hypertrophy due to osteoarthritis, or fractures involving the lesser trochanter. The quadratus femoris muscle originates at the anterior portion of the ischial tuberosity and inserts on the posteromedial aspect of the proximal femur, and its main role is to assist in external rotation and adduction of the hip. Ischiofemoral impingement is more common in women and affects individuals of all ages.

Clinical Presentation

Patients with ischiofemoral impingement present with chronic pain deep in the buttock, usually without a precipitating injury. Given the proximity of the quadratus femoris muscle to the sciatic nerve, the pain may radiate distally to the posterior thigh and leg. Bilateral involvement has been observed in 25–40% of patients. On physical examination, patients may report pain during hip range of motion, and symptoms may be reproduced by a combination of hip extension, adduction, and external rotation or with hip flexion and internal rotation.

Differential Diagnosis

The differential diagnosis for ischiofemoral impingement includes proximal hamstring tendinopathy or hamstring strain, lumbosacral radiculopathy, piriformis syndrome, or intra-articular hip pathology with posterior radiation to the buttock.

Diagnostic Testing

Plain radiographs may be helpful to evaluate for other entities such as intra-articular hip pathology which may mimic ischiofemoral impingement. Thereafter, both ultrasound and MRI have utility in evaluating this difficult clinical entity. MRI may reveal edema within the quadratus femoris muscle, indicative of repetitive impingement and focal inflammation. Additionally, ultrasound may be useful in offering the ability for dynamic assessment, noting soft tissue impingement between the ischial tuberosity and lesser trochanter when the hip is brought into external rotation. With ultrasound assessment, side-to-side comparison is critical for determining whether any noted impingement might be pathologic versus a normal variant dependent on the patient's anatomy.

Nonoperative Management

Treatment of ischiofemoral impingement is nearly entirely conservative, and there is little indication for surgical intervention, unless a true bony defect or structural abnormality is noted. Rehabilitation should be focused on optimizing hip biomechanics through a progressive core and lumbopelvic stabilization program, as well as education that shows patient how to avoid movement patterns which may exacerbate symptoms. In refractory cases, ultrasound-guided injection into the ischiofemoral space (with care to avoid the sciatic nerve) may be helpful for both diagnostic and therapeutic purposes.

Expected Outcomes

Treatment outcomes are typically quite favorable with the use of a multifaceted and comprehensive rehabilitation program, as outlined above.

Table 6.1 shows a summary of soft tissue disorders of the hip with synopsis of presentation, diagnostic testing, and suggested management options.

Table 6.1 Summary of soft tissue disorders of the hip with synopsis of presentation, diagnostic testing, and suggested management options

Clinical Entity	Presentation	Diagnostic testing	Conservative management	Surgical indications and operative management
Osteitis pubis	– Insidious midline groin pain – Tender to palpation over pubic symphysis	– Primarily clinical – MRI—periarticular edema at symphysis pubis	– Rest, ice, NSAIDs – PT – Image-guided injection	– Rarely indicated – Pubic symphysis debridement; symphyseal joint fusion
Athletic pubalgia	– Groin pain over pubic tubercle – Negative tests for true hernia	– Primarily clinical – MRI—increased signal intensity at anteroinferior pubic ramus	– Rest, ice, NSAIDs – PT – Image-guided injection	– Hernia repair if indicated – Repair of abdominal wall in cases of breach of rectus abdominis aponeurosis
Adductor strain	– Acute onset groin pain – Tenderness to palpation of injured myotendinous region	– Primarily clinical – U/S—defect of muscle or tendon, associated hematoma – MRI—obtain if tendon avulsion or complex injury is suspected	– Protected weight bearing, rest, ice, NSAIDs – PT	– Reserved for complete avulsions of adductor insertion
Iliopsoas disorders	– Insidious onset anterior hip or groin pain – Pain with activities requiring hip flexion or adduction	– X-ray (AP pelvis and hip) – U/S	– PT – U/S-guided steroid injection	– Endoscopic release or lengthening of iliopsoas tendon
Greater trochanteric pain syndrome (GTPS)	– Slow-onset dull pain at lateral hip – Point tenderness over greater trochanter GT	– Primarily clinical – MRI or U/S—gluteus minimus/medius tendinopathy or tear, associated bursitis	– Activity modification, ITB stretching – PT – U/S-guided steroid injection	– Endoscopic repair

(continued)

Table 6.1 (continued)

Clinical Entity	Presentation	Diagnostic testing	Conservative management	Surgical indications and operative management
Hip pointer	– Acute, traumatic onset of pain at iliac crest – Localized tenderness over iliac crest	– X-ray (AP pelvis)—rule out fracture – MRI—evaluate for bone or soft tissue edema	– Protected weight bearing, rest, ice, NSAIDs – PT	None
Proximal hamstring strain	– Acute onset sharp posterior thigh pain – Provoked with resisted knee flexion, hip extension	– Primarily clinical – U/S—myotendinous defect or hematoma – MRI—evaluate for full avulsion of ischial tuberosity	– Protected weight bearing, rest, ice, NSAIDs – PT	– Typically reserved for complete avulsion of hamstring origin
Proximal hamstring tendinopathy	– Slow-onset of deep buttock pain over ischial tuberosity – Pain provocation with bent-knee stretch test, single-leg bridge, resisted hip extension in prone	– U/S or MRI—tendinopathy or tear of proximal hamstring tendinous insertion, intra-tendinous calcifications	– PT – U/S-guided tenotomy with injection	– Open tendon debridement or primary tendon repair
Ischiofemoral impingement	– Slow-onset of deep buttock pain +/− radiation distal posterior leg – Pain typically provoked with hip extension/ adduction/ external rotation OR hip flexion/ internal rotation	– MRI—edema within quadratus femoris muscle – U/S—dynamic evaluation of quadratus femoris impingement with hip ER/IR	– PT – U/S-guided injection into ischiofemoral space	None

P physical therapy, *U/S* ultrasound, *MRI* magnetic resonance imaging, *NSAIDs* nonsteroidal anti-inflammatory drugs

Suggested Reading

Fearon AM, Scarvell JM, Neeman T, et al. Greater trochanteric pain syndrome: defining the clinical syndrome. Br J Sports Med. 2013;47:649–53.

Grimaldi A, Mellor R, Hodges P. Gluteal tendinopathy: a review of mechanisms, assessment and management. Sports Med. 2015;45:1107–19.

Jacobson JA, Bedi A, Sekiya JK, et al. Evaluation of the painful athletic hip: imaging options and imaging-guided injections. Am J Roentgenol. 2012;199:516–24.

Rompe JD, Segal NA, Cacchio A, et al. Home training, local corticosteroid injection, or radial shock wave therapy for greater trochanteric pain syndrome. Am J Sports Med. 2009;37:981–90.

Ross JR, Stone RM, Larson CM. Core muscle injury/sports hernia/athletic pubalgia, and femoroacetabular impingement. Sports Med Arthrosc. 2015;23:213–20.

Sherry MA, Johnston TS, Heiderscheit BC. Rehabilitation of acute hamstring strain injuries. Clin Sports Med. 2015;34:263–84.

Stafford GH, Villar RN. Ischiofemoral impingement. J Bone Joint Surg Br. 2011;93-B:1300–2.

Chapter 7
Femoroacetabular Impingement, Labral Tears, Abductor Tendon Tears, and Hip Arthroscopy

Scott D. Martin

Abbreviations

FAI Femoroacetabular impingement
MRA Magnetic resonance angiography
MRI Magnetic resonance imaging

Femoroacetabular Impingement and Labral Tears

Definition and Epidemiology

Femoroacetabular impingement (FAI) and resultant labral tears are increasingly recognized as a cause of pre-arthritic hip pain, particularly in younger athletes. Indeed, 22–55% of patients presenting with hip pain have a labral tear. Tearing of the labrum is most commonly attributed to FAI, as 95% of patients with FAI will have a labral tear. Rarely, labral tears are observed in the setting of acute trauma as they can occur with hip dislocation.

Two bony abnormalities comprise FAI: cam and pincer lesions (Fig. 7.1). Cam lesions refer to an asphericity of the femoral head-neck junction, while pincer lesions result from acetabular overcoverage or retroversion. During hip flexion and rotation, FAI leads to increased contact between the femoral head and acetabular rim. Cam lesions cause shearing at the chondrolabral junction, and pincer lesions lead to direct contact between the rim and femoral neck, compressing the labrum. This repetitive trauma and loss of the labral seal is a proposed precursor to osteoarthritis.

S.D. Martin (✉)
Department of Orthopaedic Surgery, Massachusetts General Hospital and Brigham and Women's Hospital, Harvard Medical School, Boston, MA, USA
e-mail: sdmartin@partners.org

© Springer International Publishing AG 2018
J.N. Katz et al. (eds.), *Principles of Orthopedic Practice for Primary Care Providers*, https://doi.org/10.1007/978-3-319-68661-5_7

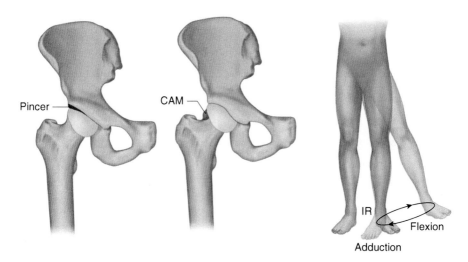

Fig. 7.1 Illustrations of the two bony abnormalities comprising FAI: cam and pincer lesions Pincer lesions refer to overcoverage or acetabular retroversion. Cam lesions represent a prominence at the femoral head-neck junction

Labral tears and FAI are more commonly recognized in an athletic population as these patients experience symptoms when loading the hip joint during practice or competition. Still an active area of research, the underlying etiology appears to be genetic, although development and activity level may contribute. The incidence of labral tears significantly increases with age. Even in an asymptomatic population, 69% of patients will have a labral tear on MRI by age 38. Additionally, in an older population, underlying arthritis may be the primary pain generator, despite a concomitant labral tear. Therefore, correlating symptoms with physical exam and imaging is crucial to providing appropriate care.

Gender-specific differences do exist. Females present with greater limitation in function, while males often have larger tears and associated chondral damage. Additionally, males are more likely to have cam lesions than females. Patients often present in the fourth and fifth decade of life. The diagnosis can be elusive, as patients may report symptoms for as long as 2 years prior to diagnosis. An awareness and understanding of the disease is essential for all providers who see patients with hip pain.

Clinical Presentation

Patients with labral tears often present with anterior hip or groin pain. Pain is characterized as deep and in a "C" distribution around the lateral aspect of the hip. Sporadic mechanical symptoms such as catching, popping, or locking are frequently reported. Symptoms frequently occur with pivoting activities or deep flexion such as rising out of a low chair and resolve quickly after cessation of an offending activity.

Complaints of a continued ache and sensitivity within the hip joint, however, are more suggestive of underlying arthritis or chondral damage. When obtaining the history, it is important to elicit symptoms that could be due to an alternate etiology. Radicular symptoms, including paresthesias and radiating pain distal to the knee, are far more suggestive of spine pathology.

On physical exam, the most sensitive test for FAI is pain with flexion, adduction, and internal rotation while the patient is lying supine. This movement is most likely to cause anterior impingement, with compression of the labrum. While most tears are located anterosuperior on the acetabulum, posteroinferior labral tears can also occur, although they are rare. Symptoms resulting from a posteroinferior tear can be elicited by abducting the patient's leg off the exam table while applying slight flexion and external rotation.

Symptoms may also be reproduced by having the patient squat deeply. Observing the patient's gait can also be helpful, as labral tears rarely lead to an antalgic gait. Full assessment of the patient's hip range of motion, strength, and neurovascular function is important in ruling out alternate diagnoses.

Differential Diagnosis and Suggested Diagnostic Testing

Symptomatic labral tears can be difficult to diagnose and require careful consideration of the patient's history, physical exam findings, and results of imaging. Other common conditions that must be excluded are osteoarthritis, spine and lower back pathology, sacroiliac joint dysfunction, abductor tendon tears, internal coxa saltans, and external coxa saltans. In females, similar symptoms can result from gynecologic pathology in certain situations.

Imaging should begin with plain radiographs, including anteroposterior (AP) view of the pelvis, and dedicated AP and lateral views of the affected hip. A Dunn lateral radiograph is easiest to view the junction of the femoral head and neck. A false profile view can also be obtained to assess acetabular coverage of the femoral head. Cam lesions can often be visualized on lateral hip radiographs (Fig. 7.2). A crossover sign, in which the anterior wall of the acetabulum is observed crossing over the posterior wall in a more lateral location, is indicative of acetabular retroversion, an anatomic finding that increases the risk of FAI (Fig. 7.3). Additional radiographic measurements, including the lateral center edge angle and alpha angle, are frequently used by orthopedic surgeons in their evaluation of patients with FAI. Radiographs should also be closely evaluated for signs of arthritis such as decreased joint space, osteophytes, subchondral cysts, and sclerosis.

Given the high prevalence of labral tears even in an asymptomatic population, MRI/MRA should be used with caution and only when there is high suspicion that a labral tear is the source of pain. While MRI and MRA are both sensitivity for labral tears, in our opinion, MRA allows for easier visualization (Fig. 7.4). Careful attention should be paid to the chondrolabral junction, as tearing beyond this region may be irreparable. In addition to assessing the labrum, the cartilage within the joint

Fig. 7.2 Frog-leg lateral
image of the left hip
demonstrating a cam lesion

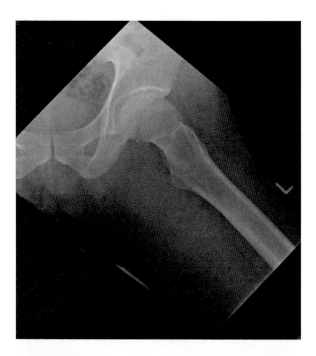

Fig. 7.3 AP pelvis in a
patient with bilateral hip
pain. Bilateral pincer
lesions as identified by a
crossover sign. Coxa
profunda is also present

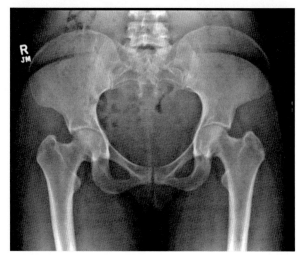

should be evaluated, and the subchondral bone should be assessed. Subchondral cysts and edema have been associated with worse outcomes following arthroscopy.

An intra-articular anesthetic arthrogram with additional steroid can serve both diagnostic and therapeutic purposes and is often performed simultaneously with an MRA. An improvement in pain shortly after the injection is thought to be more suggestive of intra-articular pathology such as a labral tear. A negative response indicates

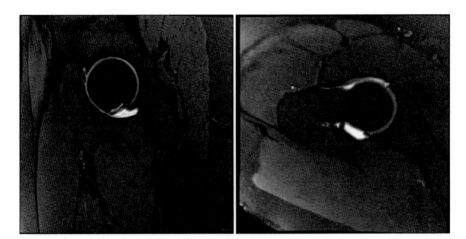

Fig. 7.4 An anterosuperior labral tear can be seen on the MRA sagittal (*left*) and axial oblique T1 FS (*right*) views. Dye has filled in the area between the labrum and acetabular rim, indicating a tear

that further evaluation is needed. However, false negatives are seen with this test and are thought to be due to overexpansion of the joint capsule due to excessive fluid within the joint. Therefore, a false test should not definitively rule out the diagnosis.

Non-operative Management

Non-operative management is typically the first-line treatment for all patients with FAI and labral tears, except in rare cases of severe FAI in a young patient when there is significant concern for rapid joint destruction. Non-operative management consists of an intra-articular steroid injection followed by physical therapy. The intra-articular injection can also be used as a diagnostic tool to localize the source of pain when an anesthetic is included. Oral nonsteroidal anti-inflammatories and acetaminophen are recommended for pain relief and to reduce inflammation until the steroid injection takes effect.

Patients with hip pain often compensate by loading other areas of the pelvis, sacroiliac joint, spine, and knee. Therefore, physical therapy should focus on all these areas with an emphasis on regaining range of motion, strength, and dynamic stability. Patient should be allowed to slowly increase activities as tolerated, with the goal of returning to most activities by 6 months. All patients are advised to temporarily limit activities involving impact loading, frequent pivoting, and extreme range of motion. Specifically, squats, lunges, deadlifts, and distance running are strongly discouraged as the patient recovers from an acute episode of hip pain.

While greater than 85% of patients respond well to therapy, some will report continued symptoms and dissatisfaction with their activity limitations. Injections can be administered 4 months apart in the event of a recurrent flare, if significant pathology is not observed on imaging. Initial non-operative management is stressed in the majority of patients with symptomatic labral tears as they often improve without need for further intervention. At this time, prophylactic surgery for asymptomatic FAI or labral tears is not indicated.

Indications for Surgery

One of the key indicators to pursue surgical intervention is failure of non-operative management. A significant proportion of patients treated with intra-articular injections, PT, and activity modification report improvement in their pain and symptoms. However, if symptoms persist, surgery may be warranted.

Due to the proposed association with joint destruction and subsequent arthritis, surgical intervention can be considered a joint preservation procedure. Therefore, more aggressive surgical treatment should be considered in younger patients and those with more severe signs of impingement on X-ray. Ideal candidates for surgery are those with minimal arthritis, age under 40, clear impingement and tearing on imaging, and failure of non-operative management.

Operative Management

Surgical intervention entails arthroscopic labral repair with acetabular or femoral osteoplasty (removal of the offending structures causing impingement) as indicated based on imaging. Upon entry into the joint, the labrum, chondrolabral junction, and cartilage are evaluated. The degree of arthritis can be more accurately assessed arthroscopically than with imaging.

The quality of the labral tear is evaluated and repaired if possible. Given the key functions of the labrum in sealing the joint and joint stability, it is our opinion that as much of the labrum should be preserved as possible. Anchors are placed into the acetabular rim, and the labral tear is repaired with suture (Fig. 7.5). Various augmentation procedures have also been described. If ultimately irreparable, the labrum may be debrided to prevent continued symptoms. However, it is thought that these patients will proceed to arthritis and total joint replacement more rapidly.

The acetabular rim and femoral head-neck junction are both inspected. Bony abnormalities are removed with a burr, and fluoroscopy is used to ensure adequate resection. Additionally, hip motion is observed during surgery to ensure that all sources of impingement have been addressed.

Typically, in an outpatient procedure, the patient is allowed immediate weight-bearing with a foot-flat gait on crutches. Patients use crutches for a minimum of 6 weeks to protect the repair by preventing the pelvis from tilting or lurching. A graded protocol is initiated with the patient first regaining motion on a stationary bike with low resistance, followed by swimming and elliptical machine. Physical

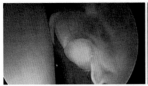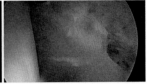

Fig. 7.5 These images demonstrate a labral tear as viewed during arthroscopic repair. For orientation, the femoral head is *left*, and acetabulum is to the *right*. *From left*: the labral tear can be identified by the wavy and frayed tissue. The capsular side of the labrum is elevated off the acetabulum, and an anchor is placed behind the labrum. Suture is then passed through the area of the tear. Once secured, the tissue returns to its anatomical location, and the knots are hidden as they lie on the capsular side

therapy may not be necessary, as aggressive treatment can irritate the hip. The objective is to return all patients to full activity 6 months after surgery.

Expected Outcomes

Patients commonly report an improvement in pain and symptoms after surgery, with most returning to pre-injury activity level. Competitive athletes are often able to return to sport and are satisfied with the results. Surgery primarily impacts the symptoms of acute pain and locking; however, achiness of the hip attributed to osteoarthritis is difficult to alleviate. Treatment of FAI and labral tears is thought to be a joint-preserving procedure that can prolong the development of arthritis and subsequent hip replacement. Factors that have been associated with worse outcomes include age over 40 and signs of advanced arthritis. At this point in time, the only surgical treatment for advanced arthritis is total hip replacement. Complications are rare but can include infection, bleeding, and paresthesias that are rarely permanent. Additionally, not all patients may feel that their symptoms have improved with surgery, and some may still go on to a total hip replacement later in life.

Abductor Tendon Tears

Definition and Epidemiology

The abductor tendons of the hip can be considered analogous to the rotator cuff of the shoulder. These large muscles travel laterally from the ilium to attach at specific sites on the greater trochanter. Tears of the abductor tendons increase in prevalence with age, and females are more commonly affected than males. These injuries can be both a significant source of pain and dysfunction and may be present in as many as 20% of individuals with hip degeneration. Occasionally attributed to an acute injury, tears are often degenerative in nature with an insidious onset. Patients will report symptoms that fail to resolve, or slowly increase, over an extended period of time despite rest or therapy regimens. As the abductors of the hip are crucial to the stability of the pelvis and gait, patients may note symptoms with daily activities.

Clinical Presentation

Patients with tears of the abductor tendons most commonly report pain located laterally over the greater trochanter. Pain in the groin is more indicative of an intra-articular process. The area over the greater trochanter may be tender to palpation, as this is the attachment site for these tendons. Pain may also be exacerbated by activity, as patients notice slight alterations in gait or weakness with activities requiring hip abduction.

While patients often report pain and dysfunction, the physical exam is important in determining the competency of the musculotendinous unit. Observing the patient's gait, the physician should pay close attention for a contralateral pelvis drop as the patient balances on the injured leg while walking (Trendelenburg gait). Similarly, the physician should stand behind the patient with one hand on each iliac crest as the patient flexes their leg to 90° while balancing on the other. If the contralateral pelvis drops while standing on the injured leg, this is considered a positive Trendelenburg sign suggesting impairment of the gluteal tendons. A worse indicator is if the patient cannot balance at all. If untreated, these deficits may become slowly progressive and less likely to resolve with surgical intervention.

Other physical examination maneuvers of the hip, including range of motion, strength, and provocative testing, should be performed to verify that the source of pain is not intra-articular. Intra-articular abnormalities can present as lateral hip pain. Additionally, the lower spine and neurovascular function should be evaluated.

Differential Diagnosis and Suggested Diagnostic Testing

On presentation, all patients should undergo standard radiographs of the hip including an anteroposterior (AP) and lateral view of the hip, in addition to an AP pelvis. The integrity of the joint, lumbosacral spine, and sacroiliac joint should be assessed for pathology as they may all contribute to lateral hip pain. Arthritis of these areas can produce pain radiating around the outside of the hip. Iliotibial band syndrome may also cause lateral hip pain but would not result in the same functional deficits seen with gluteal tendon tears.

Magnetic resonance imaging (MRI) is the definitive test to identify abductor tendon tears (Fig. 7.6). On MRI, the tendon can be seen separated from the greater trochanter as the muscles tend to retract superiorly. Inflammation within the tendon, and in the bony attachment site, may be observed. The size and thickness of the tear can also be appreciated. An angiogram is not needed given the extra-articular nature

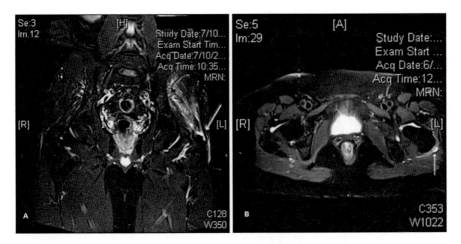

Fig. 7.6 Gluteal tendon tears are best evaluated on MRI. Here is a T2 coronal (**a**) and axial (**b**) view. When comparing the *left* to the *right* side, a hyperintense space can be seen between the greater trochanter and gluteal tendons indicating a tear (*white arrow*). The tendon tends to retract superiorly

of the injury. If there is concern for intra-articular pathology, an anesthetic arthrogram may be performed. Patients with gluteal tears typically do not report improvement with intra-articular injection.

Anesthetic and steroid injections into the tendon attachment site should be performed with caution. Pain relief with an injection suggests that the gluteal tendon is the source of pain.

Non-operative Management

Gluteal tendon tears should be treated with an initial trial of non-operative management that may entail physical therapy, activity modification, steroid injections, and nonsteroidal anti-inflammatories as needed. Many of these injuries, particularly small partial tears, respond well to conservative therapy. However, if patients fail to respond, or exhibit worsening of symptoms, early surgical intervention may allow patients to regain function.

Indications for Surgery

Surgery can be recommended if patients fail conservative therapy. Larger, full-thickness tears are likely to be more amenable to repair with a consequent greater improvement in symptoms. However, once significant functional deficits are noted on physical exam, such as Trendelenburg sign, the likelihood of regaining that

Fig. 7.7 The gluteal
tendons have distinct
insertion sites on the
greater trochanter. When
repaired, the natural
anatomy should be
restored, so awareness of
these footprints is
essential. *Top*:
Arthroscopic view of tears
of the gluteus medius
(*arrows*) and gluteus
minimus (*asterisk*) *Bottom*:
Arthroscopic view of the
repair

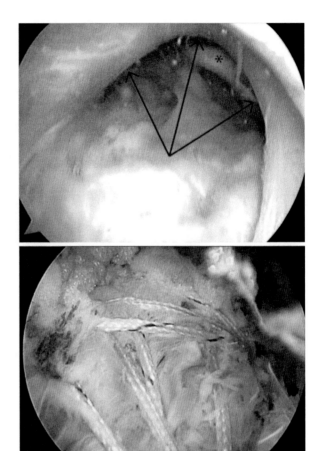

strength diminishes. Surgical repair may still improve pain; however, it may not
restore function to the desired level. This is important when counseling patients on
management options and for referring providers so that timely work-up and referral
can be pursued if needed. Without surgical intervention, these tears do not appear to
heal spontaneously, but patients may be able to compensate with surrounding musculature and strengthening of the remaining intact tissue. The tissue quality should
also be evaluated as those with more severe retraction, and fat atrophy are less likely
to experience significant functional improvement. Patients with significant fat atrophy and functional deficits at presentation should not be considered viable surgical
candidates.

Table 7.1 Summary of femoroacetabular impingement (FAI), labral tears, and abductor tendon tears of the hip with synopsis of presentation, diagnostic testing, and suggested management options

Clinical entity	Presentation	Diagnostic testing	Conservative management	Indications for surgery	Operative management
FAI and labral tear	– Hip pain with flexion and internal rotation – Catching, popping, locking – Exacerbated with pivoting	– MRI or MRA	– Steroid arthrogram – Physical therapy – NSAIDs – Activity modification	– Failure of conservative management – Significant FAI on imaging – Younger age	– Arthroscopic femoroacetabular osteoplasty with labral repair – Labral debridement and/or augmentation
Abductor tendon tear	– Lateral hip pain localized over greater trochanter – Pain exacerbated with activity or direct pressure – Trendelenburg gait or stance	– MRI	– Steroid injection – Physical therapy – NSAIDs – Activity modification	– Failure of conservative management – Full-thickness tear	– Endoscopic gluteal tendon repair

NSAIDs nonsteroidal anti-inflammatory drugs, *MRI* magnetic resonance imaging, *MRA* magnetic resonance angiography

Operative Management

Gluteal tendon tear repairs can be performed endoscopically. The patient is placed in the lateral decubitus position for the procedure. The deep peritrochanteric space is entered with trocars in four locations to allow for scope and instrument access. The tear is then visualized. An anchor is placed in the gluteal tendon insertion site on the greater trochanter, and the suture is subsequently passed through the intact portion of the tendon (Fig. 7.7). Care is taken to appropriately place the anchors so that the natural anatomy is restored for optimal function. The tendon is then securely tied back down to its anatomical insertion site. Postoperatively, patients are advised to use a progressive foot-flat weight-bearing gait with crutches. By 3 months, they may begin to return to all normal activities.

Expected Outcomes

A relatively new procedure, endoscopic repair of the gluteal tendons, has gained significant traction recently with studies reporting good to excellent results. Most reliably, surgical intervention provides pain relief and functional improvement. If significant functional deficits were present prior to surgery, postoperative resolution is variable. Additionally, patients with poor tissue quality, indicated by fat atrophy and retraction, are less likely to experience functional benefits. Complications are rare with this procedure but can include nerve palsy, infection, and bleeding.

Table 7.1 shows a summary of femoroacetabular impingement (FAI), labral tears, and abductor tendon tears of the hip with synopsis of presentation, diagnostic testing, and suggested management options.

Suggested Reading

Alpaugh K, Chilelli BJ, Xu S, Martin SD. Outcomes after primary open or endoscopic abductor tendon repair in the hip: a systematic review of the literature. Arthroscopy. 2015;31:530–40.

Byrd JW. Hip arthroscopy. J Am Acad Orthop Surg. 2006;14:433–44.

Mosier BA, Quinlan NJ, Martin SD. Peritrochanteric endoscopy. Clin Sports Med. 2016;35:449–67.

Nepple JJ, Byrd JW, Siebenrock KA, Prather H, Clohisy JC. Overview of treatment options, clinical results, and controversies in the management of femoroacetabular impingement. J Am Acad Orthop Surg. 2013;21(Suppl 1):S47–52.

Safran MR. The acetabular labrum: anatomic and functional characteristics and rationale for surgical intervention. J Am Acad Orthop Surg. 2010;18:338–45.

Chapter 8
Total Hip Arthroplasty and the Treatment of Hip Osteoarthritis

Michael J. Weaver

Abbreviations

AP	Anteroposterior
AVN	Avascular necrosis
DMARDs	Disease-modifying antirheumatic drugs
NSAIDs	Nonsteroidal anti-inflammatory drugs
OA	Osteoarthritis
RA	Rheumatoid arthritis
THA	Total hip arthroplasty

Definition and Epidemiology

Hip osteoarthritis represents one of the most common conditions within the US population, with an estimated prevalence of 10% in individuals 45 and over. Clinically symptomatic arthritis, where hip pain due to degenerative changes impairs daily activities and quality of life, remains one of the most frequent conditions prompting presentation to an orthopedic surgeon. The cost of managing hip arthritis exceeds $13 billion per year in terms of surgical treatment alone. Total hip arthroplasty (THA) remains the most common surgical intervention for primary hip osteoarthritis. THA is a resurfacing procedure of the hip joint: diseased bone and cartilage of the hip are removed and replaced by implants made of metal, plastic, and occasionally ceramic. The new articulation allows for painless motion and weight bearing. At 10-year follow-up, over 90% of patients can expect to have a well-functioning joint without the need for revision surgery. Over 300,000 hip replacement procedures are performed in the United States every year. As the baby boomer generation ages and as people continue to be more active later in life, the demand for hip replacement surgery is expected to increase over the coming decades.

M.J. Weaver (✉)
Department of Orthopaedic Surgery, Brigham and Women's Hospital, Harvard Medical School, Boston, MA, USA
e-mail: mjweaver@partners.org

© Springer International Publishing AG 2018   111
J.N. Katz et al. (eds.), *Principles of Orthopedic Practice for Primary Care Providers*, https://doi.org/10.1007/978-3-319-68661-5_8

Clinical Presentation

The primary complaint of patients with hip arthritis is pain. Typically they present with pain in their groin. The pain can also occur in the buttock, laterally over the greater trochanter, or in the anterior thigh. Occasionally patients will have referred pain down the thigh into the knee. Interestingly, a small minority of patients with hip arthritis will present with knee pain only. Pain is exacerbated by activity and relieved with rest. Occasionally patients may complain of trouble sleeping due to the pain.

Hip arthritis patients also present with stiffness in their hip. Hip flexion and particularly internal rotation can become limited and may interfere with many activities of daily living. For example, many patients complain of difficulty donning socks and tying shoes and getting into and out of a car.

The pain associated with hip arthritis typically progresses over the course of several months to a year. It often begins as an intermittent ache that evolves into a constant bother. Some patients may have occasional flare-ups associated with minor injuries that can be managed with anti-inflammatory pain medications. The pain and stiffness typically progress until patients are extremely limited in their ability to walk and perform normal daily activities.

Differential Diagnosis

Hip arthritis results from degeneration of the hip joint and its articular cartilage. This process can result from a number of factors—including genetic predisposition, congenital abnormalities of the hip, or traumatic injury. The normal hip is a ball-and-socket joint lined by smooth articular cartilage. This structure allows the hip to have a wide range of motion while being inherently stable and capable of withstanding body weight during normal activities. As the arthritic process progresses, the cartilage in the hip frays and begins to thin out. When the subchondral bone beneath the cartilage begins to wear down, inflammation, pain, and stiffness result.

Osteoarthritis

Osteoarthritis is the most common cause of musculoskeletal pain and disability. Hip osteoarthritis is thought to be due to subtle mechanical deficiencies within the hip joint. Due to slight problems in the development of the hip joint, the hip may be more susceptible to wear and damage from normal activities. As the patient ages, damage accumulates and the cartilage of the hip slowly degenerates. This is manifested by pain and stiffness in the hip and limited mobility. Osteoarthritis may affect either one or both hips and can be synchronous or asynchronous.

Patients are commonly in their fifth, sixth, or seventh decade of life and present with progressive groin pain and stiffness. Factors associated with the development of hip arthritis include age, diabetes, family predisposition, and hypertension. Patients with developmental anomalies of their hips, including Perthes disease or hip dysplasia, are also at risk. Interestingly, unlike knee arthritis, obesity does not appear to be associated with the development of hip arthritis.

Inflammatory Arthritis

Rheumatoid arthritis (RA) is the most common inflammatory arthritis that affects the hip. The synovial lining of the hip joint becomes hypertrophic and inflamed, infiltrated by mononuclear cells, polymorphonuclear leukocytes, and macrophages. Initially synovitis is primarily responsible for hip pain. Untreated, the inflamed synovium leads to irreversible cartilage destruction and damage to periarticular bone. The treatment for rheumatoid arthritis has evolved significantly over the last 10–20 years. With the advent of disease-modifying antirheumatic drugs (DMARDs), severe joint disease and end-stage arthritis as a result of rheumatoid arthritis are now much less common. Once the disease has progressed to cartilage and bone destruction, medical management alone is often ineffective, and a hip replacement may be indicated.

Seronegative spondyloarthropathies including ankylosing spondylitis, psoriatic arthritis, and Reiter syndrome can also affect the hip. These are a group of interrelated inflammatory arthritides that are often associated with the HLA-B27 gene. Ankylosing spondylitis affects the spine, sacroiliac joints, and peripheral joints. Inflammation primarily involves the entheses—the attachments of ligaments to bone. The hip is often one of the earlier joints effected. Psoriatic arthritis involves an inflammatory arthritis in association with classic psoriatic lesions. Patients also typically present with nail involvement, including hyperkeratosis or pitting of the nail bed. Reiter syndrome represents a reactive arthritis in association with eye, skin, and mucous membrane inflammation. Regardless of the underlying etiology, once advanced, the degeneration associated with these entities is best treated with total hip replacement.

Avascular Necrosis

Avascular necrosis (AVN) is a common cause of hip pain and disability that often requires treatment with a hip replacement. AVN can be associated with chronic alcohol abuse, steroid use, some viral infections such as HIV, and trauma. The bone of the femoral head dies due to microvascular damage and ischemia. As the bone is resorbed and repaired, it is weakened and slowly collapses, leading to degeneration of the hip joint. Patients typically complain of groin pain. Initially, plain radiographs may be normal. MRI is useful in this situation to evaluate for the possibility of AVN. As the disease progresses, the femoral head begins to flatten, and severe arthritic changes occur. There may be a role for observation or core decompression of the femoral head in the early stages of the disease, but once a subchondral fracture or deformation of the femoral head occurs, patients are best treated with a total hip replacement.

Posttraumatic Arthritis

Some patients who sustain a fracture of the pelvis around the hip joint or the proximal femur may develop posttraumatic arthritis as a consequence of their injury. This may be due to disruption of the blood supply to the femoral head (avascular necrosis), failure of the fracture to heal, implant failure, or simply a result of the chondral injury sustained at the time of injury. Patients with previous fractures and surgery who develop posttraumatic arthritis are at slightly higher risk for perioperative complications due to the scar tissue and altered anatomy resulting from their initial trauma as well as prior surgeries.

Suggested Diagnostic Testing

Arthritis of the hip is best diagnosed with plain radiographs. Typically three views are obtained. An anteroposterior (AP) radiograph of the pelvis, to allow for evaluation and comparison to the contralateral hip, as well as AP and lateral views of the affected hip should be obtained.

The four cardinal signs of osteoarthritis are loss of joint space, osteophyte formation, subchondral sclerosis, and subchondral cyst formation. Figure 8.1 shows an AP pelvis radiograph demonstrating the comparison of a normal hip with preserved joint space and an arthritic hip showing signs of advanced degeneration. Inflammatory arthritis often presents with a different pattern. Initially the joint changes are more subtle, but, as the disease progresses, the bone of the femur or acetabulum can become osteopenic and erosions of bone may appear. The femoral head often exhibits a more medial and central loss of joint space and, in extreme cases, can protrude into the pelvis.

Computed tomography (CT) and magnetic resonance imaging (MRI) are not generally useful in the work-up of typical patients with hip arthritis. MRI may be indicated in patients with hip pain where radiographs are normal, in order to assess for lesions of the articular cartilage and labrum or to investigate the possibility of AVN. CT is occasionally used preoperatively in some complex and revision cases to assist with preoperative planning but is generally not useful in the diagnosis and initial management of hip arthritis.

Fig. 8.1 Anteroposterior radiograph of a patient with a normal *right hip* and advanced arthritis of their *left hip*. There is complete loss of the superior joint space, osteophyte formation, and subchondral sclerosis

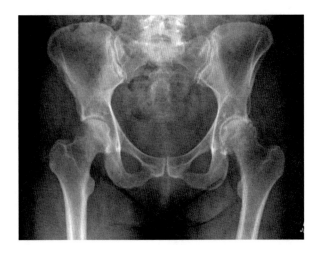

Non-operative Management

The primary treatment for hip arthritis is over-the-counter pain medications. Nonsteroidal pain medications (NSAIDs) such as naproxen and ibuprofen often provide excellent relief of mild to moderate pain-related symptoms. Some patients have difficulty tolerating NSAIDs due to stomach upset or bleeding episodes. Acetaminophen is widely tolerated and also provides excellent pain relief without the gastrointestinal or hematologic side effects associated with NSAIDs. Generally speaking, it is best to avoid narcotic pain medication in the treatment of long-term arthritis pain.

Some patients benefit from a nonimpact exercise program focused on strengthening the muscles around the hip—particularly the gluteus medius muscle and other hip abductors. While therapy and exercise do not alter the natural course of arthritis, they may provide some symptomatic relief. Impact exercise, such as jogging, is often poorly tolerated and can exacerbate symptoms.

While not associated with the risk of developing hip arthritis, obesity may exacerbate or potentiate symptoms. Weight loss can improve the painful symptoms associated with hip arthritis. The mechanical environment around the hip magnifies body weight, leading to forces across the hip joint of many multiples of total body weight during activities such as running and stair climbing. Preoperative weight loss also reduces the risk of complications in the perioperative period, speeds recovery, and reduces the postsurgical risks of infection and dislocation.

Weight loss in the setting of hip arthritis can be challenging as the pain associated with arthritis often limits patients capacity to perform vigorous exercise. Nonimpact exercise programs including cycling or water aerobics may be beneficial as they tend to aggravate hip arthritis to a lesser extent. Involving a nutritionist to make dietary changes is also useful.

While steroid injections are often used in the management of knee arthritis, they are infrequently used in the setting of hip arthritis. The hip joint is much less accessible and requires the use of either fluoroscopy or ultrasound to accurately place medication into the joint itself. There is little role for visco-supplementation with hyaluronic acid in the management of hip arthritis.

Injections can be helpful from a diagnostic perspective when they are used to tease out how much of a patient's symptoms can be attributed to their hip arthritis. For example, in a patient with lumbar stenosis and moderate hip arthritis, an injection of local anesthetic into the hip joint—a diagnostic injection—that alleviates most of the patient's pain will confirm that the hip is the primary pain generator.

Indications for Surgery

The indications for hip replacement surgery are multifactorial and patient dependent. Patients with significant limitations to their activities of daily living, quality of life, and employment who also have radiographic signs of moderate to severe hip arthritis are generally considered to be good candidates for hip replacement surgery. However, the severity of arthritis, patient age, medical comorbidities, and tolerance for surgical risk all play a role in the decision-making process.

As progress has been made in hip replacement surgery and the recovery and complication profile has improved, younger and more active patients are undergoing such procedures. However, the risks associated with surgery are real, and only patients with significant functional limitations should be considered for total hip replacement.

Perioperative complications as well as the risks of infection and dislocation are higher in overweight patients. These risks are particularly elevated in patients with morbid obesity. Some orthopedic surgeons will avoid hip replacement surgery in patients with a body mass index (BMI) of over 40 or 50 kg/m^2.

Operative Management

A total hip replacement is a resurfacing procedure of the hip joint. The diseased and arthritic bone and cartilage of the hip joint are removed, and implants made of metal, plastic, and occasionally ceramic are used to create a new articulation between the femur and pelvis. This new joint glides easily and allows for painless motion and weight bearing. Figures 8.2 and 8.3 demonstrate an example of a contemporary hip prosthesis and the radiograph of a patient with a similar implant in place following their hip replacement surgery.

Fig. 8.2 A contemporary hip prosthesis with an acetabular shell, a polyethylene liner, a metallic head component, and a proximally porous-coated femoral stem. The porous coating allows for a cementless press fit into bone. The components are fit snugly into the bone creating a friction fit. The bone then grows into the porous surface of the implants

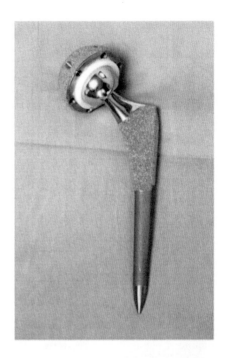

Fig. 8.3 An anteroposterior radiograph of a patient following *left* total hip replacement. The radiolucent liner of the acetabulum can be seen with the femoral head located securely within the acetabular component.

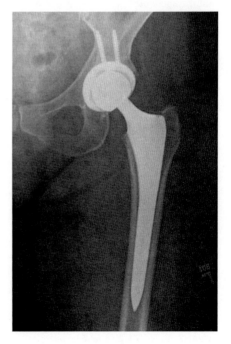

The hip joint is surgically exposed and the diseased bone removed with specialized tools that help shape the remaining bone to accept the new prosthesis (Fig. 8.4). Hip prostheses are manufactured in a wide range of shapes and sizes to match the particular anatomy of a patient. The specific implants selected for a surgery depend upon the patient's anatomy, bone quality, and the preferences of the treating surgeon.

Implant Design

Most hip replacement surgery performed in the United Sates uses cementless joint prostheses. These implants are covered in a rough, gritty surface that is biologically friendly. Once implanted into the bone, they first achieve fixation through a tight friction fit. The surrounding bone then grows into, or onto, the prosthesis to create a durable biologic bond.

Occasionally bone cement may be used to fix either or both the femoral and acetabular components to bone. Bone cement is a polymer of methyl methacrylate that acts as a grout to affix the components to the host bone. The advantage of bone cement is that it achieves an immediate and strong bond. The bone cement does not require strong host bone, and if a patient has particularly poor quality, bone cement may be selected to affix the prosthesis.

Approach

Total hip replacements may be performed through a number of approaches. Most common are the posterior approach, anterolateral approach, and direct anterior approach. All of the approaches are similar in terms of long-term outcome. Different surgeons prefer different surgical approaches for a number of reasons including training, complication profile, and patient variables. There is some emerging data that the direct anterior approach may help speed initial recovery, but there is little data to suggest that long-term results vary. There are some technical issues related to patients' specific anatomy that may cause a surgeon to favor one approach over another.

Perioperative Period

Patients are typically admitted to the hospital following the surgery and stay between 1 and 3 days. Fit and active patients are often discharged home, while more frail patients may benefit from a short stay in a skilled nursing facility to assist in their recovery.

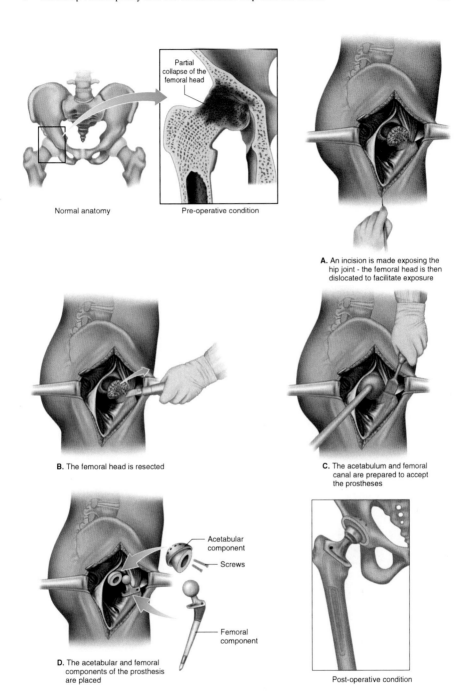

Fig. 8.4 Schematic depicting the surgical approach and procedural steps associated with a total hip replacement

Postoperative Rehabilitation

Physical therapy and exercise are critical to recovery following hip replacement surgery. In the hospital, therapists work with patients to mobilize them from bed and safely ambulate with the assistance of a walker or crutches. Generally speaking, the more active and aggressive patients are with their mobilization and exercise, the better their ultimate result.

Depending on the type of implant used, and the strength of the patient's bone, most patients will be allowed to put full weight on their affected hip immediately following surgery. Occasionally, patients may have a limitation to weight bearing for the first 1–3 months following surgery.

Hip Precautions

Following surgery and dependent upon the surgical approach and patient characteristics, surgeons may place their patients on hip precautions. These are a set of instructions regarding mobility and exercise to avoid putting the hip in a position that may lead to a dislocation. For posterior approaches, precautions typically involve avoiding flexing the hip beyond 90° or sitting in low chairs. For anterior approaches, precautions typically avoid hyperextending the hip or putting the leg in extreme external rotation. Many surgeons employ hip precautions during the immediate postoperative period but reduce or remove them once the patient has sufficiently recovered from surgery.

Expected Outcomes

The vast majority of patients who undergo total hip replacement have significant pain relief and improvement in their symptoms, with studies showing durable satisfactory outcomes achieved in greater than 90% of patients at 10 years. Once their rehabilitation is complete, most patients have little or no pain associated with their hip. Many patients have concomitant improvements in their range of motion, endurance, strength, and gait.

While patients may have activity limitations in the short term, within a few months, most patients can participate in normal activities without difficulty. Most surgeons limit their patients from impact exercise, such as running or jogging, but there is no limit on nonimpact exercise like cycling, swimming, or using an elliptical exercise machine. Sports such as downhill skiing, soccer, and tennis are also appropriate but may increase the risk of periprosthetic fracture or dislocation if the patient falls or is otherwise injured.

As technological advances have been made in materials and surgical technique, the life expectancy of hip replacements continues to improve. It is generally anticipated that approximately 90% of patients will have their hip replacement last at least 10 years without need for revision surgery, and as many as 50% will be able to extend joint longevity to 20 years post-surgery.

Wear/Longevity

Hip replacements are mechanical devices—with every step the femoral component rubs against the acetabular liner. Despite significant advancements in the design of total hip replacements, from the metallurgy of the components to the composition of the liners and heads, we still expect that hip replacements will slowly wear out over time. With current implants, the wear rates are extremely small, measured in microns per year. In the past, wear was a significant problem and the most common cause of hip replacement failure and need for revision. It appears that with contemporary implants, wear will be less of an issue than it has been previously.

Dislocation

The hip replacement allows for improved motion following surgery. However, if the patient puts their hip in an extreme position or falls poorly, it is possible for the hip to become dislocated. A periprosthetic hip dislocation affects about 1% of patients who have a hip replacement.

If a prosthetic hip becomes dislocated, the patient will have severe pain and a significant leg length inequality and will be unable to ambulate. Radiographic evaluation shows the femoral head to be dislocated from the acetabulum. The treatment for a dislocation is a reduction performed under sedation, either in the emergency department or the operating room. Most patients who have a dislocation are treated with a simple closed reduction and do not go on to have further problems. About a third of patients who do have one dislocation event go on to recurrent instability. In this case, they may be treated with a course of bracing, or potentially surgery, to try to correct the mechanical problem leading to the dislocations.

Periprosthetic Fracture

As hip replacements are increasingly performed within a more active population, the incidence of periprosthetic fractures is also growing. Periprosthetic fractures may result from high-energy trauma such as car accidents or falls from height or from ground-level falls if the patient has osteoporosis or other compromise to their bone quality.

Periprosthetic hip fractures are challenging to treat and typically involve either surgical repair of the fractured bone or removal of the previous prosthesis and revision to a new—more extensive—prosthesis. Some minor fractures, particularly those isolated to the greater trochanter, may be managed non-operatively.

Thromboembolic Disease

There is a small risk of developing a deep venous thrombosis (DVT) or pulmonary embolism (PE) following hip replacement surgery. The risk of a fatal PE is approximately 1 in 10,000. To reduce the risk of PE, most surgeons encourage rapid mobilization to promote circulation and use noninvasive measures such as compression stockings or sequential compression devices while the patient is in the hospital.

Chemical prophylaxis is also utilized. There is considerable debate as to the optimal medication and duration, but typically chemical prophylaxis is achieved with aspirin (ASA), warfarin, or low molecular weight heparin (LMWH). Prophylaxis is typically continued for 2–4 weeks following surgery.

Infection

While rare, occurring less than 1% of primary hip replacements, infection is a devastating complication. A deep infection is typically treated with surgical irrigation and debridement. The modular parts of the prosthesis are exchanged. If the infection becomes entrenched, then the prosthetic components have to be removed and exchanged with new components either at the same time or after 3 or more months of antibiotics and surveillance.

There is a slight risk of seeding bacteria onto the hip replacement components if patients develop bacteremia. For this reason, the American Academy of Orthopedic Surgeons (AAOS) recommends that patients with a hip replacement receive prophylactic antibiotics prior to any dental work or other invasive procedure for the first 2 years following their surgery. Some orthopedic surgeons recommend lifetime prophylaxis. The risk of infection following dental procedures is extremely small, but the consequences are significant. For patients with no penicillin allergy, a single dose of 1 g of amoxicillin given orally 1 h prior to a dental procedure is a common regimen. Clindamycin may be used in patients who are allergic to penicillin.

Leg Length Inequality

Hip replacement surgery alters the leg length, restoring height lost on the side of the degenerative hip joint. Occasionally leg lengths may be asymmetric following hip replacement surgery. The difference is typically small, and it is rare that patients will require a shoe lift.

Table 8.1 Summary of hip osteoarthritis with a synopsis of presentation, diagnostic testing, and suggested management options

Clinical entity	Presentation	Diagnostic testing	Conservative management	Surgical indications and operative management
Hip osteoarthritis	– groin pain – hip stiffness and limited range of motion	– plain film radiographs of affected hip and pelvis	– nonsteroidal pain medication – physical therapy and non-weight-bearing exercise – weight loss	– failure of non-operative treatment – Total hip replacement

Summary

Patients with hip arthritis typically present with progressive groin pain and stiffness in the hip that limits normal activity. Once symptoms progress to the point where they have significant limitations in activities of daily living or employment, patients may be considered good candidates for hip replacement surgery. Most patients can expect to have a significant improvement in their symptoms with a durable result that should last more than 10–20 years. Hip replacement surgery, when used appropriately, can have a massive impact on a patient's life, relieving pain and restoring function.

Table 8.1 is a summary of hip osteoarthritis with a synopsis of presentation, diagnostic testing, and suggested management options.

Suggested Reading

Callaghan JJ, Templeton JE, Liu SS, Pedersen DR, Goetz DD, Sullivan PM, Johnston RC. Results of charnley total hip arthroplasty at a minimum of thirty years. J Bone Joint Surg. 2004;86(4):690–5.

Ethgen O, Bruyère O, Richy F, Dardennes C, Reginster JY. Health-related quality of life in total hip and total knee arthroplasty. J Bone Joint Surg. 2004;86(5):963–74.

Hamel MB, Toth M, Legedza A, Rosen MP. Joint replacement surgery in elderly patients with severe osteoarthritis of the hip or kneedecision making, postoperative recovery, and clinical outcome. Arch Intern Med. 2008;168(13):1430–40.

Hoaglund FT, Steinbach LS. Primary osteoarthritis of the hip: etiology and epidemiology. J Am Acad Orthop Surg. 2001;9(5):320–7.

Mont MA, Jacobs JJ. AAOS clinical practice guideline: preventing venous thromboembolic disease in patients undergoing elective hip and knee arthroplasty. J Am Acad Orthop Surg. 2011;19(12):777–8.

Part VI
Shoulder

Chapter 9
Shoulder Soft Tissue Pathology

Robert C. Spang III and Courtney Dawson

Abbreviations

AC   Acromioclavicular
AP   Anterior-posterior
MRI   Magnetic resonance imaging
NSAIDs Nonsteroidal anti-inflammatory drugs

Introduction

The evaluation and diagnosis of shoulder pain is a common challenge encountered by primary care providers. The differential for shoulder pain is broad and the presentation may be varied. The patient's history and physical examination alone are often enough to reach a diagnosis; however, plain films and advanced imaging studies are frequently helpful for further confirmation and to guide decision-making. In this section, we will review several common causes of shoulder pain related to soft tissue pathology: adhesive capsulitis, biceps tendinopathy, acromioclavicular joint pain, and rotator cuff pathology (Fig. 9.1).

R.C. Spang III
Orthopedic Surgeon, Sports Medicine and Orthopedic Surgery, Brigham and Women's Hospital, 75 Francis Street, Boston, MA 02115, USA

Harvard Combined Orthopaedic Residency Program,
55 Fruit Street, Boston, MA 02114, USA
e-mail: rspang@partners.org

C. Dawson (✉)
Orthopedic Surgeon, Sports Medicine and Orthopedic Surgery, Brigham and Women's Hospital, 75 Francis Street, Boston, MA 02115, USA
e-mail: ckdawson@partners.org

© Springer International Publishing AG 2018   127
J.N. Katz et al. (eds.), *Principles of Orthopedic Practice for Primary Care Providers*, https://doi.org/10.1007/978-3-319-68661-5_9

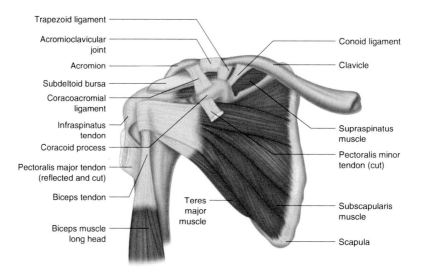

Fig. 9.1 Shoulder anatomy (anterior view)

Adhesive Capsulitis

Summary of Epidemiology

While many patients presenting with a painful and stiff shoulder are diagnosed with "frozen shoulder," adhesive capsulitis is a specific pathological condition wherein chronic inflammation of the shoulder capsule leads to capsule thickening, fibrosis, and adhesion to the humeral neck. As a result, there is decreased synovial fluid within the joint with diminished overall joint volume. This produces pain and mechanically restrains shoulder motion.

Commonly encountered in the outpatient setting, the prevalence of adhesive capsulitis ranges from 2% to 5% but can be as high as 30% in patients with insulin-dependent diabetes mellitus (IDDM). Comorbid IDDM is associated with a worse prognosis and increased likelihood for surgical intervention. While the exact pathogenesis remains unclear, other factors associated with adhesive capsulitis include female sex, age over 40 years, prolonged immobilization, sedentary lifestyle, trauma, thyroid disease, stroke, myocardial infarction, and the presence of an autoimmune disease. Most cases occur in women ages 40–60 years of age.

Clinical Presentation

Adhesive capsulitis is characterized by an insidious onset of shoulder pain for several months with a global limitation of both active and *passive* range of motion. While there may be a history of recent trauma to the shoulder, this is not always the case.

Pain is worsened with motion and may be referred to the deltoid region. Night pain is also common (difficulty sleeping on affected side). The gradual loss of motion may cause difficulty dressing, combing hair, reaching backward, or fastening a brassiere.

The disease progression of adhesive capsulitis has been described as occurring in four stages. Stage 1, the pre-adhesive stage, is characterized by a fibrinous inflammatory synovitic reaction without adhesion formation. As such, patients usually have full motion but have pain, often at night. Misdiagnosis is common at this stage. Stage 2 progresses to an acute synovitis with synovial proliferation and early adhesion formation. Pain is prominent, but loss of motion remains mild. Stage 3 is referred to as the maturation stage wherein inflammation and hence pain have decreased; however, more fibrosis is present, and range of motion becomes further limited. Stage 4, the chronic stage, is characterized by adhesions that have matured resulting in severely reduced motion. Some have likened the condition to wearing a jacket or piece of clothing that has dramatically shrunk.

Differential Diagnosis and Suggested Diagnostic Testing

Adhesive capsulitis may be challenging to diagnosis in the early phases, but more readily declares itself as the symptoms progress. Perhaps the most important consideration is the loss of *passive motion* in addition to active motion. While numerous painful conditions about the shoulder can generate pain or limit active motion, relatively few substantially limit passive motion. Glenohumeral arthritis is an additional cause of limited passive range and should be considered in the differential diagnosis.

Examination of a patient with shoulder pain should proceed in a thoughtful and systematic fashion. Inspection and palpation is followed by observation of active range of motion of the shoulder joint as well as the neck. At the shoulder, active forward flexion, abduction, functional internal rotation (reaching behind and up back), and external rotation should be assessed. To evaluate passive motion, the examiner repeats the above motions while the patient is relaxed. In adhesive capsulitis, motion restriction is most pronounced with external rotation of the shoulder with the arm at the side and elbow in 90° of flexion. Motion should be compared to the contralateral side. Typically, rotator cuff muscle strength will be preserved (although weakness may be seen due to pain inhibition), and other special tests of the shoulder will be negative.

In patients with substantially limited passive motion of the shoulder, plain radiographs (AP, lateral, and axial views) must be obtained. In patients with a history of shoulder instability, trauma, or seizure, the axial view is of particularly importance to rule out shoulder dislocation, as this can also severely limit passive motion and should not be missed. As noted above, osteoarthritis of the shoulder is common and often restricts passive shoulder motion. In patients with adhesive capsulitis, radiographs are usually normal but may show osteopenia. Magnetic resonance imaging (MRI) and other advanced imaging modalities are typically not used as initial diagnostic tools, however, can be helpful to evaluate for other structural pathologies (e.g., rotator cuff tear) and to confirm the presence of findings consistent with adhesive capsulitis such as thickening of the joint capsule and fibrosis of the axillary pouch.

Nonoperative Management

Regardless of stage, physical therapy with bridge to a home exercise program is a mainstay of treatment. The goal is gentle progressive stretching—aggressive movements are not needed and may exacerbate pain. It should be emphasized to patients that recovery can take a long period of time. While one might think the inflammatory nature of adhesive capsulitis would lend itself to successful anti-inflammatory treatments, this is frequently not the case. Nonsteroidal anti-inflammatory drugs (NSAIDs) may be used to control pain however have not been found to alter the disease course. Oral steroids and intra-articular corticosteroid injections may reduce pain but do not typically improve long-term outcome. Intra-articular injections can, however, be very helpful in allowing the patient to tolerate the advancing passive range of motion in physical therapy.

Indications for Surgery

Most patients do not require surgery for adhesive capsulitis. The conservative management strategies outlined above may continue for up to a year if slow progress is being made. Surgery is reserved for patients with persistent or intractable painful restriction despite an adequate trial of conservative management. Those who have more severe initial symptoms, are younger in age, and those who have an ongoing reduction in motion despite at least 6 months of diligent physical therapy are more likely to be considered for surgery.

Operative Management

Before widespread availability of arthroscopy, manipulation under anesthesia was the treatment of choice for cases of adhesive capsulitis refractory to conservative measures. This involves a carefully planned manipulation technique to ensure the tightened capsule is ruptured while avoiding damage to other bony or soft tissue structures such as the subscapularis or humerus. Results are generally favorable, with most patients regaining the ability to do daily tasks within days of the procedure.

More recently, arthroscopic capsular release has overtaken manipulation as the surgical treatment of choice as this allows for intra-articular inspection and confirmation of diagnosis, followed by a more precise capsulotomy. Results are generally favorable and maintained. Postoperative range of motion is important to preserve the gains made in surgery, particularly in abduction.

Expected Outcome and Predictors of Outcome

The natural history of adhesive capsulitis is not entirely understood. Some feel this is a self-limiting process and hence does not need to be treated aggressively. With minimal intervention, subjective outcomes tend to be favorable; however, objective measures show that patients do not all fully recover. Uncertainty of the natural history of adhesive capsulitis complicates studying the efficacy of various treatment options. Patients may be substantially limited for a prolonged period of time; thus, interventions typically focus on improving the speed of recovery and decreasing pain.

Biceps Tendinopathy

Summary of Epidemiology

Biceps tendon pathology is a common cause of anterior shoulder pain. This inflammatory tenosynovitis occurs as the long head of the biceps tendon courses in its relatively constrained position within the bicipital groove of the humerus. Although biceps tendonitis may exist in isolation, it is frequently associated with other shoulder pathology. This is not surprising, given the long head of the biceps has an intra-articular proximal insertion at the supraglenoid tubercle and lies in close proximity to both the supraspinatus and subscapularis tendons within the rotator interval.

Clinical Presentation

Patients with biceps tendinopathy often describe progressive anterior shoulder pain that may be associated with repetitive overhead activities. The pain may be localized to the anteromedial shoulder in the region of the bicipital groove and may radiate downward toward the biceps muscle belly. Younger overhead throwing athletes or overhead laborers may have isolated biceps tendonitis. In the instance of proximal biceps rupture, patients may describe feeling a sudden, sharp pain in the upper arm or an audible pop or snap. This may be accompanied by subtle weakness in forearm supination or elbow flexion and a prominence of the biceps musculature (i.e., "Popeye" sign).

Differential Diagnosis and Suggested Diagnostic Testing

The differential diagnosis for anterior shoulder pain is broad and includes impingement syndrome, rotator cuff tendinopathy or tears, AC joint pathology, labral pathology, subacromial bursitis, glenohumeral instability, and cervical spine pathology.

In cases of true biceps tendinopathy, physical exam may reveal point tenderness elicited with direct palpation over the bicipital groove. This should be done with the arm at the patient's side and in slight internal rotation (approximately 10°) to bring the biceps groove into a forward-facing position. Pressure approximately 5 cm below the edge of the acromion may elicit pain. The contralateral side may be tested for comparison.

Speed's test is positive if pain in the bicipital groove is elicited with resisted forward flexion of the arm with the forearm supinated, the elbow extended, and the humerus in 90° of forward flexion. Yergason's test is another special test that can be helpful in attributing a patient's pain to biceps pathology. It is important to note that the biceps muscle is a strong supinator of the arm, but a weak flexor relative to the brachialis muscle. A patient is asked to hold their elbow flexed to 90° with their arm at their side, then supinate the forearm. The examiner applies manual resistance to supination. Reproduction of a patient's shoulder pain with this test implicates the biceps as a pain generator.

As noted above, in the case of proximal biceps rupture, gross deformity of the biceps muscle may be present in the form of a "Popeye" sign. This may be made more obvious by asking the patient to contract the muscle. Bruising may be present from the upper arm down toward the elbow.

A careful and thoughtful physical examination will usually suffice in diagnosing biceps tendonitis as the source of a patient's pain and may also yield information about associated shoulder pathology. Plain radiographs (AP, lateral, and axial views) of the affected shoulder are helpful in investigating other sources of shoulder pain such as underlying bony abnormalities, particularly in the setting of recent trauma, and may show evidence of rotator cuff calcific tendonitis or suggest chronic rotator cuff insufficiency. Generally, once the diagnosis is confirmed on physical examination, conservative management may be trialed prior to obtaining advanced imaging.

In patients in whom the diagnosis is in doubt, MRI is the imaging modality of choice given its ability to evaluate soft tissue abnormalities of the shoulder. When multiple potential pain generators or abnormal findings are present, local injection to the bicipital groove with short-acting analgesics and corticosteroids may be used (typically guided by ultrasound) to gain valuable diagnostic information regarding the primary pain generator, while also providing therapeutic relief.

Nonoperative Management

The vast majority of patients with biceps tendinopathy will be successfully managed with nonoperative treatment. This includes a brief period of rest and activity modification. The use of NSAIDs can be helpful for analgesia. This should be followed by formal physical therapy to optimize scapular biomechanics and address any concomitant issues such as muscle imbalance. As biceps pathology is most often seen with concomitant shoulder dysfunction, the goal of physical therapy is to restore proper shoulder biomechanics rather than focusing solely on the biceps tendon. As opposed to other joints in the body (such as the hip joint), which have deep sockets and much inherent bony stability, the shoulder is more akin to a golf ball on a relatively shallow tee. As such, soft tissue and muscle balance is crucially important. Explaining to patients the logic behind targeted physical therapy may help optimize nonoperative results and improve adherence to a program, as it may take weeks to see improvements.

In most cases, nonoperative treatment is similarly pursued for complete tears of the long head of the biceps tendon. In such an instance, referral to an orthopedic surgeon is warranted to discuss the risks and benefits of surgery versus nonoperative treatment. Surgery is most beneficial for higher-demand patients such as athletes or manual laborers.

Indications for Surgery

Indications for surgical management include partial-thickness tears of the long head of the biceps tendon involving more than 25–50% of the tendon thickness, full-thickness tears in high-demand patients, medial subluxation of the tendon out of the bicipital groove, and/or subluxation in the setting of a tear of the subscapularis tendon or biceps sling. Relative indications include certain types of SLAP (superior labrum anterior-posterior) tears, and persistent pain despite an aggressive trial of nonoperative treatment.

Operative Management

Optimal surgical management of proximal biceps tendon pathology remains controversial. The two most common procedures performed are biceps tenotomy and biceps tenodesis. Tenotomy is a simple procedure wherein the proximal biceps is cut, usually arthroscopically, without subsequent repair. This provides predictable pain relief without the need for postoperative rehabilitation. However, cosmesis and fatigue discomfort are potential challenges, as the "Popeye" deformity may be noted. Biceps tenodesis involves cutting the biceps tendon with subsequent reattachment/anchoring of the tendon at a more distal point to maintain the length-tension relationship, strength, and contour. Surgeons frequently prefer this method in younger, more active patients.

Expected Outcome and Predictors of Outcome

Nonoperative management of biceps tendinopathy is often successful; however, data supporting the efficacy of specific treatment modalities is lacking. In operative cases, biceps tenotomy typically results in high patient satisfaction with reliable pain relief; however, approximately 70% of patients show the classic "Popeye" sign, and approximately 38% show fatigue discomfort with resisted elbow flexion. As such, this would not be the treatment of choice for young laborers. In these cases, biceps tenodesis has been shown to be a relatively effective and safe procedure.

Acromioclavicular Joint Pain

Summary of Epidemiology

The acromioclavicular (AC) joint is a relatively frequent source of anterior shoulder pain, often in the setting of primary osteoarthritis or posttraumatic arthritis. The AC joint is a diarthrodial joint which supports the shoulder girdle through the clavicular "strut." The convex distal clavicle articulates with the concave acromial facet, with a fibrocartilaginous meniscal disc between the articular surfaces. Degeneration of the AC joint is a natural consequence of the aging process, and the AC joint is vulnerable to the same processes affected other joints in the body, such as degenerative arthritis, infections, and inflammatory or crystalline arthritis. Its relationship to the shoulder and superficial location makes it susceptible to traumatic injury. Moreover, the biomechanics of the shoulder girdle leads to large loads across a small AC joint surface area, which predisposes to degeneration with overuse. An increased emphasis on weight training and upper extremity strengthening adds stress to the AC joint.

Clinical Presentation

Patients with AC joint pathology often present with aching pain or discomfort over the anterior and superior aspect of the shoulder. The pain may radiate to the neck or deltoid region. It is often worsened by activities such as reaching across body while driving, washing the opposite axilla, reaching behind one's back, or rolling onto the affected side while sleeping. Pushing, exercises such as push-ups or bench presses, or overhead activities also may exacerbate the pain. It is important to inquire about history of prior acute shoulder injuries, as instability following AC joint trauma may alter treatment.

Differential Diagnosis and Suggested Diagnostic Testing

The differential for anterior superior shoulder pain includes AC joint pathology (osteoarthritis, sprain or fracture, instability, dislocation), rotator cuff impingement, biceps tendinopathy, and cervical spine pathology. As with other conditions of the shoulder, a comprehensive physical exam often reveals the diagnosis, with imaging used as confirmation.

The exam begins with inspection, which may show prominence or asymmetry over the AC joint. Direct palpation may elicit tenderness. The most reliable provocative maneuver is the cross-body adduction test. The arm of the affected side is elevated to 90°. The examiner then grasps the elbow and passively adducts the arm across the body. Reproduction of pain is suggestive of AC joint pathology. Stability of the clavicle at the AC joint may be evaluated by holding the distal clavicle in one hand while stabilizing the acromion with the other and testing translation. Examination should also evaluate for other diagnosis such as rotator cuff pathology or biceps tendon pathology, which may coexist.

Following examination, radiologic evaluation should include bilateral AP shoulder plain films (for side to side comparison) and axillary views, particularly in the setting of trauma. Adding a Zanca view is frequently helpful because this offers an unobstructed view of the distal clavicle and AC joint. Patients with degenerative AC joint arthritis will have changes such as joint space narrowing, marginal osteophytes, and sclerosis. MRI may be obtained if the diagnosis remains in doubt or if associated pathology, such as rotator cuff tear, is suspected. MRI should be obtained only after a careful history and physical exam. Reactive bone edema on MRI is a more reliable predictor of symptomatic AC joint pathology than degenerative changes on x-ray or MRI. However, a patient's clinical symptoms may not correlate with changes on MRI—it has been shown that up to 82% of patients with AC joint arthritis based on MRI are asymptomatic. Similar to the evaluation of other suspected soft tissue pathologies of the shoulder, advanced imaging does not obviate the need for careful history and physical exam.

Nonoperative Management

Initial treatment of AC joint pain is conservative, including activity modification, nonsteroidal anti-inflammatory medications, corticosteroid injections, and physical therapy. For some patients, particularly younger athletes, activity modification may involve decreasing exercises such as bench presses, dips, and push-ups. Physical therapy is useful for treating concomitant soft tissue shoulder issues such as impingement or restricted motion; however, its role is typically limited in most cases of isolated AC arthritis.

Intra-articular corticosteroid injections are an important tool for the clinician caring for a patient with AC joint pain. While history, physical exam, and imaging often point to the correct diagnosis, many patients have vague anterior shoulder pain that is not easily localized to one pain generator. An intra-articular lidocaine injection provides important diagnostic information and can confirm the diagnosis if the patient experiences pain relief shortly thereafter. Corticosteroid may additionally provide longer-lasting relief.

Indications for Surgery

Surgery is considered for patients who have failed nonoperative treatment and who have history, physical exam, and radiographic evidence confirming AC joint pathology. Prior to surgery, the patient should experience pain relief after a focal AC joint injection for further confirmation of the AC joint as the source of pain.

Operative Management

Options for surgical management of AC joint pain include open versus arthroscopic distal clavicle resection. Open resection allows for direct visualization of the resected and remaining clavicle to ensure adequate bone removal. Disadvantages of this approach include interfering with the deltoid and trapezius muscles, with associated time to heal these structures. Active shoulder flexion, elevation, and abduction are avoided in the immediate postoperative period. Arthroscopic resection may be performed via either subacromial (indirect) versus superior approach. One advantage of the arthroscopic approach is the opportunity to diagnose and address concomitant pathologies at the time of surgery, as well as shorter recovery time. Arthroscopic techniques avoid injury to the deltoid but are more technically demanding than an open approach and may have somewhat higher risks of inadequate resection.

Expected Outcome and Predictors of Outcome

Outcomes after distal clavicle resection are generally positive, but there is much variability in patient response. Those with posttraumatic arthritis or AC instability may have a worse prognosis. Most patients are able to return to their prior activity after distal clavicle resection. Continued pain postoperatively should raise concern for diagnostic error, which again underscores the importance of detailed history, examination, and judicious use of diagnostic and therapeutic injections.

Rotator Cuff Pathology

Summary of Epidemiology

The evaluation and management of rotator cuff tears differ according to the patient (young vs. older, athlete vs. nonathlete) and mechanism (acute traumatic vs. chronic atraumatic). Rotator cuff pathology accounts for a significant portion of shoulder-related complaints presenting to the primary care physician. The rotator cuff consists of four muscle-tendon units. The supraspinatus abducts, the infraspinatus and teres minor externally rotate, and the subscapularis internally rotates the shoulder at the glenohumeral joint. These muscles are also important for maintaining the humeral head's concentricity within the glenohumeral joint—in cases of chronic "massive" rotator cuff tears, the powerful deltoid muscle causes superior migration of the humeral head and resultant rotator cuff arthropathy (arthritic narrowing of the subacromial space) over time.

Rotator cuff pathology may occur due to trauma or may occur gradually over time. While shoulder dislocations in younger patients more commonly result in labral pathology, in older patients, dislocations are more likely to result in traumatic rotator cuff tears. Tendinopathy and tears may also occur gradually due to overuse, such as with overhead laborers or athletes.

Subacromial impingement syndrome is a common cause of shoulder pain and also represents a spectrum ranging from subacromial bursitis and rotator cuff tendinopathy to partial-thickness rotator cuff tears. While the exact pathophysiology of impingement and partial-thickness rotator cuff tears is not entirely understood, it is thought to be due to external compression from the acromion.

Calcific tendinopathy is another common cause of shoulder pain. Calcium deposits can be seen within the substance of the rotator cuff tendons, but only about one-third of patients are symptomatic. The exact etiology remains unclear. Most cases of shoulder pain due to calcific tendinitis gradually improve over time as the deposit often resorbs.

Clinical Presentation

Rotator cuff pain can present acutely in the setting of trauma, chronically in the absence of trauma, or in an acute-on-chronic fashion. Trauma may occur as a result of heavy lifting, falls, or dislocations. Acute injuries to the rotator cuff are usually accompanied by pain and a significant decline in function. Conversely, in the case of overuse injuries, older patients or overhead athletes/laborers tend to present with a more gradual onset of pain. In these patients, functional decline may be more subtle, with a gradual decrease in strength and functionality affecting activities of daily living.

Rotator cuff pathology usually presents as a dull, aching pain over the anterior and lateral aspect of the shoulder. The pain is often worsened by overhead activities, such as washing one's hair, dressing, or reaching overhead. Night pain is a common complaint, and the patient may have difficulty sleeping on the affected side.

As with any patient presenting with shoulder pain, the physical exam is critical. Upon inspection, the examiner may be able to appreciate an asymmetry over the posterior scapular region, particularly in the setting of chronic rotator cuff tears wherein tendon/muscle retraction and atrophy occur. Patients with rotator cuff tears, impingement, and calcific tendinopathy may have decreased active range of motion due to pain and, in cases of rotator cuff tears, often have adjusted their shoulder mechanics in order to compensate for the lost rotator cuff strength. The examiner should stand behind the patient to observe scapular motion with forward flexion at the shoulder, in order to assess for scapulothoracic dyskinesia or scapular winging, which may contribute to altered shoulder biomechanics and thus worsen pain.

Rotator cuff strength should be evaluated. To test the supraspinatus, the examiner asks the patient to hold their arms abducted to 90°. The patient's arms are then brought forward approximately 30°, to align their arms with the anatomic position of the scapula. A complete inability to maintain the arm elevated against gravity may produce a "drop arm" sign, which is consistent with a significant rotator cuff tear. Resisted abduction strength—referred to as Jobe's supraspinatus test—is then tested in this position (Fig. 9.2), to evaluate the integrity of the supraspinatus tendon.

The infraspinatus is tested by having the patient flex their elbows to 90°, with the elbow tucked at their sides, in neutral position. The patient is asked to externally rotate from a neutral position while the examiner resists (Fig. 9.3).

Subscapularis strength is assessed by evaluating the patient's ability to push the back of the hand off the lower back (the lift-off test) or by asking the patient to bring both their elbows forward against resistance while the hands are held pressed against the abdomen (belly-press test) (Fig. 9.4a, b).

In addition to rotator cuff strength testing, examination should also include special tests specifically looking for impingement signs. The Neer impingement test (Fig. 9.5) involves the examiner passively flexing the patient's shoulder forward while using the other hand to stabilize the scapula. Pain with this maneuver, while not specific, may be indicative of shoulder impingement. The Hawkins test (Fig. 9.6) entails forward flexion of the shoulder to 90°, followed by elbow flexion and internally rotating at the shoulder. Again, pain with this test suggests impingement syndrome.

The examiner should also consider alternative painful pathologies of the shoulder and investigate for evidence of AC joint pain (cross-body adduction test) and biceps tendinopathy (bicipital groove tenderness, Speed's test, Yergason's test). The possibility of cervical spine pathology should also be considered in appropriate patients.

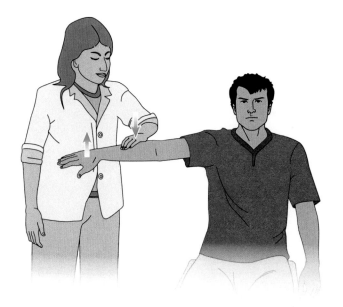

Fig. 9.2 Jobe's supraspinatus test

Fig. 9.3 Infraspinatus test

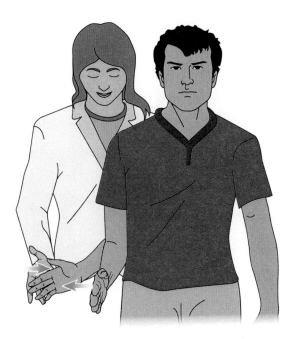

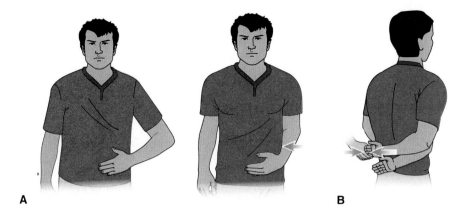

Fig. 9.4 Subscapularis tests. (**a**) Belly press test; (**b**) Lift-off test

Fig. 9.5 Neer
impingement test

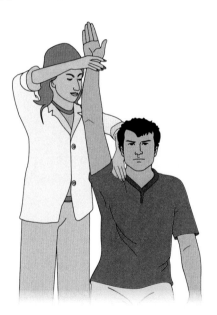

Differential Diagnosis and Suggested Diagnostic Testing

The differential diagnosis for shoulder pain is broad and depends largely on patient age and history. For young patients, the rotator cuff tendons are typically robust and pain results from acute trauma or repetitive activity. For middle-age patients, rotator cuff pathologies are a common source of pain; however, glenohumeral arthritis and adhesive capsulitis should also be considered. Biceps tendinopathy and AC joint arthritis are other common sources of pain.

Fig. 9.6 Hawkins
impingement test

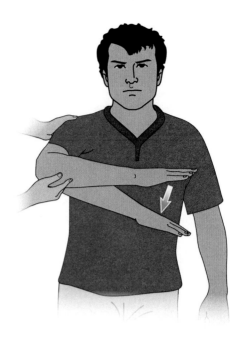

Shoulder imaging does not substitute for a thoughtful history and comprehensive physical examination, as these are frequently sufficient for accurate diagnosis. For patients in whom the diagnosis is in doubt, or for whom multiple associated pathologies are suspected, imaging should begin with plain radiographs including an AP, Grashey (true AP), axillary lateral, and outlet views of the shoulder. This may reveal calcific tendonitis or other sources of pain such as glenohumeral or AC joint arthritis or rotator cuff arthropathy.

MRI is the modality of choice for imaging the soft tissue structures of the shoulder, including the rotator cuff tendons, and has been shown to reliably diagnose rotator cuff pathology. In addition to cost, an important consideration is the high false-positive rate in older patients. MRI abnormalities including rotator cuff tears are very frequently detected in older patients who are otherwise asymptomatic, and as such, MRI should be used judiciously in correlation with clinical exam to avoid overly aggressive treatment. Ultrasound is another noninvasive alternative imaging technique and allows for dynamic assessment of the rotator cuff tendons. It is frequently limited by the availability and skill of the radiologists interpreting these studies.

Nonoperative Management

The initial nonoperative treatment of rotator cuff pathology, including rotator cuff tears, calcific tendinopathy, and impingement, is generally similar and includes NSAIDs, activity modification, physical therapy, and injections.

Physical therapy is the mainstay of treatment in most cases. A comprehensive exercise program should focus on rotator cuff strengthening using resistance bands, the "sleeper stretch" for posterior capsular tightness, progressive range of motion in all planes, and scapular stabilization techniques. These can be done at home, but it is often recommended that the patient learns the correct technique under the guidance of a physical therapist to avoid further injury. Once pain is better controlled, the focus of conservative treatment is on strengthening and normalizing scapulothoracic motion.

Subacromial corticosteroid injections are often used in cases of severe pain that is limiting range of motion or activities of daily living and can be used to supplement the therapy program. Most clinicians prefer to limit the total number of injections to three per year in a given shoulder due to the potential risk of tissue degeneration and tendon weakening or rupture, although the evidence for this is lacking. Subacromial injections can be performed in the office with relative ease using the posterior and lateral acromion as bony landmarks. Patients with underlying diabetes should be cautioned to monitor their blood sugars carefully after a corticosteroid injection as values can become transiently elevated in some cases. Additional treatment modalities for calcific tendinopathy include needling, image-guided aspiration/lavage of the calcium deposit, or extracorporeal shock wave therapy.

Indications for Surgery

As with other etiologies of shoulder pain, surgery is reserved for patients who have failed to improve despite a comprehensive conservative treatment program. Acute, traumatic rotator cuff tears are the exception. These tears generally occur after a specific traumatic event and should be easily identified based on the patient's history. Acute pain, weakness, and limited active range of motion after a traumatic event should raise suspicion and guide the diagnostic workup. Plain films are used to rule out a fracture, and an MRI can be used to confirm the diagnosis of a tear (Fig. 9.7). In cases of acute, traumatic rotator cuff tears in healthy individuals, surgery is often considered; therefore, early referral to an orthopedic surgeon is warranted. A delay in treatment may lead to chronic changes which cause the tear to be irreparable.

Chronic, massive, retracted rotator cuff tears with associated muscle atrophy are usually treated conservatively and may yield good results in lower-demand individuals. Some of these patients progress to rotator cuff arthropathy, at which point a reverse total shoulder arthroplasty may be considered.

Fig. 9.7 Coronal STIR
MRI: Full-thickness
supraspinatus tear

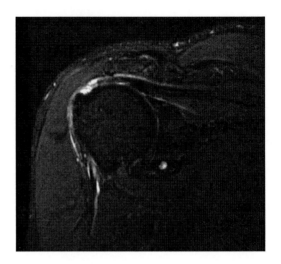

Operative Management

Rotator Cuff Tear

Rotator cuff repair can be performed either arthroscopically or open, depending on the size of the tear and surgeon preference. The main goal is reattachment of the torn, retracted tendons back to the humerus. Specific techniques can vary but include single- vs. double-row repairs and suture anchors vs. transosseous techniques. Biomechanical studies have shown double-row repairs to have a higher load to failure and possible improved tendon healing; however, these advantages have not been matched clinically as outcomes have been similar when compared to single-row repairs. Advances in arthroscopic instrumentation have led to better visualization and potentially faster recovery without the risk of postoperative deltoid dysfunction.

Calcific Tendinopathy

Calcific tendinopathy that is recalcitrant to conservative treatment may be treated surgically with an arthroscopic debridement of the calcium deposit under direct visualization. After debridement, the void in the rotator cuff left by the calcium deposit may require direct repair if greater than 50% of the tendon substance is affected. In these cases, the postoperative recovery is similar to a standard rotator cuff repair, requiring protection in a sling and a guided therapy program to allow for tendon healing.

Impingement Syndrome

The surgical management of impingement syndrome is somewhat controversial as most patients improve with conservative treatment. Arthroscopic subacromial decompression with or without acromioplasty is the mainstay for patients who fail to improve. There has been some debate among orthopedic surgeons as to the role of the acromioplasty as there is more recent data showing no long-term benefit when compared to a structured exercise program.

Expected Outcome and Predictors of Outcome

Outcomes after rotator cuff repair are generally favorable. The re-tear rate at 6 months is approximately 20%; however, this is usually atraumatic and often associated with massive initial tears and lower quality tissue. Despite this, the majority of patients still report clinical improvement at long-term follow-up. There is a risk of developing adhesive capsulitis postoperatively, often resolving with formal physical therapy and rarely requiring a manipulation or arthroscopic release. This is more common in diabetics or with prolonged immobilization. Arthroscopic debridement of calcific tendinopathy can yield high patient satisfaction and excellent functional results with minimal downtime. Slings are used for comfort, and physical therapy is initiated to avoid persistent stiffness. Outcomes after subacromial decompression for impingement syndrome are positive but likely no better than conservative treatment in many cases.

Summary

Shoulder pain is a common yet challenging entity presented to primary care providers. The differential is broad, and there is considerable overlap between the various etiologies of pain. Obtaining a thorough history and careful physical exam will help the provider more clearly identify the specific diagnosis in almost all cases. Advanced imaging can be reserved for cases where the diagnosis is less clear or if the patient fails to respond to initial conservative treatment methods. Referral to an orthopedic surgeon is recommended in cases of acute traumatic rotator cuff tears, fractures, considerable weakness, concerning physical exam findings, or if there is a question as to the appropriate treatment in a given patient. In most cases, a trial of conservative treatment is warranted and is often successful.

Table 9.1 shows a standard algorithm for the evaluation and treatment of common soft tissue shoulder pathology. Note that there is considerable overlap in the initial conservative treatment of many of these common diagnoses.

Table 9.1 Summary of common soft tissue shoulder pathology, evaluation, and treatment

Clinical entity	Presentation	Diagnostic testing	Conservative management	Indications for surgery	Operative management
Adhesive capsulitis	Insidious onset, pain, limited AROM[a] and PROM[b]	Plain films	NSAIDs, PT focusing on aggressive PROM then AROM, intra-articular injection	Failure to respond to conservative treatment	Manipulation under anesthesia, arthroscopic capsular release
Biceps tendinopathy	TTP at the bicipital groove, positive Speed's and Yergason's tests	Clinical diagnosis often sufficient, MRI or ultrasound to confirm	NSAIDs, PT, ultrasound-guided bicipital sheath injection	Failure to respond to conservative treatment	Biceps debridement or tenotomy (older, less active), biceps tenodesis (younger, more active)
Long head biceps tendon rupture	Acute traumatic event, usually a "pop" or "snap," ecchymosis, swelling, "Popeye" sign	Clinical diagnosis often sufficient, plain films to rule out fracture if needed	NSAIDs, PT, or home exercises	None except for rare cases of young, active patients/laborers	None except possible biceps tenodesis in young, active patient
AC joint pain	TTP at the AC joint, positive cross-body adduction maneuver	Plain films, MRI to evaluate for concomitant pathology if needed	NSAIDs, PT, image-guided AC joint or subacromial injections	Failure to respond to conservative treatment	Arthroscopic or open distal clavicle excision
Rotator cuff tear	Pain, weakness in rotator cuff testing, "drop arm" sign, positive Jobe's test	Plain films, MRI to confirm diagnosis	NSAIDs, PT, subacromial injections	Acute, traumatic tear with weakness, Failure to respond to conservative treatment	Arthroscopic or open rotator cuff repair, subacromial decompression
Calcific tendinopathy	Often severe pain, AROM may be limited due to pain, positive Neer and Hawkins tests	Plain films, occasional MRI to evaluate integrity of tendon	NSAIDs, PT, injections; if persistent consider needling, aspiration/lavage, extracorporeal shock wave therapy	Failure to respond to conservative treatment	Arthroscopic debridement of the calcium deposit, possible rotator cuff repair

(continued)

Table 9.1 (continued)

Clinical entity	Presentation	Diagnostic testing	Conservative management	Indications for surgery	Operative management
Impingement syndrome	Pain with overhead activity, positive Neer and Hawkins tests	Plain films, clinical exam often sufficient	NSAIDs, PT, injections	Limited, failure to respond to conservative treatment	Arthroscopic subacromial decompression

[a]AROM = active range of motion
[b]PROM = passive range of motion
NSAIDs = nonsteroidal anti-inflammatory drugs
PT = physical therapy
TTP = tenderness to palpation

Suggested Reading

Bishay V, Gallo RA. The evaluation and treatment of rotator cuff pathology. Prim Care. 2013;40(4):889–910.

Harrison AK, Flatow EL. Subacromial impingement syndrome. J Am Acad Orthop Surg. 2011;19(11):701–8.

Levine WN, Kashyap CP, Bak SF, Ahmad CS, Blaine TA, Bigliani LU. Nonoperative management of idiopathic adhesive capsulitis. J Shoulder Elb Surg. 2007;16(5):569–73.

Neviaser AS, Neviaser RJ. Adhesive capsulitis of the shoulder. J Am Acad Orthop Surg. 2011;19(9):536–42.

Nho SJ, Strauss EJ, Lenart BA, Provencher MT, Mazzocca AD, Verma NN, Romeo AA. Long head of the biceps tendinopathy: diagnosis and management. J Am Acad Orthop Surg. 2010;18(11):645–56.

Simovitch R, Sanders B, Ozbaydar M, Lavery K, Warner JJ. Acromioclavicular joint injuries: diagnosis and management. J Am Acad Orthop Surg. 2009;17(4):207–19.

Suzuki K, Potts A, Anakwenze O, Singh A. Calcific tendinitis of the rotator cuff: management options. J Am Acad Orthop Surg. 2014;22(11):707–17.

Chapter 10
Shoulder Instability

Marie E. Walcott and Arnold B. Alqueza

Abbreviations

CT Computed tomography scan
MDI Multidirectional instability
MRI Magnetic resonance imaging
PT Physical therapy
RTC Rotator cuff

Introduction

The stability of the shoulder joint depends primarily on the surrounding soft tissue structures and secondarily on bony architecture. The bony glenoid does provide stability in the short arc of motion of the shoulder, whereas static stabilizers provide stability in the medium arc of motion. Finally, muscles and tendons provide stability in the extreme ranges of motion. The soft tissue structures are divided into static stabilizers (labrum and glenohumeral ligaments) and active stabilizers (rotator cuff, deltoid, biceps, and periscapular muscles) (Fig. 10.1). The bony anatomy of the shoulder provides stability in a small range of motion, since the large humeral head articulates with the small, shallow glenoid. This lack of bony constraint allows for the shoulder to move through a wide range of motion.

 Shoulder instability can be due to a single traumatic injury, repetitive activities causing microtrauma, or an imbalance of the shoulder stabilizers. Shoulder instability represents a spectrum of pathology from traumatic unidirectional instability to atraumatic multidirectional instability. For the purposes of this chapter, we group shoulder instability into three categories: unidirectional anterior, unidirectional posterior, and multidirectional. There is certainly pathology that does not strictly fit into these categories; however, this is beyond the scope of this chapter.

M.E. Walcott • A.B. Alqueza (✉)
Department of Orthopedics, Brigham and Women's Hospital, Harvard Medical School,
75 Francis St, Boston, MA 02115, USA
e-mail: mwalcott@gmail.com; aalqueza@bwh.harvard.edu

© Springer International Publishing AG 2018   147
J.N. Katz et al. (eds.), *Principles of Orthopedic Practice for Primary Care
Providers*, https://doi.org/10.1007/978-3-319-68661-5_10

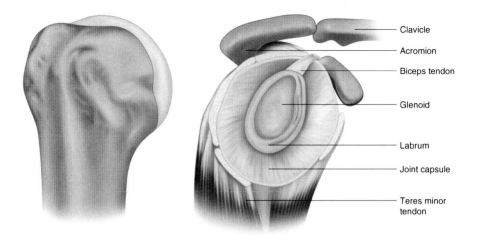

Fig. 10.1 Pertinent shoulder anatomy

Anterior instability, commonly seen with an anterior shoulder dislocation, tends to be of traumatic origin and occurs from an anterior force on an abducted, externally rotated arm. Similarly, posterior instability can result from a posterior shoulder dislocation, caused by a seizure, electrical shock, or posterior-directed force on a forward flexed, adducted, and internally rotated arm, such as seen in blocking in football or in a motor vehicle accident. For this reason, offensive linemen have a higher incidence of posterior shoulder instability than other positions.

Multidirectional instability (MDI) is defined as symptomatic shoulder instability in two to three directions with or without hyperlaxity. Similar to the other forms of shoulder instability, MDI can result from a significant traumatic event or recurrent microtraumas, or can even be atraumatic. Patients with multidirectional instability tend to have generalized, congenital ligamentous laxity. It is important to differentiate laxity from instability when evaluating a patient's shoulder. A shoulder with hyperlaxity will typically have signs of MDI, such as a positive sulcus sign, but be completely asymptomatic. When the patient presents with both symptoms and physical findings of laxity, this is defined as instability.

Summary of Epidemiology

Anterior Shoulder Instability

In the general population, the incidence of traumatic anterior shoulder instability is approximately 1.7%. The majority of recurrences happen within the first 2 years after the initial anterior dislocation. The most important risk factor for recurrence is

Fig. 10.2 A Bankart tear is a tear of the anterior/inferior labrum. Sometimes this is associated with a Hill-Sachs lesion

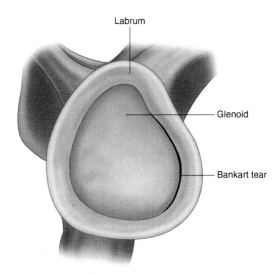

Labrum

Glenoid

Bankart tear

age. For patients under 20 years old, research shows a >90% rate of recurrent instability. For 20- to 40-year-olds, this rate drops slightly to approximately 80%. For patients over 40, there is <20% risk of recurrent instability, but a 30% risk of concurrent traumatic rotator cuff tears. In patients over 60, the rate of concurrent traumatic rotator cuff tears increases to approximately 80%. In this group of patients, there is also an increased risk of associated greater tuberosity fracture. A particularly high-risk group is contact athletes who return to contact sports after experiencing an anterior shoulder dislocation, wherein the recurrence rate is as high as 80%.

There are several associated lesions that are seen in cases of traumatic anterior shoulder dislocation. For example, Bankart lesions (a tear of the anterior/inferior labrum) and Hill-Sachs lesions (impression fracture of the posterior humeral head) have been reported in nearly 100% of patients with an anterior shoulder dislocation (Figs. 10.2 and 10.3). Bony Bankart lesions (avulsion fracture of the anterior/inferior glenoid) are also seen frequently (Fig. 10.4). While there are other lesions associated with traumatic anterior shoulder instability, these are the most common.

Posterior Shoulder Instability

Posterior instability comprises only a minority of all cases of shoulder instability, but the incidence is increasing as it is now more recognized. In posterior instability, approximately 50% of cases are traumatic. This can be due to an isolated trauma such as frank dislocation; however, this can also be seen in cases of recurrent subtle subluxation events. Atraumatic posterior shoulder instability can be associated with a bony defect of the glenoid; thus, careful review of imaging is important.

Fig. 10.3 A Hill-Sachs lesion is the result of the humeral head recoiling into the anterior glenoid when the shoulder is dislocated

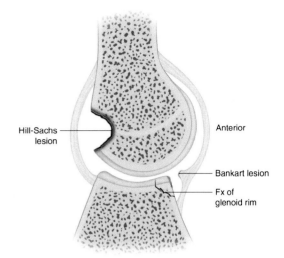

Similar to anterior dislocations, there are associated lesions commonly seen in cases of posterior shoulder dislocation. In contrast, however, posterior shoulder dislocations result in an associated lesion only 65% of the time. These include fractures of the lesser or greater tuberosity, reverse Hill-Sachs lesions (impression fracture on the anterior aspect of the humeral head), and fractures of the posterior glenoid rim (the reverse of Fig. 10.3).

Multidirectional Instability

Multidirectional instability has an increased incidence in the second and third decades of life and an increased incidence in overhead athletes such as those who participate in volleyball, swimming, or gymnastics. Multidirectional instability can also be associated with generalized hyperlaxity.

Clinical Presentation

In cases of shoulder pain, the localization of symptoms is helpful in determining the source of the patient's pathology. For example, pain at the posterior joint line may be attributable to a posterior labrum or infraspinatus injury, while anterior shoulder pain suggests involvement of the subscapularis, biceps, or anterior labrum. Pain over the lateral aspect of the shoulder is most consistent with superior or superior-posterior rotator cuff pathology. Patients under 40 years old, who present with shoulder pain, maintain a high level of suspicion for shoulder instability.

Fig. 10.4 A Bony Bankart lesion with the glenoid fracture segment attached to the labrum

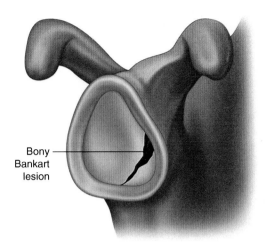

Bony
Bankart
lesion

Anterior Shoulder Instability

Anterior shoulder instability typically presents after a distinct dislocation event or in cases of recurrent subluxations, with asymptomatic periods in between. Many patients report an unstable feeling of their shoulder in the position of abduction and external rotation.

Posterior Instability

Posterior shoulder instability can present with symptoms of subtle instability or pain and, however, often without obvious symptoms of instability. For example, an athlete may complain of posterior shoulder pain at the end of a sporting event due to fatigue of the dynamic shoulder stabilizers (e.g., rotator cuff), thus unveiling pain due to injury to the static stabilizers. For patients involved in a trauma, there needs to be a high level of suspicion for posterior shoulder dislocation, as this is commonly missed at initial presentation.

Multidirectional Instability

The diagnosis of multidirectional shoulder instability is less straightforward. Patients frequently present with the insidious onset of activity-related shoulder pain rather than a sense of instability. Symptoms are often vague and not localizable. Due to this insidious onset, patients may compensate by avoiding certain shoulder positions that provoke symptoms. A thorough history should be obtained, including assessment of other joint problems (such as patellofemoral instability) and/or a family history of collagen disorders.

Essential History

In all cases of shoulder instability, obtaining a focused history is essential. This history should include focused questions related to hand dominance, level of athletic activity, history of other joint injuries, and symptoms of generalized ligamentous laxity. Specific to the shoulder, it is important to assess factors such as direction and position of the arm at the time of initial trauma, position of arm when symptoms recur, number and types of recurrences (dislocation versus subluxation), associated neurologic symptoms, magnitude of force to cause recurrent instability, and prior treatment.

Physical Exam

A systematic and complete shoulder exam is important to fully evaluate for instability. The exam should start with examination of the skin for muscle atrophy of the supraspinatus, infraspinatus, and deltoid. The axillary nerve can be injured in traumatic anterior dislocations so motor function (manual muscle testing of the deltoid) and sensation (cutaneous distribution over the lateral deltoid) should be assessed and compared to the contralateral side. The axillary nerve can be stretched during an anterior dislocation event as it runs inferior to the glenohumeral joint from anterior to the subscapularis posteriorly to the quadrilateral space. These are mostly transient neurapraxias and resolve spontaneously. The incidence is 5%, and X-rays can show the humeral head subluxated inferiorly.

Shoulder range of motion should be evaluated with the examiner first viewing the patient from a posterior direction to evaluate for scapular dyskinesia or scapular winging, which can be compensatory in posterior shoulder instability. Range of motion should then be assessed from an anterior direction. Shoulder range of motion includes forward flexion, abduction, external rotation with the elbow at the side, and functional internal rotation behind the patient's back (measured at the spinal level, the patient can reach with his or her thumb), followed by external and internal rotation with the patient's arm abducted to 90°.

Rotator cuff testing should include external rotation strength (testing infraspinatus), belly press and liftoff tests (testing subscapularis), and abduction strength (testing for supraspinatus). It is important to note both pain and weakness with these tests. For further details on how to carry out these tests, please see the chapter on shoulder soft tissue pathology.

Special tests for shoulder instability are useful to identify more subtle findings. If the patient has recently had a shoulder dislocation, these tests should be performed cautiously to prevent re-dislocating the patient's shoulder.

Anterior Instability

The apprehension test can be done with the patient sitting or lying supine, although performing the test supine leads to less guarding. The arm is abducted to 90° and externally rotated to the patient's end range. The test is positive if the patient exhibits or reports a sense of instability or apprehension about the shoulder in this position. Of note, patients with MDI may also have a positive test. The relocation test is done with the patient in the same position as the apprehension test. The examiner applies a posterior pressure on the humerus when the patient's arm is abducted and maximally externally rotated. If the patient reports relief of the prior feeling of instability, this is considered a positive test. Pain with the apprehension or relocation test is not a positive test and may be due to other shoulder pathology.

Posterior Instability

The posterior drawer test or posterior stress test is done with the patient supine. The arm is forward flexed to 90° and adducted. A posterior load is applied at the elbow in line with the humerus. A click or a clunk is indicative of a positive test. The jerk test is performed with the patient seated and the arm supported abducted to 90° in neutral position. A load is applied at the elbow in line with the humerus, while stabilizing the patient's scapula. The arm is then moved into adduction. A painful click or clunk as the humeral head subluxates is indicative of a positive test. The Kim test is similar to the jerk test but is more specific for inferior labral lesions. The arm is supported and abducted to 90°, and a posterior and axial load is applied to the humerus as the arm is flexed diagonally upward 45°. A positive test is sudden onset of posterior shoulder pain.

Multidirectional Instability

The sulcus sign is done with the patient seated. With the forearm in neutral and the arm adducted, an inferior force is applied to the humerus. A positive test is noted as reproduction of the patient's pain with inferior translation of the humerus. This should be repeated in external, internal, and neutral rotation, as well as 90° of abduction. This test is graded on a 0 to +3 scale. Of note, this test can be positive in patients with asymptomatic ligamentous laxity. The load-and-shift test is done with the patient supine. The examiner applies a gentle axial load to center the humeral head in the glenoid, followed by an anterior and posterior translational force to test the degree of laxity in different degrees of abduction. If the patient is guarding, the examiner may not be able to fully evaluate the shoulder. Of note, signs of rotator cuff impingement in a young adult (<20 years old) is also suggestive of MDI.

Fig. 10.5 True AP
(Grashey) radiograph of a
63-year-old male status
post reduction of right
shoulder dislocation. One
may be able to see an
irregularity of the anterior/
inferior glenoid

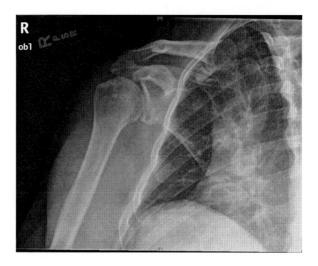

Differential Diagnosis and Suggested Diagnostic Testing

In cases of traumatic shoulder injury, it is important to assess for other bony injuries involving the clavicle, scapula, and proximal humerus. An acromioclavicular joint injury can also present similarly. In patients over 40, it is important to also assess for a rotator cuff tear. SLAP lesions can also present in the overhead throwing athlete population; these may occur via an overuse or traumatic mechanism. The differential diagnosis of shoulder instability should also include cervical disease and thoracic outlet syndrome. Several types of imaging can be helpful in the diagnostic work-up of shoulder instability.

Radiographs (X-Ray)

Evaluation of shoulder instability starts with X-rays, to include true AP (or Grashey) and axillary lateral views (Fig. 10.5). Axillary views are critical to confirm that the shoulder is indeed reduced given that shoulder dislocations are commonly missed, particularly those in the posterior direction. Shoulder X-rays are helpful to evaluate for bony lesions of the glenoid, Hill-Sachs lesions of the humeral head, and overall glenohumeral and acromioclavicular joint alignment. Additional views specific to shoulder instability include the West Point axillary view (evaluation for a bony Bankart lesion) and Stryker notch view (evaluation for a Hill-Sachs lesion).

Further imaging is usually necessary to fully evaluate the shoulder. There are different benefits to computed tomography (CT) scan versus magnetic resonance imaging (MRI), and careful thought should be given to determine which imaging modality to choose. While general guidelines are noted below, selecting the type of advanced imaging is typically left to the discretion of the orthopedic surgeon,

Fig. 10.6 MRI axial T2
image with a bony Bankart
lesion

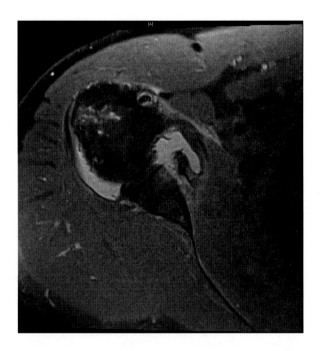

particularly for cases in which the patient will likely be having surgery and preoperative planning is required.

CT Arthrogram

A CT arthrogram is ideal for evaluating the bony anatomy of the glenoid and the humeral head as well as to evaluate for a bony Bankart lesion. This test tends to be ordered in cases of chronic shoulder instability, especially posterior instability, or when a patient has history of multiple shoulder dislocations or subluxations. The use of the arthrogram is surgeon specific and should be left to the treating surgeon as to whether the advanced imaging should be done with joint contrast.

MRI Arthrogram

An MRI arthrogram is ideal for evaluating the soft tissues of the shoulder including the rotator cuff, labrum, glenohumeral ligaments, and capsular attachments (Figs. 10.5 and 10.6). This is the imaging of choice for evaluating traumatic unidirectional instability in absence of a bony Bankart lesion or MDI. The use of the arthrogram is surgeon specific and should be left to the treating surgeon as to whether the advanced imaging should be done with joint contrast.

Nonoperative Management

Patients presenting for the first time with symptoms of shoulder instability may benefit from an initial course of nonoperative management. After a traumatic event, rest, ice, and anti-inflammatories can help control symptoms. Then physical therapy is the mainstay of nonoperative treatment of shoulder instability.

Traumatic Anterior Shoulder Instability

There is no consensus for how long to immobilize a patient after a shoulder dislocation. Furthermore, the literature does not show any decrease in recurrence with immobilization. Thus, it is currently recommended to immobilize patients in a regular sling for 1–3 weeks for comfort only. Nonoperative management can be successful in treating many isolated causes of traumatic anterior shoulder dislocation, particularly in older adults. In these cases, short-term immobilization should be followed by a focused physical therapy program.

Posterior Shoulder Instability

The majority of patients with posterior shoulder instability can be managed with physical therapy. The program should consist of posterior rotator cuff and deltoid strengthening, along with periscapular stabilization exercises. Nonsurgical management is successful in 65–80% of cases.

Multidirectional Instability

The mainstay of treatment for MDI is physical therapy. The physical therapy protocol should focus on a periscapular stabilization program, as well as including a rotator cuff strengthening program and proprioceptive training. A prolonged course of up to 6 months of physical therapy is sometimes necessary, and research supports an even longer trial before surgical options are considered.

Indications for Surgery

First-Time Traumatic Shoulder Dislocation

Patients who are at high risk for recurrent shoulder instability should be strongly encouraged to discuss treatment options with an orthopedic surgeon. Patients in this higher-risk category include age <30, glenoid bone loss, large Hill-Sachs lesion

(>5/8 of humeral head), presence of ALPSA lesion (anterior labroligamentous peri-osteal sleeve avulsion), contact athlete, male, and positive anterior apprehension test. The data is strongest for young, athletic males, who have the highest recurrence rate with conservative management.

Posterior Instability

In cases of posterior instability, patients who fail a course of physical therapy and continue to have symptoms that interfere with daily life or sporting activities are candidates for arthroscopic labral repair. Patients who present with multidirectional instability that have gone through a complete physical therapy program and have ongoing unidirectional posterior instability may be surgical candidates.

Multidirectional Instability

In cases of multidirectional instability, only patients who have failed a prolonged course of physical therapy and continue to have symptoms that interfere with daily life and sporting activities should be considered for surgery.

Operative Management

Arthroscopic Labral Repair

Arthroscopic labral repair consists of diagnostic arthroscopy to evaluate the anterior and posterior labrum, as well as the other interarticular structures. If indicated, the labrum is then most commonly repaired with suture anchors (smaller anchors than in rotator cuff repair) placed at the rim of the glenoid. The labrum is then sutured back to the glenoid. This process is similar whether the anterior or posterior labrum is torn (please see Figs. 10.5, 10.6, 10.7, and 10.8 for clinical cases).

Latarjet

The Latarjet procedure is commonly performed via an open approach, although it can be done arthroscopically. The coracoid is cut at its base and moved with the attached conjoined tendon to the anterior rim of the glenoid, in order to provide a soft tissue sling and more glenoid surface area to prevent recurrent anterior stability. It is then attached with one or two metal screws.

Fig. 10.7 MRI sagittal oblique T1 image showing the glenoid with a bony Bankart lesion anteriorly

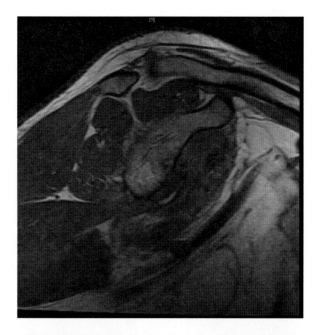

Fig. 10.8 Arthroscopic repair of a bony Bankart lesion using the double bridge technique. The humeral head is at the *top left*, and glenoid is to the *right*. The inferior glenohumeral ligament with labrum and fracture is centered

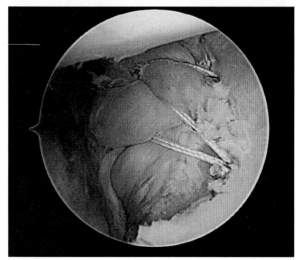

Arthroscopic Capsular Plication

Arthroscopic capsular plication is performed by suturing the capsule to the labrum in order to reduce the volume of the joint space. Depending on the direction of instability, the posterior, inferior, and/or anterior capsule can be plicated.

Table 10.1 Three general categories of shoulder instability with presenting symptoms, clinical exam findings, and a basic treatment algorithm

Clinical entity	Presentation	Diagnostic testing	Conservative management	Indications for surgery	Operative management
Traumatic anterior instability	– Dislocation or subluxation event(s)	+ Apprehension/relocation tests – X-ray – MRI if older than 40 y/o	– Sling for comfort for 1–3 weeks – PT: Scapular stabilization, RTC strengthening	– <20 years old, male, athletes, large glenoid bone loss, multiple dislocations	– Arthroscopic Bankart repair – Latarjet
Posterior instability	– Dislocation or subluxation event(s) – Posterior shoulder pain	+ Jerk/Kim tests – CT arthrogram or MRI arthrogram	– PT: Scapular stabilization, RTC strengthening	– Continued pain/instability after full course of PT	– Arthroscopic labrum repair – Posterior bone block procedure
Multidirectional instability	– Insidious onset of shoulder pain and instability	+ Sulcus, load-and-shift test, symptoms of impingement in young patient – MRI arthrogram	– PT: Scapular stabilization, RTC strengthening	– Continued instability after prolonged course of PT	– Capsular plication

PT physical therapy, *RTC* rotator cuff tear, *MRI* magnetic resonance imaging, *CT* computed tomography

Posterior Bone Graft

This is similar to the Latarjet procedure in that a piece of bone is being attached to the glenoid to provide a robust bumper for the humeral head. The bone graft is most commonly taken from the iliac crest. A posterior bone graft can be used in the setting of posterior shoulder instability with glenoid bone loss or significant glenoid retroversion.

Expected Outcome and Predictors of Outcome

The rate of recurrent anterior shoulder instability is quite high in young, active males after their first dislocation. Older patients and those not involved in contact sports usually do well with conservative management. In posterior shoulder instability, conservative treatment is reportedly successful in 65–80% of patients. For patients with a frank posterior dislocation, however, the risk of recurrence is 18%. Risk factors to having recurrence include age <40, presence of a large reverse Hill-Sachs lesion, and seizure disorder. Finally, in multidirectional instability, one study reported that 83% of patients with traumatic or atraumatic MDI had good-to-excellent results with conservative treatment. A recent study in a carefully selected population of athletes with MDI who underwent capsular plication procedure showed an 85% return to sport at their prior level.

Table 10.1 shows the three general categories of shoulder instability with presenting symptoms, clinical exam findings, and a basic treatment algorithm.

Summary

In summary, shoulder instability can be generally grouped into three categories: anterior, posterior, and multidirectional. The cause of instability may be due to trauma such as a dislocation, to repetitive microtraumas, or atraumatic. A careful history and physical exam are important to correctly identify shoulder instability. In traumatic anterior dislocations, there is a very high risk of recurrence with young (<20-year-old), contact athletes, and these patients may benefit from early surgical intervention. Patients over 40 years old with a shoulder dislocation should be carefully evaluated for a concurrent rotator cuff tear. Posterior shoulder instability can be difficult to diagnose. High clinical suspicion for posterior instability is important in patients under age 40 with shoulder pain. Perhaps with the exception of young contact athletes, patients with shoulder instability benefit from starting with conservative management with a course of physical therapy. For those who fail nonoperative management, surgical management depends on the direction of the instability and if there is bone loss on the glenoid. Arthroscopic surgery can repair the static stabilizers of the shoulder, but open surgery is usually necessary if there is associated bone loss.

Suggested Reading

Gaskill TR, Taylor DC, Millett PJ. Management of multidirectional instability of the shoulder. J Am Acad Orthop Surg. 2011;19(12):758–67.

Kane P, Bifano SM, Dodson CC, Freedman KB. Approach to the treatment of primary anterior shoulder dislocation: a review. Phys Sportsmed. 2015 Feb;43(1):54–64. https://doi.org/10.1080/00913847.2015.1001713.

Schepsis A, Busconi B, editors. Sports medicine (Orthopaedic surgery essentials series) second edition. Philadelphia, PA: Lippincott Williams & Wilkins; 2006.

Chapter 11
Glenohumeral Osteoarthritis

Michael J. Messina and Laurence D. Higgins

Summary of Epidemiology

Arthritis represents a significant burden to the healthcare system in the United States. It is projected that by 2030, 67 million adults, or 25% of the adult population, will experience some form of physician-diagnosed arthritis. Currently, nearly 50% of persons age greater than 65 are diagnosed with arthritis. Similar to other joints such as the hip and knee, arthritis of the shoulder glenohumeral joint can have a variety of underlying etiologies. These include osteoarthritis, rheumatoid arthritis, posttraumatic arthritis, instability arthritis, capsulorrhaphy arthritis, osteonecrosis, and rotator cuff arthropathy. For the purposes of this chapter, we will focus discussion primarily on osteoarthritis, although it should be noted that many of the diagnostic and treatment approaches presented here may also apply to varied types of shoulder arthritis.

Glenohumeral osteoarthritis can affect a wide range of patients and however is most commonly associated with an age greater than 60 and is more common in women than men. The specific incidence and prevalence of shoulder osteoarthritis in the United States are not well documented, but it is estimated that osteoarthritis of the glenohumeral joint is generally underdiagnosed. This is likely due to the fact that glenohumeral arthritis, involving a non-weight-bearing joint, is often less symptomatic than arthritis of the hips and knees. Thus, patients are able to tolerate

M.J. Messina • L.D. Higgins (✉)
Sports Medicine and Shoulder Service, Brigham and Women's Hospital, Harvard Medical School, 75 Francis St, Boston, MA 02115, USA
e-mail: mjmessina3@gmail.com; ldhiggins@partners.org

© Springer International Publishing AG 2018   163
J.N. Katz et al. (eds.), *Principles of Orthopedic Practice for Primary Care Providers*, https://doi.org/10.1007/978-3-319-68661-5_11

cartilage loss and degradation in the shoulder for a longer period of time, often resulting in more severe radiographic disease at the time of initial diagnosis. Despite this, given the aging of our population combined with an expectation of higher activity levels, the need for shoulder replacement surgery continues to grow at a rapid pace and is currently the third most common arthroplasty performed, second only to hip and knee replacement.

Clinical Presentation

Patients presenting with osteoarthritis of the glenohumeral joint predominantly complain of shoulder pain that can vary in location, however, is most typically described as deep within the shoulder. When asked to point to where they feel pain, patients often will use more than one finger and point to the anterior aspect of the shoulder as well as reach underneath the axilla in order to point directly to the posterior aspect of the glenohumeral joint. This is in contrast to the common presentation of a patient with rotator cuff pathology or subacromial bursitis, which is typically localized to the lateral or posterosuperior aspect of the shoulder, consistent with the course of the supraspinatus and infraspinatus musculotendinous units. It should be noted, however, there is considerable variability in how patients perceive and describe pain referral patterns around the shoulder.

Pain attributable to glenohumeral osteoarthritis is often described as deep, constant, and achy. Patients may or may not ever have complete relief from the pain but typically have alleviation with rest and exacerbation with increased activity and demand on the shoulder. It is common for patients to have pain at night, specifically if they prefer to sleep on the side ipsilateral to their arthritis. Sleep disturbance is a common complaint that ultimately pushes patients to proceed with surgical treatments when nonoperative treatments have failed. Crepitus is common with advancing severity of disease and is usually described as "catching," "clicking," "popping," or "grinding" inside the joint, associated with motion. As seen in hip and knee osteoarthritis, patients with glenohumeral osteoarthritis usually will also have some degree of stiffness. The degree to which patients perceive stiffness can vary, and many times it is most apparent during the physical examination.

Physical examination should follow a standard progression including inspection, palpation, range of motion, strength testing, and special tests. Osteoarthritis is not usually associated with abnormalities on inspection; thus, the changes such as significant deformities or muscle atrophy may suggest another diagnosis. Likewise, the value of palpation is to rule out other pathologies such as acromioclavicular (AC) joint pain due to AC arthritis or bicipital groove pain stemming from biceps tendinopathy. Given the proximity of the biceps tendon to the anterior aspect of the glenohumeral joint, it is not uncommon for palpation over the bicipital groove to elicit pain, which can be either referred pain from the underlying osteoarthritis or concomitant biceps tendon disease, not uncommon in a multitude of shoulder pathologies.

Depending on the severity of the disease, the most apparent physical exam finding for patients with glenohumeral osteoarthritis is loss of motion. Patients frequently have a loss of terminal active forward elevation, which is associated with pain and discomfort when further passive elevation is attempted. They also have stiffness in internal and external rotation, the latter of which is most apparent with the arm at the side and the elbow flexed to 90°. Keeping the elbow firmly adducted to the body, the patient is asked to rotate the forearm and hand externally. The degree of external rotation on the affected side will be significantly less than the contralateral side, unless the patient has stiffness bilaterally (normal external rotation is from approximately 40°–90°). Many times, patients with advanced osteoarthritis will have a complete loss of external rotation such that they are unable to actively or passively externally rotate the arm beyond the neutral position. Internal rotation is assessed by asking the patient to place their hand behind their back, reaching their thumb as high up the spine as is possible. Again, the hand on the affected side will usually reach lower along the spine than the contralateral side. With more advanced disease, the patient may be unable to position the hand much past the greater trochanter or sacrum. In severe cases, the examiner can often hear or palpate crepitus with range of motion, particularly in forward elevation and external rotation.

As is routine for any shoulder examination, rotator cuff strength testing should be performed, although routine examination maneuvers may need to be modified secondary to a loss of motion. For the supraspinatus, this is most easily accomplished by placing the arm in the empty can position (90° of elevation in the plane of the scapula with the thumb pointing down) and asking the patient to resist a downward force placed on the arm by the examiner. For the infraspinatus, the elbow should be bent to 90° and adducted against the body (similar to examining external rotation motion as described above). Beginning with the forearm in neutral rotation, the patient is asked to resist an internal rotation force. Depending on the degree of motion loss, evaluation of subscapularis strength can be difficult, as the most common techniques for this require some capacity to internally rotate the hand, such as the liftoff test and belly press. One solution for this is to place the arm at the side in the same neutral rotation position as used to evaluate external rotation strength and instead have the patient resist an external rotation force. This maneuver, however, also engages the pectoralis muscles and does not isolate the subscapularis.

Classic osteoarthritis is associated with a tear of the rotator cuff less than 10% of the time, and thus rotator cuff strength should be preserved. It should be noted, however, that all of these strength tests will result in a compressive load on the shoulder joint and thus may elicit osteoarthritis pain resulting in decreased effort, which can inaccurately be perceived as weakness. Similarly, patients will often times have other associated positive special tests due to provocation of arthritis pain with certain maneuvers, such as a Hawkins test, Speed's test, or O'Brien's test. In completing the shoulder examination, a neurovascular assessment of the upper extremity should be performed with particular attention paid to confirming intact function of the axillary nerve, including an assessment of sensation over the deltoid as well as appropriate deltoid contraction force.

Differential Diagnosis and Suggested Diagnostic Testing

A patient presenting with a primary complaint of shoulder pain can have a very broad differential diagnosis; however, the most common etiologies include rotator cuff disease, glenohumeral arthritis, AC joint arthritis, biceps tendon disease, adhesive capsulitis (frozen shoulder), and various types of labral tears. Correctly diagnosing glenohumeral osteoarthritis requires careful consideration of the history, physical exam, and imaging studies. Imaging studies play an integral role in the work-up and diagnosis of glenohumeral arthritis. It should be noted, first and foremost, that advanced imaging such as a computed tomography (CT) scan or magnetic resonance imaging (MRI) are NOT required in the initial and routine work-up of glenohumeral arthritis. As with nearly all musculoskeletal complaints, appropriate work-up should begin with plain film radiography, which in this case is all that is needed to confirm the diagnosis.

There are numerous described techniques for obtaining shoulder radiographs, and it is worthwhile to not only spend some time reviewing what findings are consistent with arthritis but also which views are most useful and how they are obtained. Most traditional shoulder series include approximately two to five views of the shoulder, the specifics of which can vary. It should be noted, however, that at least two orthogonal views are required to adequately assess the glenohumeral joint. Thus, at the minimum, each patient should have some type of AP view (preferably a Grashey AP) as well as an axillary lateral.

There are multiple types of AP shoulder films that can be obtained, and the differences between these types are notable. In a standard AP view of the shoulder, the X-ray beam is oriented perpendicular to the transverse axis of the patient. However, because the scapula is oriented at an angle approximately 30°–45° anterior to this transverse axis, the resulting film does not produce a view parallel to the glenoid face, which is most ideal to assess for osteoarthritis. In order to obtain a truly orthogonal view to the glenohumeral joint, the beam must be oriented at an angle perpendicular to that of the scapula on the chest wall. This view is called a "Grashey" view or a "true" AP (Fig. 11.1a). The value of this in assessing glenohumeral osteoarthritis is that it produces a direct view in line the glenohumeral joint space, which is essential for evaluating many of the classic associated findings such as joint space narrowing, osteophyte formation, subchondral cyst formation, and sclerosis.

Likewise, there are different ways of obtaining a "lateral" view of the shoulder, which include, most commonly, either a "scapular Y" or an "axillary lateral." In most cases of shoulder pathology, including glenohumeral arthritis, the axillary lateral view is far superior and should be obtained as part of the initial screening series. A well-positioned axillary lateral provides a second look parallel to the glenoid face in line with the glenohumeral joint (Fig. 11.1b). From a surgical perspective, this view also yields valuable information in determining the glenoid orientation and how well the humeral head is centered on the glenoid. This is important because often times more severe osteoarthritis is associated with some degree of asymmetric posterior glenoid wear and posterior subluxation of the humeral head. The scapular Y view adds very little to the work-up and evaluation for glenohumeral osteoarthritis and is unnecessary.

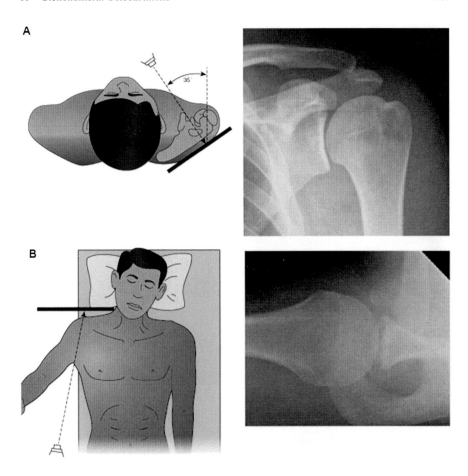

Fig. 11.1 (a) Proper X-ray technique and corresponding radiographic result to obtain "true AP" or "Grashey AP" view of the shoulder, which provides a view directly parallel with the glenoid face, essential for evaluating for arthritic changes. (b) Proper X-ray technique and corresponding radiographic result to obtain axillary lateral view of the shoulder, which provides a view directly parallel with glenoid face and orthogonal to the true AP. (Adapted from Matsen FA http://shoulderarthritis. blogspot.com/2011/03/plain-x-ray-key-to-diagnosing-arthritis.html)

Similar to the clinical course, radiographic evaluation of osteoarthritis demonstrates a wide range of severity from subtle findings associated with mild, early arthritis to more severe, advanced changes. With an increasing degree of severity, the findings become more obvious, thus making the diagnosis more apparent. However, certain more subtle findings can be helpful in diagnosing the disease at an earlier time point. One such finding is the inferior humeral head osteophyte. The inferior humeral head osteophyte, or "goat's beard," is the most classic X-ray finding associated with glenohumeral arthritis and is also one of the earliest. Its presence (even when small) is highly associated with at least some degree of full-thickness cartilage loss, even with generally well-persevered

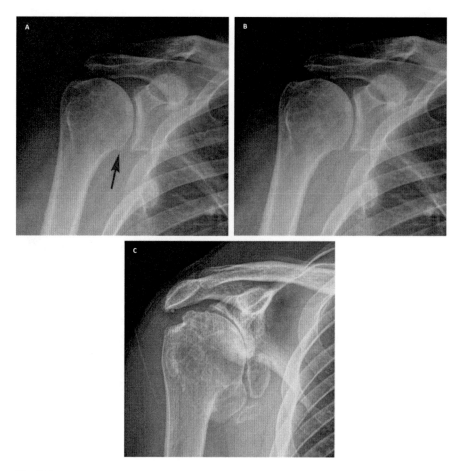

Fig. 11.2 AP shoulder X-rays demonstrating varying sizes of inferior humeral head osteophyte in shoulder osteoarthritis. (**a**) Patient with very early and subtle radiographic changes with a small osteophyte (*red arrow*). This patient underwent arthroscopy and was found to have large areas of full-thickness cartilage loss despite well-preserved joint space and ultimately required shoulder replacement surgery soon after this image was taken. (**b**) Patient with severe osteoarthritis with moderate-sized osteophyte. (**c**) Patient with severe osteoarthritis with large inferior osteophyte

joint space (Fig. 11.2a). Over time, the size of this osteophyte can become quite large, which in and of itself may restrict motion (Fig. 11.2b, c).

As noted previously, there is typically no role for ordering advanced imaging beyond the X-ray images discussed above once the diagnosis of osteoarthritis has been made, unless there is a concern for a concomitant symptomatic rotator cuff tear, which is associated with osteoarthritis <10% of the time. CT and MRI imaging may be required for surgical planning in the event that the patient ultimately elects to proceed with shoulder replacement surgery. However, these tests should be ordered by the treating surgeon, as specific protocols to allow for 3D modeling may be required for surgical planning.

Nonoperative Management

Osteoarthritis is a dynamic and progressive process in which ongoing cartilage degradation almost always leads to worsening of symptoms, particularly pain, over time. To date, there remains no effective treatment option that can reverse the loss of cartilage or even slow down the progression to any clinically relevant degree. Thus, the mainstay of nonoperative treatment remains focused on symptom management. The primary goals are to minimize pain while preserving function. The classic techniques used to achieve these goals in management of lower extremity arthritis include activity modification, weight loss, nonsteroidal anti-inflammatory drugs (NSAIDs), physical therapy, and injections. The majority of these can be applied to the treatment of arthritis of the shoulder as well.

Activity modification is a simple and straightforward strategy to decrease symptoms by avoiding the particular tasks that bring about the most pain. This can be effective for patients who are accustomed to high demand use of their shoulder, but they must be willing to alter their lifestyle, which many are not. Furthermore, this becomes a less effective strategy as arthritis worsens and minimal use of the shoulder still results in significant pain. Given the fact that the shoulder is not a weight-bearing joint in most individuals, weight loss has less of an impact on alleviating arthritis pain.

NSAIDs can be a useful adjunct to nonoperative treatment of glenohumeral osteoarthritis via both a direct analgesic effect and by decreasing the production of inflammatory cytokines over time. NSAIDs have a long track record of safety; however, caution should be exercised with prolonged chronic use and in patients with a history of gastritis or gastric ulcers or kidney disease or in patients who require concomitant anticoagulation. For patients who cannot tolerate NSAID therapy, alternative options include acetaminophen as well as tramadol, which are favorable alternatives to stronger opioids. While opioids are occasionally used in the short-term management of arthritis pain, there are high risks associated with their use, and they should therefore be reserved for only unique situations.

Physical therapy is a common treatment in the nonoperative management of many musculoskeletal complaints including various types of osteoarthritis. Unfortunately, physical therapy plays a less significant role in the treatment of glenohumeral osteoarthritis compared to other joints, such as knee osteoarthritis. One possible explanation for this could be that while knee osteoarthritis patients benefit greatly from muscle strengthening techniques to serve as a type of "shock absorber" for the joint during weight bearing, muscle strengthening in the shoulder often leads to increased compressive loads across the joint and can exacerbate pain. The primary role for therapy in glenohumeral osteoarthritis is more so geared toward maintaining motion, and thus function, through various gentle muscular and capsular stretching techniques as well as symptom management through pain relief modalities such as electrical stimulation, iontophoresis, ultrasound, and others.

The use of injections in the treatment of many different types of shoulder pathologies is common, especially for conditions such as subacromial bursitis or rotator

cuff tears, where subacromial injections can be readily performed in the office setting. It is critical to note, however, that in the presence of an intact rotator cuff, the
subacromial space does not communicate with the intra-articular joint space, and
thus subacromial injections are not indicated in the treatment of glenohumeral
osteoarthritis. While intra-articular injections can be used successfully in the management of glenohumeral osteoarthritis, there are considerations to keep in mind.
First and foremost, glenohumeral joint injections are more technically challenging
to perform in the office without the use of image guidance. In fact, prior studies have
shown a success rate of only 47.5% for fellowship-trained orthopedic sports/shoul-
der specialists. As a result, it is recommended that these injections are administered
using ultrasound or fluoroscopic imaging guidance, both of which have been shown
to be highly effective but frequently require a second visit or referral to interventional radiology. Additionally, most evidence suggests that injections are more
effective when used for mild to moderate radiographic arthritis. As mentioned earlier in this chapter, glenohumeral arthritis patients are commonly diagnosed at a
more advanced stage when injections may have a less dramatic effect.

Despite the above considerations, intra-articular glenohumeral injections do
have a role in the nonoperative management of glenohumeral osteoarthritis. Most
commonly these injections are performed with corticosteroids, although recently
there has also been interest in the use of viscosupplementation in the management
of shoulder osteoarthritis. Despite a relative lack of high-level evidence to support
the use of glenohumeral injections, they remain a widely accepted treatment option
for patients with osteoarthritis. In the appropriately selected patient, injections can
provide meaningful pain relief and improve function. Additionally, despite often
diminishing returns over time, injections can be repeated, making them a particularly attractive option for long-term pain management in patients who are poor surgical candidates. We recommend injections no more frequently than every 3 months.
Despite local delivery and limited systemic effects, intra-articular steroid injections
can lead to increased glucose levels, and, as such, blood sugars should be closely
monitored in diabetic patients following injections. While viscosupplementation
appears to offer a safe, effective alternative to steroid injections, it is not currently
FDA approved for use in the shoulder, and its specific role in the management of
glenohumeral osteoarthritis requires further study.

Indications for Surgery

Simply stated, the indication for surgical treatment of glenohumeral osteoarthritis is
failure of nonoperative treatment, defined as persistent pain and dysfunction despite
use of modalities listed above, to the point where activities of daily living and quality of life are significantly affected. Ultimately, a shared decision-making process is
essential, involving a thorough discussion about the risks and benefits of surgery.
Patients must ultimately decide for themselves when their symptoms warrant more
aggressive treatments.

Operative Management

Operative management of glenohumeral osteoarthritis can be divided into two general groups: arthroscopic/joint preserving surgery and joint replacement surgery. Indications for arthroscopic treatment of the osteoarthritic shoulder are few and, however, may show benefit in properly selected patients. Typically these are younger patients (less than 55 years of age) with advanced osteoarthritis and significant symptoms and, however, with high risk for failure of arthroplasty due to young age and high demands on shoulder use. Generally, this procedure involves lavage and extensive debridement with some degree of osteophyte removal and axillary nerve decompression. The goals are to provide pain relief, restore motion, and improve function in order to ultimately prolong time until shoulder replacement is needed. Developed by Millet and Gaskill[9], this procedure has been termed comprehensive arthroscopic management (CAM) of glenohumeral osteoarthritis. They have reported a high level of patient satisfaction with decreased pain and increased range of motion up to 2.7 years postoperatively and, however, with high rates of early failure and conversion to arthroplasty in patients with less than 2 mm of joint space preoperatively. In these patients, further evaluation will certainly be needed to assess for long-term success. Other joint preserving surgical techniques such as microfracture of contained lesions and bulk osteochondral allografts have also been described but are used less frequently and are beyond the scope of this chapter.

Shoulder replacement surgery remains the gold standard for operative treatment of glenohumeral osteoarthritis. The primary indications are severe pain and dysfunction with loss of quality of life and failure of nonoperative treatment. The two most commonly used techniques are anatomic total shoulder arthroplasty (TSA) and reverse shoulder arthroplasty (RSA). As the name implies, anatomic TSA involves reconstruction of the glenohumeral joint to restore normal anatomical relationships typically with a metal humeral head component and an all-polyethylene glenoid component (Fig. 11.3). Success of anatomic TSA is highly reliant upon an intact and well-functioning rotator cuff. Given the low prevalence of rotator cuff tears in patients with true glenohumeral osteoarthritis (<10%), these patients are frequently ideal candidates for anatomic TSA.

Anatomic TSA is performed through a deltopectoral approach from the front of the shoulder which requires reflection of subscapularis for complete exposure and commonly also involves concomitant tenodesis of the biceps tendon at the time of surgery. Historically, humeral components have involved the use of a stem in the humeral intramedullary canal that is fixed either with or without the use of cement. Recently, a stemless humeral component has been approved for use in the United States as well, with advantages of preserving bone stock and facilitating easier removal in the event revision surgery is required (Fig. 11.4). The polyethylene glenoid component is cemented, and, upon satisfactory placement of all implants, the subscapularis is repaired. Healing of the subscapularis is critical for proper function and stability following surgery, and as such, protection of the repair is a major driving force that dictates postoperative restrictions and speed of recovery. Specifically,

Fig. 11.3 Components of
anatomic total shoulder
arthroplasty. Image
courtesy of Arthrex Inc.
Used with permission

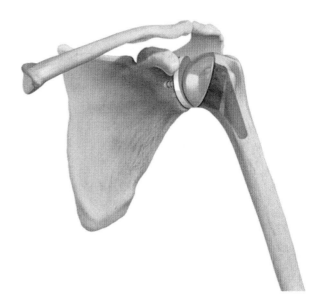

Fig. 11.4 Example of
components in stemless
anatomic shoulder
arthroplasty. Published
with permission from
Tornier, Inc., an indirect
subsidiary of Wright
Medical Group N.V.

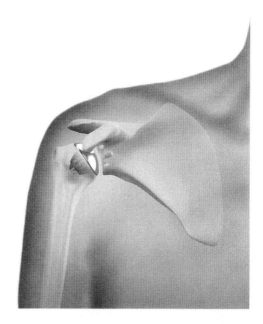

it is critical to avoid any external rotation (passive and active) beyond 0°–30°, as
well as any active internal rotation for up to 4–6 weeks after surgery.

The alternative to anatomic TSA is reverse shoulder arthroplasty in which the
"ball and socket" parts of the prosthesis are switched such that the glenoid side now
consists of a spherical metal component, or glenosphere, and the humeral side consists of a stemmed, cupped, metal component. A polyethylene insert then fits

Fig. 11.5 Example of
components of reverse
shoulder arthroplasty.
Image courtesy of Arthrex
Inc. Used with permission

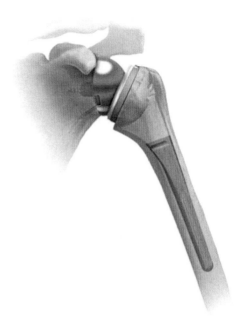

between the two metal components (Fig. 11.5). The most classic indication for RSA
is rotator cuff deficiency leading to rotator cuff arthropathy, which is a separate
process from glenohumeral osteoarthritis and outside the scope of this chapter.
However, there are certain instances in which RSA is indicated in patients with
glenohumeral osteoarthritis as well. These instances include patients with osteoarthritis with intraoperative findings of significant concomitant rotator cuff tears,
severe glenoid wear and bone loss, and overall poor bone quality typically associated with older patients. Postoperative recovery does not differ significantly from
anatomic TSA, and because the healing of the subscapularis tendon is far less integral to function, patients may recover slightly faster after RSA.

Expected Outcomes and Predictors of Outcome

While specific postoperative recovery and rehab protocols vary by surgeon preference, most patients can expect to spend some length of time after surgery immobilized in a sling; typically this phase lasts 4–6 weeks. Patients may start therapy prior
to having their sling discontinued to begin working on pendulums and passive range
of motion. For patients who have an anatomic TSA, careful attention is paid during
the initial recovery period to protect the repair of the subscapularis tendon, and as
such, they are strictly cautioned against any active internal rotation as well as passive external rotation beyond 0°–30°. As patients begin to wean from their sling at

Table 11.1 Clinical management of glenohumeral osteoarthritis

Clinical entity	Presentation	Diagnostic testing	Conservative management	Surgical indications and operative management
Glenohumeral osteoarthritis	– Gradual onset and worsening of deep shoulder pain; dull and aching – Loss of shoulder range of motion—Particularly in internal and external rotation – Pain with shoulder motion and pain at night	– X-RAY (Grashey AP and axillary lateral)—Joint space narrowing, inferior humeral head osteophyte, subchondral sclerosis, and cystic changes – MRI and CT scan are not needed	– Begins with lifestyle modification – Analgesics including NSAIDs, Tylenol, and tramadol in more severe cases – Limited role for physical therapy – Injections can be helpful—must be given with image guidance to localize within glenohumeral joint (subacromial not effective)	– Mainstay of surgical treatment is shoulder replacement – Shoulder replacement is associated with significant pain relief and increased function as well as high patient satisfaction

NSAIDS nonsteroidal anti-inflammatory drugs, *MRI* magnetic resonance imaging, *CT* computed tomography, *AP* anteroposterior

around 4–6 weeks postoperatively, they are permitted to begin active ROM and use the arm for daily activities. Strengthening begins at 2–3 months postoperatively.

Shoulder replacement surgery has a complication profile similar in many ways to lower extremity joint replacement, with some very pertinent differences. The common risks include bleeding, infection, nerve injury, instability, stiffness, loosening of implants, and venous thromboembolism (VTE). Blood transfusion following shoulder replacement is less common than in lower extremity joint replacement and is required in only approximately 5% of patients. One of the most dramatic differences between shoulder and lower extremity joint replacement is the higher risk for infection with *Propionibacterium acnes* (*P. acnes*) in shoulder surgery. This is due to the difference in normal skin flora of the shoulder compared to the hip or knee. Specifically the chest and back contain a higher density of oily sebaceous glands, which harbor the growth of *P. acnes*. The clinical relevance is that *P. acnes* is a low virulence organism that can sometimes exist in the shoulder for years prior to development of symptoms, and, as such, there should always be a high index of suspicion for infection in a patient who presents with pain, stiffness, or evidence of component loosening after total shoulder replacement surgery.

Shoulder replacement surgery for patients who have failed conservative treatment of osteoarthritis has proven to be a highly successful operation with high patient satisfaction and long-term durability rivaling that of knee or hip arthroplasty. Shoulder replacement has consistently led to improvements in both subjective, patient-reported outcomes and objective clinical outcomes. Shoulder replacement is most reliable at relieving pain; however, most patients can additionally expect to achieve improved range of motion in forward elevation and external rotation as well as improved overall function after surgery. Given that the natural course of glenohumeral osteoarthritis is a slow progression of pain and declining function over time, shoulder replacement offers an excellent long-term solution by providing pain relief and restoring quality of life in patients who are appropriate surgical candidates. Table 11.1 shows a brief description of the clinical management of glenohumeral osteoarthritis.

Suggested Reading

Gross C, Dhawan A, Harwood D, Gochanour E, Romeo A. Glenohumeral joint injections: a review. Sports Health. 2013;5(2):153–9. https://doi.org/10.1177/1941738112459706.

Hootman JM, Helmick CG. Projections of US prevalence of arthritis and associated activity limitations. Arthritis Rheum. 2006;54(1):226–9. https://doi.org/10.1002/art.21562.

Hsu JE, Bumgarner RE, Matsen FA. Propionibacterium in shoulder arthroplasty: what we think we know today. J Bone Joint Surg Am. 2016;98(7):597–606. https://doi.org/10.2106/JBJS.15.00568.

Kidd BL, Langford RM, Wodehouse T. Arthritis and pain. Current approaches in the treatment of arthritic pain. Arthritis Res Ther. 2007;9(3):214. https://doi.org/10.1186/ar2147.

Kircher J, Morhard M, Magosch P, Ebinger N, Lichtenberg S, Habermeyer P. How much are radiological parameters related to clinical symptoms and function in osteoarthritis of the shoulder? Int Orthop. 2010;34(5):677–81. https://doi.org/10.1007/s00264-009-0846-6.

Millett PJ, Gaskill TR. Arthroscopic management of glenohumeral arthrosis: humeral osteoplasty, capsular release, and arthroscopic axillary nerve release as a joint-preserving approach. Arthroscopy. 2011;27(9):1296–303. https://doi.org/10.1016/j.arthro.2011.03.089.

Millett PJ, Gobezie R, Boykin RE. Shoulder osteoarthritis: diagnosis and management. Am Fam Physician. 2008;78(5):605–11. http://www.ncbi.nlm.nih.gov/pubmed/18788237. Accessed 6 April 2016.

Millett PJ, Horan MP, Pennock AT, Rios D. Comprehensive arthroscopic management (CAM) procedure: clinical results of a joint-preserving arthroscopic treatment for young, active patients with advanced shoulder osteoarthritis. Arthroscopy. 2013;29(3):440–8. https://doi.org/10.1016/j.arthro.2012.10.028.

Prevalence of doctor-diagnosed arthritis and arthritis-attributable activity limitation–United States, 2010–2012. MMWR Morb Mortal Wkly Rep. 2013;62(44):869–73. http://www.ncbi.nlm.nih.gov/pubmed/24196662. Accessed 6 April 2016.

Padegimas EM, Clyde CT, Zmistowski BM, Restrepo C, Williams GR, Namdari S. Risk factors for blood transfusion after shoulder arthroplasty. Bone Joint J. 2016;98-B(2):224–8. https://doi.org/10.1302/0301-620X.98B2.36068.

Rutten MJCM, Collins JMP, Maresch BJ, et al. Glenohumeral joint injection: a comparative study of ultrasound and fluoroscopically guided techniques before MR arthrography. Eur Radiol. 2009;19(3):722–30. https://doi.org/10.1007/s00330-008-1200-x.

Tobola A, Cook C, Cassas KJ, et al. Accuracy of glenohumeral joint injections: comparing approach and experience of provider. J Shoulder Elb Surg. 2011;20(7):1147–54. https://doi.org/10.1016/j.jse.2010.12.021.

Part VII
Elbow

Chapter 12
Elbow Osteoarthritis and Soft Tissue Injuries

George S.M. Dyer and Stella J. Lee

Introduction

This chapter discusses various common inflammatory, traumatic, and arthritic conditions of the elbow region of the upper extremity. In each case, we have tried to address common presentation, diagnosis, options for management, and outcomes.

Elbow Septic Arthritis and Olecranon Bursitis

Septic arthritis involving the elbow is an infection within the joint resulting in inflammation of the joint synovium and painful distension of the joint capsule, followed by progressive destruction of cartilage and ultimately leading to arthritis. The pathogen is usually bacterial, most commonly *Staphylococcus aureus*. Etiologies of septic arthritis include hematogenous spread from bacteremia, direct inoculation from trauma or surgery, or local spread from adjacent cellulitis or osteomyelitis. Olecranon bursitis does not involve the joint itself but rather the olecranon bursa, a synovial-lined, fluid-filled sac overlying the triceps tendon insertion onto the olecranon. This bursa can become inflamed and filled with aseptic synovial fluid, causing discomfort at the elbow. It is important to differentiate these two conditions as one may be treated with observation, whereas the other requires urgent surgical intervention.

G.S.M. Dyer (✉) • S.J. Lee
Department of Orthopedic Surgery, Brigham and Women's Hospital,
75 Francis St, Boston, MA 02115, USA
e-mail: gdyer@partners.org; slee81@partners.org

© Springer International Publishing AG 2018
J.N. Katz et al. (eds.), *Principles of Orthopedic Practice for Primary Care Providers*, https://doi.org/10.1007/978-3-319-68661-5_12

Summary of Epidemiology

Septic arthritis more commonly occurs in weight-bearing joints, and infections of the elbow account for only 3–9% of cases. Risk factors for septic arthritis include previous trauma, immunosuppression, rheumatoid arthritis, hemophilia, and history of intravenous drug use. Aseptic olecranon bursitis is typically associated with gout, rheumatoid arthritis, other inflammatory conditions, or intensive physical labor. Anatomic variances such as a prominent olecranon process or bone spurs are associated with higher occurrences of bursitis. Although olecranon bursitis is typically aseptic, the most common cause of septic bursitis is iatrogenic infection from attempts to aspirate or drain the collection. Aseptic olecranon bursitis should never be drained.

Clinical Presentation

Septic arthritis of the elbow presents with fever, erythema, edema, and pain with range of motion of the elbow. Olecranon bursitis, on the other hand, typically presents as a non-tender fluctuant mass overlying the proximal olecranon. It may be asymptomatic until the bursa is quite distended. Alternatively, in the case of gouty or septic olecranon bursitis, the bursa can be painful and tender, and there may be overlying hyperemia or erythema.

Differential Diagnosis and Suggested Diagnostic Testing

The differential diagnoses for septic elbow include crystalline arthropathies such as gout and pseudogout, trauma, hemarthrosis, and abscess not involving the joint. An elevated ESR and CRP are suggestive of infection but are not diagnostic. Imaging such as X-ray, CT, or MRI can be helpful in detecting an effusion or ruling out other diagnoses; however, it is not diagnostic of an infection. The definitive diagnosis of septic arthritis is made with joint aspiration; this should be completed prior to the initiation of antibiotics and performed using sterile technique. The needle is placed into the soft space at the center of a triangle formed by the olecranon, radial head, and lateral epicondyle. Samples should be sent to the laboratory for Gram stain, culture, cell count, and crystal analysis. A cell count of greater than 50,000/mm^3, as well as neutrophils greater than 90%, is indicative of infection.

Aseptic olecranon bursitis should be distinguished from septic bursitis, which accounts for 20% of cases. If septic bursitis is suspected, a needle aspiration should be performed. To avoid creating a chronically draining sinus, it is recommended to use a long spinal needle, entering the bursa from proximally on the radial side at a

Fig. 12.1 Aspiration of the olecranon bursa. The patient is positioned with the elbow flexed at approximately 90°. The needle is placed obliquely through the triceps muscle into the olecranon bursa. The clinician should avoid inserting the needle directly into the skin overlying the olecranon bursa as this can lead to the formation of a chronically draining sinus tract

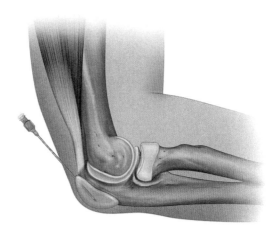

very acute angle, so that the needle traverses a long path of skin and soft tissue. With this technique, elbow flexion will collapse and seal the resulting aspiration tract, rather than stretching it open. Care should also be taken not to enter the joint space during bursal aspiration. A white blood cell count of greater than $10,000/mm^3$ with predominantly polymorphonuclear cells is concerning for septic bursitis.

Non-operative Management

There is no role for non-operative treatment of septic arthritis—antibiotic therapy is an adjunct to surgical debridement. Empiric antibiotic therapy based on patient risk factors should be initiated after joint aspiration, followed by a long-term course of intravenous antibiotic therapy based on culture data. The non-operative management of aseptic olecranon bursitis consists of a combination of compressive dressings, avoidance of pressure to the area, nonsteroidal anti-inflammatories (NSAIDs), and padded splinting, usually with resolution over a period of months. Persistent bursitis is sometimes treated via serial aspirations performed under sterile technique; however, this procedure may lead to the formation of a chronically draining sinus tract. The recommended technique in this case involves placing a needle proximally through the triceps muscle and then aiming distally into the bursal sac (Fig. 12.1). Given the specificity of these procedures, it is recommended that diagnostic and therapeutic injections for olecranon bursitis be performed with the care of an orthopedic specialist.

Indications for Surgery

Surgical debridement of the elbow joint should be performed if diagnostic aspiration shows frankly purulent fluid, cell count greater than $50,000/mm^3$, or positive culture. Bursectomy is a treatment option for chronic symptomatic bursitis. It is also recommended for septic bursitis that is not responsive to needle aspiration and antibiotic treatment.

Operative Management

Elbow irrigation and debridement consists of either open or arthroscopic debridement of inflamed synovium, removal of any cartilage or bony debris, and irrigation with several liters of normal saline. In open bursectomy, a longitudinal incision is made over the olecranon bursa. The bursal sac is completely excised, hemostasis is achieved, and the dead space is obliterated. A drain is placed prior to wound closure.

Expected Outcomes and Predictors of Outcome

Both open and arthroscopic debridements are effective in treating septic elbow. It should be noted, however, that there is a high mortality rate associated with septic arthritis—one study showed a 50% mortality rate after the diagnosis of septic elbow. Postoperatively, the best functional outcomes are seen in patients without preexisting elbow pain who undergo debridement within 2 days of presentation. Most patients with olecranon bursitis are successfully treated with non-operative therapy. Bursectomy results in long-term pain relief but is much less effective in patients with gout.

Tendinopathies: Lateral Epicondylitis and Medial Epicondylitis

Lateral epicondylitis, or "tennis elbow," and medial epicondylitis, or "golfer's elbow" are degenerative tendinopathies of the tendon origins at the lateral and medial epicondyles of the elbow. Lateral epicondylitis most commonly affects the extensor carpi radialis brevis (ECRB) and less commonly the extensor digitorum communis (EDC). Medial epicondylitis affects the pronator teres and flexor carpi radialis (FCR) tendons. Although the background cause of tendinopathy is poorly understood, in many cases it is believed to be caused by repetitive microtrauma to the tendons.

Summary of Epidemiology

The prevalence of lateral and medial epicondylitis is 1.3% and 0.4%, respectively. Epicondylitis most often presents in patients in their 30s to 50s, favors the dominant arm, and affects men and women equally. It is associated with smoking, obesity, and forceful repetitive activities and as such may be considered a work-related condition in some cases. Medial epicondylitis in particular may affect young throwing athletes.

Clinical Presentation

In cases of lateral epicondylitis, patients complain of pain at the region of the lateral epicondyle which is aggravated by wrist extension. On exam, pain is elicited with resisted wrist extension with the forearm pronated and elbow extended, as well as with resisted extension of the long finger. In cases of medial epicondylitis, patients complain of pain at the region of the medial epicondyle. On exam, pain is elicited with resisted wrist flexion and resisted pronation. Medial epicondylitis is often associated with ulnar neuritis, and ulnar nerve dysfunction should be tested. With ulnar neuritis, patients may report pain or paresthesias with tapping the ulnar nerve at the elbow (Tinel's sign) or with cubital tunnel compression. In cases of medial epicondylitis, the elbow should also be evaluated for ulnar collateral ligament (UCL) insufficiency resulting in valgus instability. The "milking maneuver" is performed by flexing the elbow to 90° and supinating the forearm, while the examiner then pulls on the thumb radially to produce valgus stress. The test is positive with pain or instability when compared to the contralateral side.

Differential Diagnosis and Suggested Diagnostic Testing

Lateral epicondylitis and medial epicondylitis are clinical diagnoses. Plain films and magnetic resonance imaging (MRI) may be obtained to evaluate for other disorders, such as arthritis, osteochondral defects, or ligamentous injuries, but are not required for diagnosis. If obtained, MRI may reveal increased signal within the common extensor or common flexor tendons on T1 and T2 sequences. In the presence of a partial tear, it may show tearing of the muscle from bone, noted as a focal area of high T2 signal intensity. It is also important to note that lateral epicondylitis has a similar presentation to radial tunnel syndrome (i.e., entrapment of the deep radial or posterior interosseous nerve in the lateral forearm); however, the location of pain in radial tunnel syndrome is approximately 2 cm more distal when compared to lateral epicondylitis.

Non-operative Management

For both lateral and medial epicondylitis, watchful waiting and activity modification with avoidance of exacerbating activities is the first step of treatment and is effective for most. A counterforce brace may be used if it provides symptomatic relief. This should be followed by physical therapy and gradual return to resistive activities. Local corticosteroid injections have been shown to provide a benefit in the short term but not in the long term and are thus discouraged. Up to 90% of patients experience symptom resolution with non-operative treatment, but it is important to counsel patients that this may take up to a full year.

Indications for Surgery

Surgery for epicondylitis can be considered in cases that fail to improve with non-operative treatment for more than 12 months.

Operative Management

Surgical treatment for epicondylitis may be performed open or percutaneously. The affected area of tendon is sharply excised, the surrounding area debrided, and the tendon reattached to the epicondyle as necessary. If there is progressive ulnar neuritis associated with medial epicondylitis, ulnar nerve decompression is recommended. Please refer to Chap. 15 for further information on upper extremity compression neuropathies and ulnar nerve decompression.

Expected Outcomes and Predictors of Outcome

It is important to note that most patients experience resolution of symptoms in 8–12 months simply with activity modification. For the 10% of patients who do not improve with non-operative treatment, surgical management has a success rate of approximately 97% in lateral epicondylitis and 87–100% in medial epicondylitis.

Biceps and Triceps Tendon Ruptures

Triceps tendon injuries are generally traumatic and result from rapid eccentric muscle contraction. Distal biceps tendon ruptures also occur after an acute traumatic event, usually forced elbow flexion and supination, but can also occur in the setting of chronic tendon degeneration with chronic elbow pain. Avulsions are defined as injuries at the osseous surface, whereas ruptures are defined as injuries at the intra-substance of the muscle or the musculotendinous junction. Tendon ruptures may be partial or complete, involving all the tendon fibers.

Summary of Epidemiology

Triceps ruptures are quite rare, accounting for less than 1% of all tendon ruptures. About 3% of biceps injuries occur at the distal biceps tendon. Both triceps and distal biceps ruptures usually occur in men, and avulsion and musculotendinous ruptures in particular are associated with anabolic steroid use. Renal failure and hyperpara-thyroidism are also risk factors for tendon injuries. Spontaneous tendon injuries are higher after total elbow arthroplasty.

Clinical Presentation

In cases of complete triceps rupture, patients present with pain at the posterior elbow and loss of active elbow extension. Physical exam reveals a palpable defect at the triceps tendon. Partial tendon ruptures result in some active elbow extension, however often with decreased strength and an extensor lag (inability to actively bring the elbow into full extension). In cases of distal biceps rupture, patients complain of pain at the antecubital fossa that is worsened with supination. On exam, there is often ecchymosis over the antecubital fossa and asymmetry of the biceps muscle belly when compared to the contralateral side. Pain is elicited with resisted elbow flexion and forearm supination. The examiner should perform the "hook test" to attempt to palpate and pull on the distal biceps tendon in the antecubital fossa with the elbow in 90° of flexion, using a hooked index finger. With a complete rupture, the distal biceps tendon is not palpable.

Differential Diagnosis and Suggested Diagnostic Testing

The diagnosis of triceps tendon injuries may be made clinically, but plain films should be obtained to evaluate for olecranon fracture or bony avulsion which may also result in an extensor lag. MRI may also be useful for distinguishing between partial and complete tendon ruptures. Plain films are generally not useful in suspected biceps tendon ruptures as associated bony injuries are rare. MRI is helpful when the diagnosis of biceps injury is unclear and can distinguish between complete and partial ruptures.

Non-operative Management

Partial triceps tendon ruptures may be treated non-operatively. Both partial and complete distal biceps ruptures may be treated non-operatively. The principal flexor muscle of the elbow is the brachialis, not the biceps, thus flexion strength is typically only diminished by 20–40%, even in cases of complete biceps rupture. Forearm supination strength, however, is often greatly diminished. Non-operative treatment consists of splint immobilization in 30° of flexion for triceps ruptures and simple sling immobilization for biceps ruptures. Patients should receive regular follow-up to ensure that partial ruptures do not progress into complete ruptures.

Indications for Surgery

Surgical repair is indicated for acute complete triceps ruptures. It may also be considered for residual weakness with non-operative treatment, although surgical repair is more difficult in a chronically injured elbow, in which case the tendon may become retracted. Surgical repair for distal biceps ruptures may be considered for patients with high functional demands.

Operative Management

In cases of triceps rupture, the triceps tendon is attached to the olecranon via nonabsorbable sutures passed through drill holes in the olecranon. Large bony fragments may be attached with additional hardware. Postoperatively, the patient is made non-weight-bearing through the arm, and the elbow is initially immobilized in partial flexion. Patient should undergo physical therapy for gradual range of motion and progression to active extension. In a distal biceps rupture, the distal biceps tendon is mobilized and then reattached to the biceps tuberosity. The repair is completed with the elbow in slight flexion in order to maximize flexion and supination strength; as the tendon attenuates, the patient can then achieve full extension. A variety of methods are used to attach the tendon to bone, including suture anchors and bone tunnels with interference screws. For both biceps and triceps injuries, acute repair is recommended over delayed repair before significant tendon retraction occurs.

Expected Outcomes and Predictors of Outcome

Most patients regain satisfactory function following triceps tendon repair—one study reported 92% of peak strength compared to the uninjured side. Outcomes are poorer following repair of chronic tendon injuries. The most common postoperative complications include olecranon bursitis, flexion contractures up to 20°, and, rarely, re-rupture. Following non-operative treatment of distal biceps ruptures, there is an approximately 30% loss of flexion strength and 40% loss of supination strength. Most patients report satisfactory outcomes following distal biceps repair, although similar to triceps repair, there may be slight deficits in strength and endurance. Risks of a distal biceps repair include radial nerve palsy with a single-incision approach and heterotopic ossification or synostosis—fusion of the proximal ulna and radius—with a two-incision approach.

Elbow Arthritis

Elbow osteoarthritis primarily affects the ulnohumeral joint and less commonly the radiocapitellar joint. Due to the high congruence of this articulation, bony changes first occur at the margins of the joint—the tips of the olecranon and coronoid processes—and complete loss of articular cartilage does not occur until advanced stages of the disease (Fig. 12.2). Rheumatoid arthritis, by contrast, is an inflammatory disease of the soft tissue surrounding joints. The development of an inflammatory pannus ultimately results in erosion of cartilage and subchondral bone, attenuation of ligaments, and progressive joint deformity.

Summary of Epidemiology

Primary osteoarthritis of the elbow is fairly rare compared to osteoarthritis of other major joints, affecting 2% of the population. It is seen in relatively young men involved in manual labor or throwing sports and more commonly affects the dominant arm. It can also follow elbow injury such as fracture or dislocation. Elbow involvement is common in rheumatoid arthritis, affecting about 50% of the patients affected with this systemic disorder. Patients with elbow rheumatoid arthritis are generally older than those with osteoarthritis.

Clinical Presentation

Elbow arthritis presents with pain and progressive stiffness of the elbow. In the early stages of osteoarthritis, patients complain of pain only at terminal flexion or terminal extension. As the disease progresses to involve the entire ulnohumeral joint, there is pain throughout the arc of range of motion. In radiocapitellar arthritis, there is lateral elbow pain with forearm rotation. Due to posterior osteophyte formation, some patients present with associated ulnar neuropathy, complaining of medial-sided elbow pain along with paresthesias in the ulnar digits. Patients should be

Bony anatomy of the elbow

Anterior view

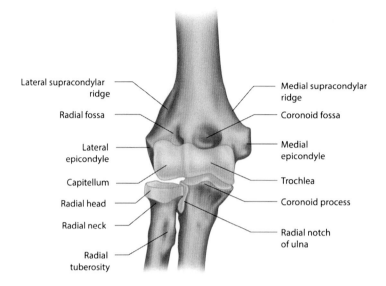

Lateral supracondylar ridge

Radial fossa

Lateral epicondyle

Capitellum

Radial head

Radial neck

Radial tuberosity

Medial supracondylar ridge

Coronoid fossa

Medial epicondyle

Trochlea

Coronoid process

Radial notch of ulna

Medial view

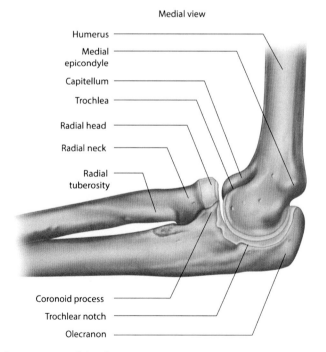

Humerus

Medial epicondyle

Capitellum

Trochlea

Radial head

Radial neck

Radial tuberosity

Coronoid process

Trochlear notch

Olecranon

Fig. 12.2 Bony anatomy of the elbow

examined for sensory deficits in the ulnar nerve distribution and intrinsic hand weakness. The physical exam should also include elbow varus and valgus stress tests for instability.

Differential Diagnosis and Suggested Diagnostic Testing

In the evaluation of arthritis, plain films of the elbow, including AP, lateral, and oblique views, should be obtained. In osteoarthritis, X-rays usually show preservation of joint spaces with anterior and posterior osteophytes at the coronoid and olecranon processes and its associated fossae. Loss of joint space does not occur until advanced stages of the disease. In rheumatoid arthritis, X-rays may be normal in early stages as pure synovitis has few radiographic correlates. As the disease progresses, X-rays may show bony erosions, joint space narrowing, and, ultimately, significant joint destruction. Regarding other imaging modalities, obtaining a computed tomography (CT) scan can be helpful in cases of osteoarthritis to evaluate for loose bodies, which is important in planning for surgical debridement. MRI is usually not helpful unless soft tissue pathology is suspected, such as involvement of the MCL in cases of instability.

Non-operative Management

In the early stages of elbow osteoarthritis, activity modification, for example, avoidance of terminal flexion and extension, can be effective. Non-operative treatments including use of NSAIDs, intra-articular corticosteroid injections, and neoprene elbow sleeves (used for comfort) may help. Hyaluronic acid injections may be helpful in the short-term but do not provide long-term benefit. The mainstay of treatment for rheumatoid arthritis of the elbow is medical management with DMARDs (disease-modifying antirheumatic drugs). The goal of medical therapy is control of synovitis and prevention of joint destruction. Corticosteroid injections may also be helpful in the early stages of RA.

Indications for Surgery

Surgery may be considered for patients with significant pain and stiffness affecting activities of daily life despite non-operative treatment. In selecting the appropriate surgical treatment for osteoarthritis, a distinction should be made between stiffness and pain at extremes of flexion or extension, which may be treated with debridement, versus pain throughout the arc of motion indicative of total destruction of articular cartilage, treated with elbow arthroplasty. Lastly, prior to total elbow arthroplasty, the patient's current functional demands and ability to comply with postoperative activity restrictions should be assessed in order to optimize the likelihood of a successful postoperative course.

Operative Management

Surgical debridement is an appropriate choice for patients with moderate osteoarthritis complaining primarily of elbow stiffness or pain at end range of motion. Release of anterior soft tissues and removal of posterior osteophytes improve elbow extension, and similarly, release of posterior soft tissues and removal of anterior osteophytes improve elbow flexion. Debridement may be performed open or arthroscopically. An open procedure is recommended in the presence of severe contractures requiring extensive release, prior elbow operations with presumed abnormal anatomy, and associated ulnar neuropathy requiring concurrent ulnar nerve release.

For patients with severe osteoarthritis, definitive treatment consists of a total elbow arthroplasty (TEA). Following TEA, patients are subjected to lifelong weight-bearing and lifting restrictions—typically 8–10 lbs. This procedure is more suitable for older, low-demand patients. For younger patients, interposition arthroplasty poses fewer postoperative restrictions. The elbow joint should never be fused. Complete resection of the joint and a "flail" elbow is less functionally limiting than fusion in any position. Isolated radiocapitellar arthritis may be treated with radial head excision or radial head replacement.

Similar to the treatment of osteoarthritis, surgical treatment of rheumatoid arthritis depends on the stage of disease. Synovectomy is effective in earlier stages of disease marked by synovitis with some bony erosions but without significant joint destruction. Good results have been seen with both arthroscopic and open synovectomy. In some cases, synovectomy may be accompanied by radial head resection. The surgical treatment for end-stage rheumatoid arthritis is total elbow arthroplasty.

Expected Outcomes and Predictors of Outcome

Open and arthroscopic debridement for primary osteoarthritis is effective in decreasing pain and improving range of motion. However, in the long term, there is gradual loss of range of motion as arthritis progresses. Following total elbow replacement for primary osteoarthritis and rheumatoid arthritis, the most common complication is early loosening. Revision rates range from 5% to 20%. There is a higher rate of early revisions in younger patients with osteoarthritis. However, once end-stage arthritis occurs, it is favorable to proceed directly to TEA, as surgical intervention prior to TEA results in poorer outcomes. Other complications include superficial and deep infections and transient ulnar neurapraxias.

Elbow Fractures and Fracture-Dislocations

There are numerous patterns of traumatic bony and ligamentous injury to the elbow. These include simple elbow dislocations, complex fracture-dislocations with radial head fractures, olecranon fractures, coronoid fractures with their associated ligamentous injuries, and Monteggia lesions—proximal ulna fractures with radial head dislocation. In the management of these injuries, the key is to identify unstable injury patterns that lead to development of arthrosis.

The elbow is an intrinsically stable joint owing to its bony anatomy. There are three main articulations: ulnohumeral, radiocapitellar, and proximal radioulnar (Fig. 12.2). The ulnohumeral joint is formed by the articulation of the coronoid process and the semilunar notch of the proximal ulna onto the spool-shaped trochlea of the distal humerus. The radiocapitellar joint is formed by the radial head and the ball-shaped capitellum of the distal humerus. There are two elements to stability: sagittal, which prevents posterior subluxation of the ulna on the distal humerus, and coronal, which counters varus and valgus stresses. Sagittal stability is conferred by the prominent coronoid process anteriorly, which remains in contact with the trochlea even in full extension. Valgus stability is provided by tension on the medial collateral ligament and the bony buttress of the radial head, and varus stability is similarly provided by tension on the lateral ulnar collateral ligament and the bony buttress of the anteromedial facet of the coronoid process. Significant disruption of any of these structures may lead to elbow instability.

Summary of Epidemiology

Most fractures of the elbow occur in the elderly, predominantly women, following a low-energy mechanism of injury such as a fall from standing position. The most common elbow fractures are radial head fractures, accounting for one-third of elbow fractures and 1–4% of all fractures. High-energy mechanism elbow fractures occur more often in young men.

Clinical Presentation

The patient with an elbow fracture presents with pain and swelling around the elbow. The skin should be carefully examined for wounds that could represent an open fracture. Certain injuries, such as elbow fracture-dislocations and posteriorly and laterally displaced Monteggia fractures, may be accompanied by a neurologic deficit, usually due to ulnar nerve injury. A complete neurovascular exam should be performed for all injury types. Escalating pain and significant swelling, especially in the setting of ipsilateral distal radius and proximal ulna fractures, raise concern for compartment syndrome. There are a few exam maneuvers that are specific to various injuries. For example, in a radial head fracture, range of motion testing should include pronation and supination to assess for a mechanical block. In a displaced olecranon fracture, patients should be examined for an extensor lag or a loss of full active elbow extension.

Differential Diagnosis and Suggested Diagnostic Testing

Plain films of the elbow should be obtained at the time of injury, followed by repeated imaging obtained after any manipulation or splinting, as needed. X-rays should be carefully examined for subtle signs of instability such as coronoid fractures, which may appear as a small fleck, or subluxation of the radial head. As the radial head normally points to the center of the capitellum on both AP and lateral views, any deviation indicates instability. Obtaining a CT scan is helpful for further evaluation of a suspected coronoid fracture or radial head fracture on plain films. CT is also used for preoperative planning of complex elbow fractures. Upon diagnosis of an elbow fracture, X-rays of the humerus and forearm are recommended in order to evaluate for ipsilateral injuries. MRI is usually not necessary.

Common Injury Patterns and Management

Simple Elbow Dislocation

In these cases, X-rays show posterior, or less commonly anterior, displacement of the ulna relative to the distal humerus. Twenty-five percent of elbow dislocations are associated with fractures. Simple elbow dislocations—those without associated fractures—are treated with closed reduction under sedation or intra-articular block. Following reduction, stability should be tested with flexion, extension, and varus-valgus stresses. The elbow is temporarily immobilized in a posterior splint for 1 week, followed by progressive range of motion exercises.

Radial Head Fracture

Patients with radial head fractures will present with tenderness to palpation over the radial head. Range of motion testing assesses for mechanical blocks to forearm pronation and supination, which can occur with displaced fractures. The elbow should also be tested for valgus instability. With a nondisplaced radial head fracture, X-rays may show an elbow effusion—displacement of the anterior fat pad and visualization of the posterior fat pad—without obvious fracture. X-rays should also be examined for an associated coronoid fracture, indicating instability. CT scan is helpful for identifying subtle associated injuries and for preoperative planning. Isolated nondisplaced or minimally displaced radial head fractures without block to motion can be immobilized very briefly in a sling for comfort, with early return to activity. Immobilization for more than a week can may cause permanent loss of motion in the elbow—move it early! Displaced radial head fractures should be splinted, followed by surgical treatment with open reduction and internal fixation versus radial head replacement.

Olecranon Fracture

The olecranon is a subcutaneous structure, and injury often results from direct trauma. On exam, patients should be examined for skin wounds indicative of an open fracture. The integrity of the extensor mechanism should be evaluated. Patients should be examined for an extensor lag, presenting as an inability to actively extend the elbow into full extension. X-rays of the elbow are evaluated to characterize the fracture as nondisplaced versus displaced and simple versus comminuted. Imaging should be reviewed for ipsilateral injuries such as coronoid fractures, radial head fractures, ulnohumeral dislocation, and proximal radioulnar joint dislocation. Isolated olecranon fractures do not cause the elbow to dislocate, even if they are displaced.

Nondisplaced or minimally displaced olecranon fractures are treated non-operatively with a posterior splint in extension. Displaced olecranon fractures are usually associated with disruption of the extensor mechanism on exam and require surgical fixation. They may initially be splinted with a posterior slab and then fixed on a non-urgent basis. Simple fractures are treated with a tension band construct, whereas comminuted fractures or those associated with other elbow injuries are treated with plates and screws. Very distal fractures may be treated with excision of the small proximal fragment and repair of triceps onto the distal fragment.

Elbow Fracture-Dislocations

There are several patterns of elbow fracture-dislocation: trans-olecranon fracture-dislocation, Monteggia injuries, and posteromedial and posterolateral rotatory fracture-dislocations. Trans-olecranon fracture-dislocation is a displaced olecranon fracture combined with ulnohumeral dislocation. Monteggia injury is a proximal ulna fracture with proximal radioulnar dissociation, which is apparent on X-rays as a radial head dislocation. Posteromedial and posterolateral rotatory fracture-dislocations should be suspected on X-rays with small coronoid fractures or radial head fractures. Rotatory fracture-dislocations range in severity—the most severe pattern is the "terrible triad" with elbow dislocation, radial head fracture, and coronoid fracture. It is also associated with injury to the lateral collateral ligament. Dislocation is not always seen on X-ray because the elbow may "snap back" and come to rest in a congruent position, but on exam there will be anterior-posterior ulnohumeral instability and valgus or varus instability. All of these injuries should be initially splinted, then referred to an orthopedic surgeon for further evaluation. CT is used to further characterize the injury, and management consists of surgical fixation of all bony injuries as well as repair of the lateral collateral ligament as necessary.

Expected Outcomes and Predictors of Outcome

The most common complication of elbow fractures is stiffness. Extension is typically more limited than flexion, and a flexion contracture of as much as 30°–40° may be present. Fractures of the radial head may lead to loss of forearm rotation. Other complications include (1) heterotopic ossification, which occurs more often with associated head trauma or burns; (2) ulnar neuropathy, both subacute and chronic; (3) loss of fixation, which occurs with inadequate fixation of a complex elbow injury; or (4) recurrent instability, which can occur with malreduction of proximal ulna fractures or an unrecognized LCL injury. Finally, post-traumatic arthritis may occur after high-energy mechanism injuries.

Ulnar Collateral Ligament Injuries and Valgus Instability

The medial ulnar collateral ligament (UCL) of the elbow is the primary restraint to valgus stress. There are three bundles of the UCL: anterior, posterior, and oblique (Fig. 12.3). The anterior bundle arises from the medial epicondyle of the humerus and inserts onto the sublime tubercle of the proximal ulna; this structure is the most significant contributor to valgus stability.

Summary of Epidemiology

Injuries of the UCL are most commonly seen in adult throwing athletes, such as baseball pitchers. The late cocking and early acceleration phases of throwing place the most valgus stress on the elbow. In children who participate in throwing sports, medial-sided elbow pain is more commonly a result of medial epicondyle apophysitis, or Little Leaguers' elbow, rather than UCL injury.

Clinical Presentation

Patients typically present with medial-sided elbow pain. In acute injury, patients recall a "popping" sensation in the elbow during a throwing event. In chronic injury, patients complain of a dull pain associated with decreased pitching strength or

Ligamentous anatomy of the elbow

Medial view

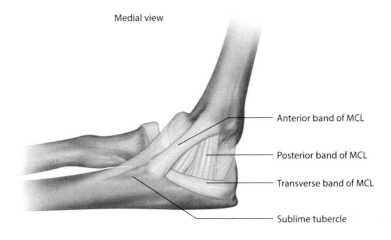

- Anterior band of MCL
- Posterior band of MCL
- Transverse band of MCL
- Sublime tubercle

Lateral view

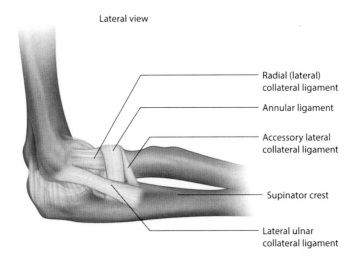

- Radial (lateral) collateral ligament
- Annular ligament
- Accessory lateral collateral ligament
- Supinator crest
- Lateral ulnar collateral ligament

Fig. 12.3 Ligamentous anatomy of the elbow

accuracy. There is tenderness along the flexor-pronator origin in acute injuries, but often no tenderness in chronic injuries. Pain with resisted wrist flexion indicates a flexor-pronator tendon injury, either in isolation or in conjunction with UCL injury. There may also be associated ulnar nerve symptoms. This should be further evaluated with Tinel's sign at the elbow and assessing for motor or sensory deficits. The physical exam should include evaluation of the entire upper extremity, including the shoulder and wrist. In the throwing athlete, there is often an associated deficit in glenohumeral internal rotation (GIRD), which may affect elbow mechanics.

Several tests are used to determine valgus stability. The valgus stress test is performed with the elbow in 30° of flexion, and laxity is compared to the contralateral side. However, this finding may also be positive in asymptomatic throwing athletes. The milking maneuver is performed by abducting the shoulder to 90°, flexing the elbow to 90°, and then supinating the forearm. The examiner pulls on the patient's ipsilateral thumb—like milking a cow—to produce a valgus stress. Pain, apprehension, or instability is indicative of UCL injury. A third test, the moving valgus stress test, is designed to recreate valgus stress during the late cocking and early acceleration phase of throwing motion. The shoulder is abducted to 90°, the elbow is placed in full flexion, and then a valgus stress is applied to the elbow. The test is positive if pain is most severe between 70° and 120° of flexion.

Differential Diagnosis and Suggested Diagnostic Testing

Medial-sided elbow pain may also be the result of flexor-pronator injuries or ulnar neuritis in the absence of a UCL injury; however, these conditions often appear in conjunction with one another. X-rays of the elbow should be obtained to evaluate for elbow osteoarthritis, bony UCL avulsions, and posterior olecranon osteophytes that may result in impingement. A valgus stress X-ray of the elbow can be used to supplement the physical exam. MRI is reliable for diagnosing full-thickness UCL tears, which are apparent as a discontinuous ligament surrounded by edema. The "T-sign," a continuation of T2-intense joint fluid along the undersurface of the UCL, may indicate a partial-thickness tear but may also represent an anatomic variant in which the UCL inserts more distally along the ulna.

Non-operative Management

Non-operative management consists of a 6-week period of rest, followed by gradual return to throwing sports accompanied by appropriate rehabilitation, including addressing shoulder motion deficits, pitching kinematics, and flexor-pronator mass strengthening. Primary prevention of injuries by promoting rest during off-season and regulating the number of pitches thrown per year is also important in addressing this problem.

Indications for Surgery

Surgical intervention is favored for high-performing throwing athletes. With the popularization of "Tommy John surgery" or UCL reconstruction, many patients who are not professional athletes may request this operation, but this is not always appropriate. Surgical reconstruction may be considered for patients who do not improve with non-operative methods and are willing to commit to intensive postoperative physical therapy.

Operative Management

Operative management consists of reconstruction of the UCL with an allograft, usually the palmaris longus tendon of the forearm. In this procedure, an incision is made along the medial elbow, and the injured UCL is dissected and removed. The tendon allograft is attached to the medial epicondyle and the sublime tubercle via bone tunnels, resulting in an anatomic reconstruction. This is often accompanied by ulnar nerve release. Postoperatively, early range of motion exercises are initiated, followed by strengthening at 4–6 weeks. Return to competitive sports is deferred until 9–12 months post-op.

Expected Outcomes and Predictors of Outcome

Results are very favorable with UCL reconstruction, with about 80–90% of patients eventually returning to prior level of sports at the major league or collegiate level. The most common complication is a transient ulnar nerve neurapraxia. Other complications can include stiffness and heterotopic ossification.

Overuse Injuries: Little Leaguers' Elbow and OCD Lesions

Athletes who engage in repetitive overhead throwing activities or weight-bearing on their upper extremities (e.g., gymnasts) may be predisposed to characteristic sports-related elbow injuries. Valgus stress on the elbow results in excessive tensile forces on the medial elbow and compressive forces on the lateral elbow. At the medial elbow, this can result in injury to the ulnar collateral ligament (UCL). In children whose growth plates are open, the elbow may instead fail due to injury through the medial epicondylar apophysis. This is the bony attachment point of the flexor-pronator tendons, before it ultimately fuses with the distal humerus. Medial epicondylar apophysitis, or Little Leaguer's Elbow as it is commonly called, typically consists of mild widening of the apophysis. Occasionally patients can develop significant displacement or medial epicondylar fracture. At the lateral elbow, repetitive microtrauma to the capitellum may result in subchondral fracture, fissure and fragmentation of the overlying cartilage, and, finally, intra-articular loose bodies. This clinical entity is called osteochondritis dissecans (OCD).

Summary of Epidemiology

As more young athletes become involved in high-performance sports, overuse elbow injuries are becomingly increasingly common. OCD is typically seen in children 10–14 years old, and medial epicondylar apophysitis more frequently occurs before then. Elbow injuries most commonly affect baseball players—almost one-third of youth baseball players develop elbow pain in-season—but can also affect gymnasts, tennis players, and wrestlers.

Clinical Presentation

Patients most commonly complain of medial or lateral elbow pain, depending on the etiology. Those with medial-sided pain may have associated symptoms of ulnar nerve irritation. Patients with OCD may present with mechanical symptoms such as clicking, catching, or giving way of the elbow. Baseball players should be questioned regarding the number, frequency, and types of pitches thrown. On exam, there may be tenderness at the medial epicondylar apophysis or at the capitellum, which is most easily palpated with the elbow in hyperflexion. Testing range of motion may show a slight flexion contracture. The elbow should be tested for valgus instability indicative of ulnar collateral ligament insufficiency. The physical exam should also include evaluation of the shoulder, which may show an internal rotation deficit in throwers.

Differential Diagnosis and Suggested Diagnostic Testing

In all cases, AP and lateral X-rays of the elbow should be obtained. In medial epicondylar apophysitis, X-rays show widening of the medial epicondylar apophysis. If there is suspicion for concomitant ulnar collateral ligament insufficiency, gravity stress X-rays should also be obtained. In the evaluation for OCD, a 45° flexion AP view of the elbow may be useful for showing the OCD lesion in profile view. MRI is more helpful for localizing and staging of OCD lesions and is becoming the standard for diagnosis. In MRI evaluation, T2-weighted sequences that show fluid deep to OCD lesions are indicative of fragment instability. MRI is also helpful in evaluating for ulnar collateral ligament injury or other pathologies. In medial epicondylar apophysitis, MRI may also show increased T2-weighted signal at the medial epicondyle.

Non-operative Management

Non-operative treatment of medial epicondylar apophysitis and OCD consists of a 6–12-week period of rest, followed by physical therapy for flexor-pronator stretching and strengthening, as well as addressing any associated shoulder issues. Patients should gradually return to sports, paying close attention to activity-related pain. Young athletes and their parents should receive age-appropriate activity guidelines, as well as realistic expectations for timing of return to sports.

Indications for Surgery

Most cases of medial epicondylar apophysitis and small avulsion fractures can be treated non-operatively, but displaced fractures of the entire medial epicondyle should be treated surgically. The decision to treat OCD with or without surgery depends on the assessment of OCD lesions either via advanced imaging or arthroscopy. OCD lesions with stable bony fragments and intact overlying cartilage may be treated non-operatively, whereas lesions with unstable fragments and disrupted overlying cartilage, especially those with intra-articular loose bodies, should be treated surgically. Surgery may be considered for patients with OCD who continue to be symptomatic despite non-operative treatment.

Operative Management

The standard treatment for OCD is elbow arthroscopy and drilling. In this procedure, the OCD lesions are unroofed and debrided. Following this, many small drill holes are made in the subchondral bone. The resulting marrow stimulation is thought to promote healing of the subchondral bone. A relatively new procedure is the OATS procedure: osteochondral autogenous transplantation surgery. This procedure consists of debriding the OCD lesion, obtaining an autograft of cartilage and subchondral bone from a remote location (often the distal femur), and transplanting it into the capitellar lesion.

Expected Outcomes and Predictors of Outcome

Younger patients and those in earlier stages of disease are more likely to be treated with non-operative treatment than older patients with closed physes or severe disease. It should be noted that average healing time for OCD lesions exceed 12 months, and patients and families should be advised accordingly. After both OCD drilling and OATS, most patients report symptom improvement; however, rates of return to prior level of activity are variable. Complications of surgical interventions include neurovascular injury, donor-site morbidity following OATS, and recurrence of OCD lesions. Although data on long-term outcomes is limited, some papers suggest progression to elbow osteoarthritis despite surgical treatment. Table 12.1 shows a summary of the conditions discussed in this chapter.

Table 12.1 Diagnosis and management of common conditions

Clinical entity	Clinical presentation	Diagnostic testing	Non-operative management	Indications for surgery	Operative management
Olecranon bursitis	– Non-tender fluctuant mass overlying olecranon	– Clinical diagnosis – Needle aspiration if septic bursitis is suspected	– Compressive dressings, avoidance of pressure to area	– Chronic symptomatic bursitis	– Open bursectomy
Tennis elbow (lateral epicondylitis)	– Pain over lateral epicondyle – Pain aggravated by resisted wrist extension and supination	– Clinical diagnosis	– Activity modification – Counterforce brace – Physical therapy for stretching and gradual strengthening	– Failure of improvement with non-op therapy >12 months	– Open debridement of affected tendon origin
Distal biceps tendon rupture	– Pain at antecubital fossa – Pain or weakness with supination and elbow flexion – Positive hook test	– MRI if diagnosis is unclear and to distinguish between complete and partial tears	– Sling immobilization with close follow-up	– Biceps rupture in a patient with high functional demands	– Open tendon repair
Elbow osteoarthritis	– Pain and progressive stiffness of elbow – Evaluate for ulnar neuropathy	– Plain X-rays of elbow – CT elbow if loose bodies are suspected	– NSAIDs – Intra-articular corticosteroid injections – Activity modification	– Symptomatic arthritis affecting quality of life in an older patient with low functional demands	– Surgical debridement – Total elbow arthroplasty

Simple elbow dislocation	– Pain and deformity of the elbow	– X-rays of elbow – CT elbow if subtle coronoid or radial head fractures are suspected	– Closed reduction under sedation and/or intra-articular block – Immobilization in a splint for 1 week, followed by progressive ROM exercises	– Instability postreduction – Associated fractures	– Open reduction and internal fixation of associated fractures and ligament repair as needed
Radial head fracture	– Tenderness to palpation over radial head	– X-rays of elbow, which may show elbow effusion without obvious fracture – CT elbow to evaluate for associated fractures or for preoperative planning	– Immobilization in a sling for comfort for 1 week – Early return to activity to avoid stiffness	– Displaced radial head fracture with mechanical block to pronation or supination – Associated fractures or dislocation	– Open reduction and internal fixation of radial head – Radial head replacement
UCL injury	– Medial-sided elbow pain in a throwing athlete – Medial elbow pain or valgus elbow instability with milking maneuver	– Plain X-rays of elbow – MRI elbow shows partial- and full-thickness UCL tears – Evaluate for ulnar neuropathy	– Period of rest followed by gradual return to sports – Pitching limits for adolescents – Physical therapy for shoulder and elbow, pitching kinematics	– No improvement with non-operative management in a patient committed to intensive postoperative physical therapy	– UCL reconstruction ("Tommy John" surgery)

(continued)

Table 12.1 (continued)

Clinical entity	Clinical presentation	Diagnostic testing	Non-operative management	Indications for surgery	Operative management
Little leaguers' elbow (medial epicondylar apophysitis)	– Medial elbow pain in a young throwing athlete – Tenderness at the medial epicondylar apophysis	– X-rays of elbow – MRI elbow shows increased T2 signal at apophysis, helpful for ruling out other pathologies	– Period of rest followed by gradual return to activity – Physical therapy for flexor-pronator stretching and strengthening – Activity guidelines	– Displaced fracture of medial epicondyle	– Open reduction and internal fixation of displaced medial epicondyle fracture
Elbow OCD	– Lateral elbow pain in a young throwing athlete or gymnast – Tenderness to palpation at the capitellum	– Plain X-rays of elbow – MRI elbow for localizing and staging OCD lesions	– Same as above	– Unstable OCD lesions based on MRI or arthroscopic appearance – Failure of improvement with non-op therapy	– Elbow arthroscopy and drilling of OCD lesions – OATS procedure (osteochondral autogenous transplantation surgery)

CT computed tomography, *MRI* magnetic resonance imaging, *NSAIDS* nonsteroidal anti-inflammatory drugs, *OCD* osteochondritis dissecans, *UCL* ulnar collateral ligament

Summary

In summary, a range of common conditions may affect the upper extremity. We have tried to distinguish between conditions that may appear superficially similar. Most of these evolve slowly; there are many opportunities to make the diagnosis, and conservative measures may often be successful in management. We have tried to show when it may be appropriate to refer for surgery, and what you may tell your patient to expect when that happens.

Suggested Reading

Adams JE, Steinmann SP. Chapter 27: Elbow tendinopathies and tendon ruptures. In: Wolfe SW, Hotchkiss RN, Pederson WC, et al., editors. Green's operative hand surgery. 6th ed. Philadelphia: Elsevier; 2010.

Bruce JR, Andrews JR. Ulnar collateral ligament injuries in the throwing athlete. J Am Assoc Orthop Surg. 2014;22(5):315–25.

Canale ST, Beauty JH. Campbell's operative orthopaedics. 11th ed. Philadelphia: Elsevier; 2007. Chapter 24: Nontraumatic soft-tissue disorders (discussion of bursitis), Chapter 25: Miscellaneous Nontraumatic disorders (discussion of osteoarthritis and rheumatoid arthritis), Chapter 44: Shoulder and Elbow Injuries (discussion of tendinopathies), Chapter 46: Traumatic Disorders (discussion of tendon ruptures)

Chauhan A, Cunningham J, Bhatnagar R, et al. Chapter 62: Elbow diagnosis and decision making. In: Miller MD, Thompson SR, editors. Delee & Drez's orthopedic sports medicine: principles and practice. 4th ed. Philadelphia: Elsevier; 2015. p. 721–9.

Cheung EV, Adams R, Morrey BF. Primary osteoarthritis of the elbow: current treatment options. J Am Assoc Orthop Surg. 2008;16(2):77–87.

Dyer GS, Blazar PE. Rheumatoid Elbow. Hand Clin. 2011;27(1):43–8.

Dyer GS, Jupiter JB. Chapter 22: Complex traumatic elbow dislocation. In: Wolfe SW, Pederson WC, Hotchkiss RN, et al., editors. Green's operative hand surgery. 7th ed. Philadelphia: Elsevier; 2016; (ahead of print).

Stans AA, Heinrich SD. Chapter 16: Dislocations of the elbow. In: Bucholz RW, Heckman JD, Court-Brown C, editors. Rockwood and Wilkins' fractures in children. 6th ed. Philadelphia: Lippincott Williams & Wilkins; 2006. p. 661–701.

Van den Ende KI, Steinmann SP. Arthroscopic treatment of septic arthritis of the elbow. J Shoulder Elb Surg. 2012;21(8):1001–5.

Waters PW, Bae DS. Chapter 41: The thrower's elbow. In: Waters PW, Bae DS, editors. Pediatric hand and upper limb surgery: a practical guide. Philadelphia: Lippincott Williams & Wilkins; 2012. p. 520–36.

Part VIII
Hand

Chapter 13
Hand and Wrist Soft Tissue Conditions

Brandon E. Earp

Introduction

Soft tissue conditions in the hand and wrist are common and may lead to symptoms ranging from minor nuisance to quite severe dysfunction. The wide range of disorders afflicting the tendons, ligaments, and other soft tissues may result from traumatic and atraumatic etiologies. Benign tumors in the hand also arise with frequency in the soft tissue structures of the hand. In this chapter, the most common soft tissue disorders of the hand and wrist (excluding open injuries and skin tumors) are discussed, with a goal of aiding the treating practitioner in the diagnostic and treatment pathways for each (see Table 13.1).

Tendon Conditions of the Hand and Wrist

Trigger Finger (Stenosing Tenosynovitis)

Summary of Epidemiology

Trigger finger, also known as stenosing tenosynovitis, is most often an idiopathic condition that affects the flexor tendons to the digits. It occurs more frequently in patients with rheumatoid arthritis and diabetes mellitus. As the two flexor tendons to each finger [flexor digitorum profundus (FDP) and flexor digitorum superficialis (FDS)] or the single flexor tendon to the thumb [flexor pollicis longus (FPL)] enter the tighter flexor sheath region, the first pulley encountered is called the A1 pulley.

B.E. Earp (✉)
Department of Orthopedic Surgery, Brigham and Women's Faulkner Hospital,
75 Francis Street, Boston, MA 02115, USA
e-mail: bearp@bwh.harvard.org

© Springer International Publishing AG 2018
J.N. Katz et al. (eds.), *Principles of Orthopedic Practice for Primary Care Providers*, https://doi.org/10.1007/978-3-319-68661-5_13

It is typically here, in the palmar region by the metacarpophalangeal joints (MCP), that the pathology occurs. Either the flexor tendon becomes thickened or nodular, the sheath becomes thickened, or both. This leads to a mismatch in size, causing the tendon to get stuck on either side of the pulley, resulting in a "popping" or "triggering" sensation when the finger is flexed or extended. Tenosynovitis can also contribute to triggering in some patients.

Clinical Presentation

Trigger finger typically presents without any associated trauma, although some patients will report onset after heavy gripping or other strenuous hand use. They may describe a "clicking," "popping," or "dislocating" sensation of the finger, which is often worse first thing in the morning. There may also be a tender nodule in the palm near the distal palmar crease of the affected digit. At times, the digit can get stuck in a flexed position ("locked"), and the patient may report having to use the other hand to pull the digit straight. For other patients, the finger may be stuck in extension, and the patient may be quite reluctant or unable to flex the digit into composite flexion due to pain. Patients may complain of discomfort at the PIP joint and may develop PIP contracture with long-standing trigger finger.

Differential Diagnosis and Suggested Diagnostic Testing

Multiple conditions can cause clicking or popping with finger motion. The joints themselves, especially when arthritic, may not move smoothly due to articular incongruity, leading to mechanical symptoms. Extensor tendon snapping due to sagittal band rupture or insufficiency causing central tendon instability dorsally over the metacarpophalangeal joint should also be considered. Trigger finger is typically diagnosed clinically by physician examination and history and does not require further diagnostic workup.

Non-operative Management

Trigger finger can be treated with observation and may resolve without intervention. Oral and topical medications have not been proven effective. Extension splinting, particularly for those patients who only experience triggering first thing in the morning, may be an effective nighttime-only treatment. Full-time extension splinting is not recommended due to concern about resultant joint stiffness. Injection with cortisone is typically the first intervention recommended for treatment of trigger finger. This can be effective when injected either within the tendon sheath or around it. Many would recommend avoiding more than two injections for any given trigger digit due to concern about potential tendon rupture.

Indications for Surgery

Surgical treatment is recommended for patients with symptomatic triggering of their digits who have failed appropriate non-operative treatment options, or in cases of a locked trigger finger (digit is irreducibly "stuck" in a flexed posture).

Operative Management

Surgical treatment involves release of the A1 pulley through a small palmar incision, followed by early motion.

Expected Outcome and Predictors of Outcome

Trigger finger may resolve without invasive intervention. Cortisone injection can be curative in approximately half of patients with a single injection. This rate is lower for patients with rheumatoid arthritis or diabetes. For patients with persistent symptoms, surgical release is a low-morbidity procedure with an excellent rate of success and very low rate of recurrence.

deQuervain's Disease

Summary of Epidemiology

deQuervain's disease, or first dorsal compartment tenosynovitis of the wrist, affects the radial wrist tendons of the abductor pollicis longus (APL) and the extensor pollicis brevis (EPB). deQuervain's seems to be associated with repetitive wrist motions using the thumbs and is found more commonly in women, especially in mothers with infants. The tendon anatomy in this compartment is variable; the APL commonly has several slips of tendon and there is often a subcompartment between the two tendons. These anatomic differences may contribute to the development of symptoms in patients performing repetitive motions, as the increased bulk of the tendons with multiple slips, and the potentially more restricted space (due to a subcompartment), may not allow as much tolerance of thickening or swelling of the tendons and/or tenosynovium.

Clinical Presentation

deQuervain's disease typically presents without any associated trauma, but most patients will report increased activity with their wrists and thumbs in the time preceding symptom onset. Patients often notice pain along the radial side of the wrist near the base of the thumb, often associated with swelling in the region. They have difficulty with activities involving the thumb, including pinching and grasping. At times, there may be a sensation of "catching" of the tendons with certain motions of the thumb. Due to the location of the radial sensory nerve branch, which crosses just superficial to the affected tendons, at times patients will experience radial sensory nerve symptoms including numbness or tingling in the dorsal radial skin of the hand and thumb. On examination, patients typically have tenderness to palpation over the tendons at the radial styloid and also have pain with resisted radial thumb abduction. A Finkelstein test is commonly performed. The patient's thumb is opposed across the palm and the other digits closed around the thumb. The wrist is then ulnarly deviated, which causes discomfort along the tendons in patients with this disorder.

Differential Diagnosis and Suggested Diagnostic Testing

It is important to evaluate the other structures in the area, which may also produce radial wrist and thumb-base pain, including thumb carpometacarpal arthritis. Traumatic conditions such as distal radius and scaphoid fractures may also mimic symptoms. deQuervain's disease is typically diagnosed clinically by physical examination and history and does not require further diagnostic workup. At times the practitioner may obtain radiographs to assess the joints in the area for trauma or arthritis and to evaluate for other local conditions.

Non-operative Management

deQuervain's disease is most often treated non-operatively with the goals of decreasing inflammation and maintaining motion. Immobilization with a splint incorporating the thumb at and distal to the metacarpophalangeal joint is the mainstay of management. Splints may be custom-made or prefabricated and are typically called thumb spica splints or long opponens splints. Therapy may incorporate exercises to maintain motion and enhance tendon gliding in the region. Injection with cortisone into the first dorsal compartment tendon sheath is another common intervention and is particularly helpful in patients with symptoms of shorter duration.

Indications for Surgery

Surgical treatment is recommended for patients with persistent symptoms, which are functionally limiting, despite appropriate non-operative care.

Operative Management

Surgical treatment involves release of the first dorsal compartment tendon sheath through a small radial wrist incision. Care must be taken to protect the superficial radial sensory nerve in the area and to ensure the complete release of all tendon slips and any subcompartments.

Expected Outcome and Predictors of Outcome

deQuervain's disease most commonly resolves without invasive intervention via activity modification, rest, and short-term immobilization. Cortisone injection can be curative. For patients with persistent symptoms, surgical release is a low-morbidity surgery with an excellent rate of success and very low rate of recurrence.

Other Nontraumatic Tendon Disorders: Intersection Syndrome, EPL, ECU, and RA-Related Pathology

Summary of Epidemiology

Any tendon in the hand or wrist can be affected by tenosynovitis or tendinosis. Other areas of pathology which are seen with some frequency include: (1) intersection syndrome, involving the crossing of tendons of the first dorsal compartment [extensor pollicis longus (EPL) and abductor pollicis brevis (EPB)] over the second dorsal compartment [extensor carpi radialis longus and brevis (ECRL and ECRB)] approximately 4 cm proximal to the wrist, resulting in focal irritation; (2) extensor pollicis longus (EPL) irritation as it curves past Lister's tubercle at the distal radius; and (3) extensor carpi ulnaris (ECU) irritation as it passes through a sheath at the level of the distal ulna.

Some tendons are affected by inflammatory conditions such as rheumatoid arthritis (RA) and are prone to invasive tenosynovitis, which can lead to attritional ruptures. The tendons most commonly affected by RA are the flexor pollicis longus (FPL) volarly and the fourth and fifth dorsal compartments [extensor digitorum communis (EDC) and extensor digitorum quinti (EDQ)] dorsally.

Clinical Presentation

The clinical presentation of the non-RA-related tendon disorders is quite similar to that of deQuervain's disease. Patients present with localized pain, focal tenderness, and discomfort with active motion. Intersection syndrome can sometimes present with audible crepitus of the tendons.

The clinical presentation of the RA-related tendon disorders typically presents with swelling along the tendons, which is often painless however may be symptomatic at the extremes of motion. The associated tenosynovitis will often be seen to move with active motion of the tendons. There is typically underlying degenerative joint disease on radiographs. With tendon rupture, the patients will be unable to actively move their digits affected by the injury (e.g., with a rupture of the finger extensor tendon to digit 5, the patient will be unable to actively extend the small finger at the MP joint).

Differential Diagnosis and Suggested Diagnostic Testing

It is always important to assess the underlying joints for arthritis, fracture, or other pathology. Radiographs are commonly performed to assess for underlying joint pathology, which may be related to the tendon issue. At times, ultrasound or MRI may be of utility.

Non-operative Management

Non-inflammatory tendon disorders are most often treated non-operatively. Typically this involves immobilization of the affected structures with splinting and progressive return of motion and function via occupational therapy (OT). Injection with cortisone may be performed for some tendon disorders, but the practitioner should be aware that tendon rupture can occur after injection for some tendon conditions (particularly involving the EPL), and primary surgical treatment may be a safer choice. Management of RA-related tendon disorders is typically via medical management of the underlying disease process, with surgical intervention reserved for failure of that treatment.

Indications for Surgery

Failure of conservative treatment of tendon disorders, including medical management of RA-related conditions is an indication for surgery.

Operative Management

Operative management typically involves freeing the tendons of any constrictive sheaths, debriding areas of tenosynovitis, possibly transposing the tendon(s) to a new position in order to avoid tension or friction (particularly helpful for the EPL), and potentially addressing underlying joint pathology, such as in cases of RA-related distal radioulnar joint (DRUJ) involvement.

Expected Outcome and Predictors of Outcome

Most tendon disorders resolve without invasive intervention via activity modification, rest, and short-term immobilization. Medical management of underlying disease can be definitive treatment. Cortisone injection can be a valuable tool, but the practitioner should exercise caution as some tendons may be predisposed to rupture after injection. For patients with persistent symptoms, surgical release, tenosynovectomy, and surgically addressing any underlying pathology are an excellent and appropriate choice to alleviate symptoms and minimize future risks of tendon rupture.

Traumatic Tendon Ruptures

Summary of Epidemiology

Trauma can lead to rupture of tendons, often at their distal insertions. The two most common are mallet finger (terminal extensor tendon rupture) and jersey finger (flexor digitorum profundus (FDP) rupture). A mallet injury can occur on any finger and typically is related to a sudden impact to the digit. A jersey finger occurs most commonly in the ring finger and can occur when the flexed digit gets caught on an opponent's jersey and suddenly pulled into extension.

Clinical Presentation

With a mallet finger, the patient is unable to extend at the distal interphalangeal (DIP) joint of the finger and reports that the fingertip "droops" (Fig. 13.1). It can be extended passively, but the patient cannot maintain this passive extension unassisted. If the patient has laxity of their joints, they may notice a "swan-neck deformity" as the unopposed pull of the distally ruptured extensor leads to hyperextension at the PIP joint with volar plate laxity.

With a jersey finger (FDP rupture), the patient is unable to flex at the DIP joint of the finger and therefore cannot tuck the digit into full flexion actively when

Fig. 13.1 With a mallet finger, the patient is unable to extend at the distal interphalangeal (DIP) joint of the finger and reports that the fingertip "droops"

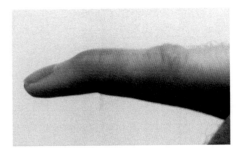

attempting to make a tight fist. The DIP joint can be passively flexed. The patient will be able to actively flex at the PIP joint due to an intact flexor digitorum superficialis (FDS) tendon.

Differential Diagnosis and Suggested Diagnostic Testing

The differential diagnosis for these injuries includes traumatic fracture and dislocation. In theory, nerve palsy could also present as weakness with certain attempted movements, and a thorough neurologic examination of the hand should always be performed. It would be exceptionally rare to have an isolated digital tendon affected due to nerve injury; however, it is important to ensure that no other weakness exists that has not yet noticed [e.g., a weak FDP to the index could be related to an anterior interosseous nerve palsy, and one would expected to also see weakness of flexor pollicis longus (FPL)].

Radiographs are typically performed to assess the underlying phalanges and articulations for fractures and/or joint incongruity. Both mallet and FDP injuries can occur in conjunction with fractures; thus, imaging is an important part of the assessment.

Non-operative Management

Mallet injuries are typically treated non-operatively with full-time (24-7) splinting or finger casting in extension for at least 6 weeks continuously. The PIP joint should be allowed motion to avoid later stiffness. Mallet injuries with fracture are also typically treated non-operatively unless the joint is incongruent due to subluxation. Patient compliance with full-time extension splinting can be challenging.

FDP ruptures are important to recognize early (within the 1st week) and are nearly always treated with surgery to reattach the tendon. At times, late presentation or patient characteristics may lead to a choice of non-operative treatment.

Indications for Surgery

Indications for surgical treatment of a mallet injury include joint subluxation and can also be considered in cases wherein a patient has an inability to comply with non-operative care. In cases of FDP rupture, surgery is the treatment of choice in nearly every patient who presents acutely. With a delay in presentation and dependent on how retracted the tendon is, the tendon may not be reparable, and the decision for or against surgical reconstruction is based on the particular patient and surgeon.

Operative Management

Operative management of a mallet finger may involve isolated extension pinning of the DIP joint or open repair of the tendon to its insertion. Both are followed by maintenance of extension and later motion. Operative treatment of an FDP rupture involves repairing the FDP tendon to its distal insertion site, most often followed by an early motion flexor tendon protocol.

Expected Outcome and Predictors of Outcome

Mallet injuries are nearly always treatable non-operatively and yield acceptable results. Many patients will ultimately have an improved extensor lag (i.e., less "droop"); however, they will regain full active extension. Most do not find this functionally limiting. FDP ruptures are typically treated early with surgery, followed by OT and an early motion therapy protocol. There are risks of re-rupture, and tendon adhesions may limit active motion. A second surgery to address adhesions can be performed if indicated.

Benign Masses of the Hand and Wrist

Ganglions

Summary of Epidemiology

Ganglion cysts are benign masses that can arise from any joint or tendon sheath. They are attached to the joint by a pedicle or stalk and are filled with gelatinous fluid that is much thicker than typical joint fluid and primarily composed of hyaluronic acid. The etiology of ganglion cysts is controversial.

Clinical Presentation

Patients present with a mass that is firm and feels tethered to the underlying tissue. Cysts can be singular or multi-lobulated. In the wrist, the two most common locations are the dorsal scapholunate region and the volar radial wrist near the radial artery. In the digits, the two most common cysts are volar retinacular cysts (cysts of tendon sheath) which are found near the bases of the fingers by the A1 and A2 pulley regions, and mucous cysts, which are found dorsally over the DIP joints.

Ganglion cysts are typically asymptomatic or mildly symptomatic but may create symptoms if they restrict motion. Mucous cysts may lead to nail plate changes due to their location near the germinal matrix of the nail (Fig. 13.2).

Fig. 13.2 Ganglion

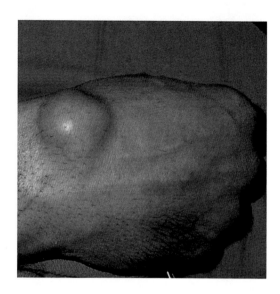

Differential Diagnosis and Suggested Diagnostic Testing

The differential diagnosis for cysts includes other common masses in the hand, such as hemangiomas, giant cell tumors, glomus tumors, nerve sheath tumors, and lipomas. Typically these can be distinguished clinically by an experienced practitioner. Radiographic evaluation is rarely necessary for diagnosis but may be used to assess for other underlying joint conditions. With a clinical concern for an occult wrist ganglion, an MRI may be indicated. For cysts in superficial locations, it is noted that they transilluminate, which can prove helpful for identifying cystic versus solid mass-like structures.

Non-operative Management

Most cysts can be treated non-operatively as they are neither dangerous nor particularly symptomatic, and it has been suggested in the literature that half will spontaneously resolve. For those that do not resolve or are symptomatic, aspiration of the cyst is highly successful at short-term alleviation of the mass and confirmation of the diagnosis due to the pathognomonic clear gelatinous fluid obtained. This said, the patient must understand that recurrence after aspiration is more likely than not. Patients may mention techniques of closed rupture of the cyst by "hitting it with a large book"; however, this is not recommended.

Indications for Surgery

Surgery is indicated for patients with ganglion cysts who are symptomatic and have not responded to or are not appropriate for an aspiration.

Operative Management

Surgical excision involves removal of the cyst, its stalk, and a small portion of the surrounding capsular (or tendon sheath) tissue. Careful dissection and avoidance of injury to nearby neurovascular and tendon structures are important.

Expected Outcomes

Postoperatively, recurrence rates for focal ganglion cysts are reported at approximately 5%.

Other Benign Soft Tissue Masses of the Hand and Wrist: Hemangiomas, Giant Cell Tumors, Glomus Tumors, Nerve Sheath Tumors, and Lipomas

Definition and Epidemiology

Benign tumors or masses of the hand and wrist are common, and appropriate recognition will often allow for diagnosis without biopsy and treatment with observation. Lesions with a rapid change in size, appearance, or symptoms warrant further evaluation and possible treatment.

The most common benign tumors of the hand and wrist, excluding ganglions, are hemangiomas (vascular masses), giant cell tumors of tendon sheath (histologically similar to pigmented villonodular synovitis), glomus tumors (arising from a glomus body, often in the periungal region of the fingertip), nerve sheath tumors including neurofibromas and schwannomas, and lipomas (fatty tumors).

Clinical Presentation

Most patients with benign hand and wrist tumors present with the discovery of a mass. Hemangiomas are often reddish or purplish in color and compressible. Giant cell tumors are typically nontender masses along the flexor tendons. Glomus tumors may demonstrate a bluish subungual mass, however also may be not visible and instead present with cold hypersensitivity and disproportionate focal finger pain. Nerve sheath tumors will often present with neurologic symptoms and demonstrate a positive Tinel's with percussion. Lipomas are soft, well-circumscribed lesions that typically present as subcutaneous masses.

Differential Diagnosis and Suggested Diagnostic Testing

The differential diagnosis includes the other masses found in the hand as well as masses related to systemic disease, such as gouty tophus, RA nodules, and xanthomas. Malignant hand tumors are rare; the most common malignancies are attributable to skin cancers followed by metastatic tumors and quite rarely primary soft tissue malignancy such as epithelioid sarcoma. Diagnostic testing may include radiographs. MRI may is not commonly indicated but should be used if uncertainty exists. Specific to glomus tumors, MRI can be helpful when a high degree of clinical suspicion exists, but no definite mass is noted clinically.

Non-operative Management

Observation is appropriate for many benign tumors of the hand and wrist which are not particularly symptomatic. Routine scheduled follow-up is common, with an understanding that the patient should call to be seen if there are changes in appearance, size, or degree of pain.

Indications for Surgical Management

Surgery is indicated for symptomatic masses or masses with features concerning for aggressive or malignant lesions.

Operative Management

Surgery typically involves an excisional biopsy. Minimizing the morbidity of the surgery is important. Nerve tumors may have unavoidable postoperative nerve deficits, and patients must be made aware of this prior to intervention. Glomus tumor surgery may lead to nail plate changes due to the often subungual location of these masses. Giant cell tumors have a high rate of recurrence, and thus adjuvant therapy may also be indicated.

Expected Outcome and Predictors of Outcome

Outcomes from treatment of benign lesions and recurrence after surgery depend on the type of lesion, the location, size, and surgery performed.

Dupuytren's Disease

Summary of Epidemiology

Dupuytren's disease is a fibroproliferative condition of the palmar fascia. It is benign, typically painless, and variably progressive. There is a genetic basis for Dupuytren's, as the condition is commonly associated with patients of northern European descent and is also found more commonly in patients with diabetes mellitus. Eighty percent of patients are men, and most patients present after the age of 50. Some patients will have associated fibromatoses, including Peyronie's disease (fibromatosis of the penis) and Ledderhose disease (plantar fibromatosis). The myofibroblast is the affected cell, and histologically, the nodules are comprised of Type III collagen.

Clinical Presentation

The typical patient presents with nodularity noted in the palm in the line of the ring and/or small fingers. There may be "pitting" or dimpling of the skin in the area. Over time, the nodule(s) can form longitudinal cords which lead to contracture of the metacarpophalangeal (MP) and/or proximal interphalangeal (PIP) joints (Fig. 13.3). At times, patients will also present with soft tissue thickenings over the

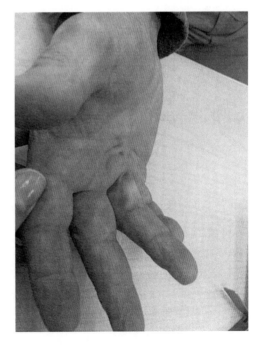

Fig. 13.3 Dupuytren's disease. The typical patient presents with nodularity noted in the palm in the line of the ring and/or small fingers. There may be "pitting" or dimpling of the skin in the area. Over time, the nodule(s) can form longitudinal cords which lead to contracture of the metacarpophalangeal (MP) and/or proximal interphalangeal (PIP) joints

dorsum of their PIP joints, called "knuckle pads." The nodules and cords are typically painless, although can be mildly tender.

Differential Diagnosis and Suggested Diagnostic Testing

The differential diagnosis of Dupuytren's disease includes other conditions causing joint contracture (arthritis, prior trauma, camptodactyly, and palmar fibromatosis, the latter of which affected all digits of both hands and can be associated with a malignancy) and other conditions causing palmar nodules. Dupuytren's disease is a clinical diagnosis and does not require further imaging or testing.

Non-operative Management

There is no data to suggest that splinting, stretching, and exercises will prevent progression of disease. Cortisone injection is not shown to affect Dupuytren's cords. There are two procedurally based non-operative treatments for Dupuytren's contractures. The first is needle aponeurotomy, which is a mechanical fasciotomy, and the second is collagenase injection/manipulation, which is a chemical fasciotomy. Both can be performed in an office-based setting and serve to disrupt the Dupuytren's cord and allow manipulation of the digit to alleviate the contracture.

Indications for Surgery

Surgery is indicated to address the contracture associated with Dupuytren's disease. There is not an exact amount of contracture that constitutes the threshold for surgical treatment, although most agree that functional impairment with greater than 30 degrees of MP joint contracture or greater than 20 degrees of PIP contracture is an indication for treatment. The type of surgery or percutaneous approach depends on the patient and surgeon preferences.

Operative Management

Surgery involves excision of the Dupuytren's cords, which is called a fasciectomy. The overlying skin may also be excised. Occasionally skin grafts are indicated, or intentional open wounds are left to heal secondarily. Joint contractures are commonly addressed simply by removing the diseased tissue, but with more advanced contractures, releases of the contracted tendon sheath or joint may be performed.

Expected Outcomes

Treatment with either percutaneous approaches (needle aponeurotomy and collagenase injection) or surgery is quite effective at improving contractures. Patients must understand that recurrence occurs after all of these treatments, and full correction of contracture may not be possible, especially with long-standing or more severe PIP joint involvement.

Soft Tissue Injuries of Wrist Joint

Scapholunate Ligament Injury

Please see chapter on "Osteoarthritis of the Hand and Wrist."

Triangular Fibrocartilage Complex (TFCC) Injury

Summary of Epidemiology

The TFCC is a localized group of soft tissue structures including cartilage and ligaments on the ulnar side of the wrist, which serves to stabilize the distal radioulnar joint (DRUJ) and the ulnar carpus. The structures comprising the TFCC include the articular disk, the meniscal homologue, the volar and dorsal radioulnar ligaments, the extensor carpi ulnaris sub-sheath, the ulnar capsule, and the ulnocarpal ligaments. Combined, these form a trampoline-like structure which extends from the distal radius to the distal ulna to the ulnar carpus, supporting the surrounding articulations. The central portion of the TFCC is avascular which leads to limited healing potential of injuries to that area. The edges of this triangular structure are perfused via their attachments, making repair possible at the periphery.

Two types of TFCC pathology exist. The first is related to a traumatic injury. These are more commonly seen in an athletic population but can also be associated with falls or injury related to manual labor. The second type is degenerative in nature. The TFCC thins with age and half of people over age 60 will have degenerative perforations of the articular disk.

Clinical Presentation

Patients with symptomatic TFCC pathology present with complaints of ulnar-sided wrist pain, often associated with clicking. Traumatic-type injuries are frequently related to a specific event leading to symptom onset. Degenerative-type injuries may be related to repetitive pulling or twisting motions, and those patients may recall a remote history of wrist injury. Symptoms typically improve with rest and are exacerbated by twisting, pushing, pulling, or lifting activities.

Common exam findings for patients with TFCC pathology include reduced grip strength, tenderness in the ulnar fovea (soft spot just distal and volar to the ulnar styloid), a click or pop with motion of the wrist, and pain with combined ulnar deviation and extension of the wrist.

Differential Diagnosis and Suggested Diagnostic Testing

There are many causes of ulnar wrist pain, which need to be distinguished from a TFCC injury. These include fractures, joint injuries or other conditions, tendon disorders, and nerve-related pain. Bony injuries may include ulnar styloid, hamate, pisiform, and metacarpal-base fractures. Joint conditions can be related to lunotriquetral ligament tear, DRUJ instability, Kienbock's disease, Madelung deformity, DRUJ arthritis, or midcarpal instability. Tendonitis can be seen in both the extensor carpi ulnaris and the flexor carpi ulnaris, both of which are localized to this region. Nerve-related pain can be caused by Guyon's canal syndrome.

Diagnostic testing should first include radiographs. Patients with ulnar positive variance on the PA view (the ulna is "longer" than the radius), whether occurring by native anatomic difference or post-traumatic malunion, are at higher risk for TFCC pathology (Fig. 13.4). The films can also evaluate for other bone/joint conditions,

Fig. 13.4 Triangular fibrocartilage complex: Patients with ulnar positive variance on the PA view (the ulna is "longer" than the radius), whether occurring by native anatomic difference or post-traumatic malunion, are at higher risk for TFCC pathology

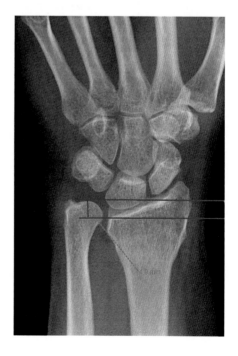

Table 13.2 Palmer classification for TFCC abnormalities

Class 1—traumatic injury
(a) Central perforation
(b) Ulnar avulsion—may involve the proximal or distal lamina (foveal or styloid attachment, respectively) or both
(c) Distal avulsion
(d) Radial avulsion
Class 2—degenerative injury
(a) TFCC wear
(b) TFCC wear with lunate and/or ulnar chondromalacia
(c) TFCC perforation with lunate and/or ulnar chondromalacia
(d) TFCC perforation with lunate and/or ulnar chondromalacia and lunotriquetral ligament perforation
(e) TFCC perforation with lunate and/or ulnar chondromalacia, lunotriquetral ligament perforation, and ulnocarpal arthritis

TFCC triangular fibrocartilage complex

such as fractures, congenital differences, and arthritis. MRI is also helpful to visualize TFCC pathology. The addition of an arthrogram to the MRI may increase both the sensitivity and specificity of the study by demonstrating the passage of dye through small perforations in the TFCC. The Palmer classification is used to stratify patients with TFCC pathology (Table 13.2).

Non-operative Management

The goals of non-operative treatment of TFCC pathology include decreasing swelling and pain, which can be accomplished by immobilization for 3–6 weeks, icing, and NSAIDs as needed. During this time, the unaffected joints of the arm and hand should be kept moving to minimize stiffness and functional loss. After this initial period, rehabilitation aims to restore motion and then strength to return the patient to function.

Indications for Surgical Management

Surgery is indicated for patients who have persistent, functionally limiting symptoms despite non-operative management or for those with an acute and unstable DRUJ injury.

Fig. 13.5 Triangular
fibrocartilage complex:
Operative management
may include arthroscopic
debridement or repair

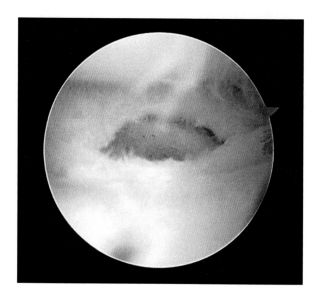

Operative Management

Operative decision-making is guided by the history, physical exam, and imaging
studies. This may include arthroscopic debridement or repair (Fig. 13.5), open
repair, and various forms of ulnar shortening, such as wafer excision or osteotomy.
The decision of whether to debride or repair is based on the location of the pathology. Due to the avascularity of the majority of the TFCC, tears in the central region
cannot heal and are treated with debridement. Peripheral tears have healing potential and should be reattached to the surrounding tissue. Ulnar shortening is performed if ulnocarpal impaction is leading to symptoms, thereby alleviating the
abutment of the distal ulna on the carpus.

Expected Outcomes

Non-operative treatment is successful at achieving symptom improvement in most
patients with ulnar wrist pain, including those with TFCC pathology. Arthroscopic
debridement of central TFCC tears can achieve full symptom resolution despite the
altered anatomy. Treatment of peripheral TFCC tears with arthroscopic or open
repair leads to symptomatic improvement in most patients, with variable rates of
success depending on the location of the tear. Ulnar shortening osteotomy or wafer
resections for ulnar positive variance also lead to alleviation of pain in the vast
majority of patients.

Table 13.1 Hand and wrist soft tissue conditions: diagnosis and management

Clinical entity	Presentation	Diagnostic testing	Conservative management	Surgical indications and operative management
Trigger finger (stenosing tenosynovitis)	– Insidious or acute onset of catching or clicking of the finger with motion – Tender to palpation (TTP) in the palm at the distal palmar crease of the affected digit – Pain with motion (may lead to decreased motion and even flexion contracture of the PIP joint)	– Primarily a clinical diagnosis – Imaging is not typically performed	– With early symptoms consider rest, ice, night extension splinting for morning-only symptoms – If persists consider cortisone injection	– Surgery indicated for persistent symptoms despite conservative treatment – Release of the A1 pulley is curative
deQuervain's disease	– Insidious or acute onset of pain at the radial wrist with thumb/wrist motion – Tender to palpation (TTP) over the first dorsal compartment tendons at the radial styloid – Pain with motion of the thumb (Finkelstein test, pain with resisted radial thumb abduction)	– Primarily a clinical diagnosis – X-ray—may be used to evaluate for other pathology in the area—fractures, CMC arthritis	– In acute phase consider rest, ice, NSAIDs, splinting (thumb spica or long opponens) – OT focused on motion/tendon glide/modalities – In persistent cases cortisone injection	– Surgery indicated for persistent symptoms despite conservative treatment – Release of the first dorsal compartment tendon sheath (and any subcompartments) is curative

(continued)

Table 13.1 (continued)

Clinical entity	Presentation	Diagnostic testing	Conservative management	Surgical indications and operative management
Other nontraumatic tendon disorders (intersection syndrome, EPL, ECU, and RA related)	– Insidious or acute onset of pain with or without swelling along the tendon sheath – Tender to palpation over the involved tendon(s) – Pain with active movement of the involved tendon(s) – Tenosynovitis may move with active motion of tendons – RA-related conditions may be painless; ruptures will lack active motion of involved tendon(s) – Intersection syndrome may have audible crepitus	– Primarily a clinical diagnosis – X-ray—may be used to assess for underlying joint pathology	– Acutely, treat with rest, ice, NSAIDs, immobilization – Corticosteroid injection can be used but be aware that rupture can occur after injection for some conditions (notably EPL) – For RA-related conditions, medical management of RA is indicated	– Surgery indicated for failure of non-operative treatment – May involve release of tendon sheath, tenosynovectomy, and tendon transposition – For RA-related conditions, surgery may need to address the underlying joint and tendon grafting or transfers may be indicated for ruptures
Mallet finger	– Usually acute onset – Frequently related to a direct impact to the digit, although many will report seemingly mild "impacts" – Extensor lag (inability to extend the DIP joint)	– Radiographs are commonly obtained to evaluate for associated fracture of the dorsal base of the distal phalanx and volar subluxation of the DIP joint	– Non-operative treatment is most common with full-time maintenance of extension at the DIP for 6 weeks (either splinting or finger casting can be used) – The PIP must be kept mobile during this time to avoid functional deficits – Six weeks of night splinting is often performed after the initial 6 weeks of full-time extension splinting	– Surgery is indicated for failure of non-operative treatment or inability to tolerate non-operative treatment – May involve extension pinning or open repair of the terminal extensor tendon to its insertion

FDP rupture (jersey finger)	– Usually acute onset		– Radiographs are commonly obtained to evaluate for associated fracture of the volar base of the distal phalanx and dorsal subluxation of the DIP joint	– Non-operative treatment is not indicated for an acute jersey finger	– Surgery involves repair of the FDP tendon to its distal insertion, followed by an early motion flexor tendon protocol
		– Most common in ring finger	– Fracture fragments that have retracted proximally may give clues as to the location of the tendon stump, although clinical examination is also required	– For chronic conditions, late presentation, or due to patient factors, non-operative treatment may be appropriate	
		– Occurs when digit tip gets caught and there is a sudden extension force against the flexed digit			
		– Inability to flex the DIP joint			
		– May be tender in the palm, depending on the degree of proximal retraction of the torn tendon stump			
Benign masses	– May present with painful or painless mass of the wrist, hand, or digit		– Radiographs are commonly performed to assess associated bones and joints for pathology	– Non-operative care with observation may be appropriate for asymptomatic classic-appearing masses	– Surgical excisional biopsy is performed for both diagnosis and treatment when appropriate
			– MRI rarely necessary but may be indicated for atypical presentations or especially to evaluate for glomus tumors	– Routine instructions to call re-changes in size, symptoms, or appearance are required.	– Type of biopsy, recurrence rate, and follow-up is dependent on the type of tumor, location, and patient characteristics
				– Aspiration can be performed for cystic masses for both diagnostic and therapeutic purposes	

(continued)

Table 13.1 (continued)

Clinical entity	Presentation	Diagnostic testing	Conservative management	Surgical indications and operative management
Dupuytren's disease	– Typically painless insidious onset – Often begins with palmar nodules that progress to cords and lead to digital contractures – Skin pitting and knuckle pads may also be seen Most commonly affects ring and small fingers	– This is a clinical diagnosis and no further testing is needed – Radiographs may be appropriate to evaluate associated joints for arthritic change	– Observation can be appropriate for isolated palmar nodules or small MP contractures that are not functionally limiting – Non-operative procedures include needle aponeurotomy to mechanical cleave the cord and alleviate the contracture, and collagenase injection/manipulation which chemically cleaves the cord	– Surgical excision of the Dupuytren cord (fasciectomy) with or without joint release may be performed to address contractures – Decision-making is based on the patient's condition and patient and surgeon preference
Triangular fibrocartilage complex (TFCC) injury	– Can be related to either acute trauma or degenerative change – Tender in the ulnar fovea – Pain may be elicited with combined ulnar deviation and extension of the wrist	– Radiographs are obtained to assess the ulnar variance – MRI +/– arthrogram may allow visualization of TFCC and other soft tissue pathology – Be aware that 50% of patients over 60 will have TFCC degenerative perorations and these are commonly asymptomatic	– Rest, ice, NSAIDs, and immobilization are appropriate for most patients without DRUJ instability	– Surgical treatment may involve debridement or repair of the TFCC tear, depending on whether it occurred in the avascular central region or along the vascularized periphery – Ulnar shortening procedures may be indicated for ulnar positive variance

Summary

In conclusion, hand and wrist soft tissue conditions are varied and extremely common. Accurate diagnosis can lead to appropriate and successful management for most of these conditions. Both the pathologic condition and various patient factors may influence decision-making and the likelihood for successful treatment.

Suggested Reading

Aggarwal R et al. Dupuytren's contracture. Up to Date; 2016.
Gude W, et al. Ganglion cysts of the wrist: pathophysiology, clinical picture, and management. Curr Rev Musculoskelet Med. 2008;1(3–4):205–11.
McAuliffe J. Tendon disorders of the hand and wrist. J Hand Surg Am. 2010;35A:846–53.
Payne E, et al. Benign bony and soft tissue tumors of the hand. J Hand Surg Am. 2010;35A:1901–10.
Pidgeon TS, Waryasz G, Carnevale J, DaSilva MF. Triangular fibrocartilage complex: an anatomic review. JBJS Rev. 2015;3(1).

Chapter 14
Hand and Wrist Osteoarthritis

Beverlie L. Ting and Barry P. Simmons

Abbreviations

CMC	Carpometacarpal joint
CPPD	Calcium pyrophosphate deposition disease
DIP	Distal interphalangeal joint
MCP	Metacarpophalangeal joint
MRI	Magnetic resonance imaging
NSAID	Nonsteroidal anti-inflammatory
PA	Posteroanterior
PIP	Proximal interphalangeal joint
SLAC	Scapholunate advanced collapse
SNAC	Scaphoid nonunion advanced collapse
STT	Scaphotrapeziotrapezoid

Introduction

Osteoarthritis is a degenerative disease of articular cartilage and can be considered either primary, wherein genetic predisposition may play a role, or secondary, in the setting of prior trauma, infection, or other identifiable events. In general, osteoarthritis is characterized by joint space narrowing, osteophyte formation, subchondral sclerosis, and cyst formation seen on plain radiographs.

The prevalence of primary osteoarthritis of the hand and wrist increases with age and is more common in women with the exception of MCP joint and wrist

B.L. Ting
Seattle Hand Surgery Group, Seattle, WA, USA
e-mail: bting@seattlehand.com

B.P. Simmons (✉)
Hand and Upper Extremity Service, Department of Orthopedic Surgery, Brigham and Women's Hospital, 75 Francis Street, Boston, MA 02115, USA
e-mail: bsimmons@partners.org

© Springer International Publishing AG 2018   231
J.N. Katz et al. (eds.), *Principles of Orthopedic Practice for Primary Care Providers*, https://doi.org/10.1007/978-3-319-68661-5_14

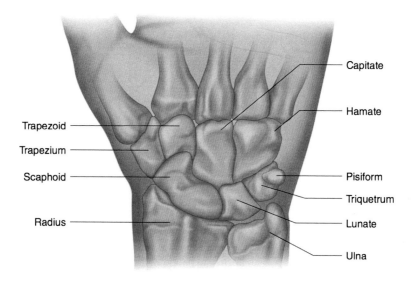

Fig. 14.1 Anatomy of the wrist joints. There are eight carpal bones, which form the radiocarpal, midcarpal, and carpometacarpal joints of the wrist

osteoarthritis. In the hand, the most common joints affected by osteoarthritis include the distal interphalangeal joint (DIP), followed by the thumb carpometacarpal joint (CMC), the proximal interphalangeal joint (PIP), and finally the metacarpophalangeal joint (MCP).

Post-traumatic Wrist Osteoarthritis: Scapholunate Advanced Collapse (SLAC) and Scaphoid Nonunion Advanced Collapse (SNAC)

The wrist is a complex arrangement of eight carpal bones that work in concert to facilitate motion in multiple planes (Fig. 14.1). Generally speaking, these carpal bones are divided into two distinct rows. The proximal row of carpal bones is comprised of the scaphoid, lunate, triquetrum, and pisiform. This proximal row articulates with the distal aspect of the forearm bones, the radius and the ulna, to form the radiocarpal joint and the ulnocarpal joint. The distal row of carpal bones is comprised of the trapezium, trapezoid, capitate, and hamate. This distal row articulates with the metacarpal bones to form the carpometacarpal joints. The interval between these two rows is referred to as the midcarpal joint. The scaphoid bone spans both rows and acts as a bridge between the proximal and distal carpal rows.

Primary osteoarthritis of the wrist is uncommon; however, secondary osteoarthritis due to trauma or vascular disease is more prevalent. The overall reported prevalence of wrist osteoarthritis is 1%, with a slight male predominance.

Fractures of the carpal bones or disruptions of the ligaments that stabilize the carpal bones and allow them to move in a coordinated fashion result in altered wrist kinematics and associated degenerative changes. Specifically, patients diagnosed with chronic scaphoid fracture nonunion or scapholunate ligament injuries are at risk of developing a characteristic pattern of wrist arthritis, known as scaphoid nonunion advanced collapse (SNAC) and scapholunate advanced collapse (SLAC), respectively. Vascular insufficiency to the lunate bone, known as Kienböck disease, can also result in degenerative changes of the wrist.

Summary of Epidemiology

In normal wrist motion, the scaphoid bone flexes with wrist flexion/radial deviation and extends with wrist extension/ulnar deviation. The scapholunate ligament stabilizes the joint between the scaphoid and the lunate, and disruption of this ligament leads to an abnormal movement pattern in which the scaphoid flexes while the lunate extends during wrist motion. These altered mechanics lead to an abnormal distribution of forces across the radiocarpal and midcarpal joints, with resultant wrist osteoarthritis known as scapholunate advanced collapse (SLAC). Acute injuries of the scapholunate ligament are distinct from degenerative tears which can be seen in >50% of patients over 80 years of age.

Scaphoid fractures are inherently at a high risk of nonunion due to the tenuous retrograde blood supply of the scaphoid bone. The more proximal the fracture location, the higher the risk for nonunion. The scaphoid bone bridges the proximal and distal carpal rows; thus, scaphoid fracture nonunion disrupts the synchronous movement of the carpal bones during wrist motion. Over time, degenerative changes of the wrist joint occur, referred to as scaphoid nonunion advanced collapse (SNAC).

Clinical Presentation

Scapholunate ligament injuries occur following a sudden impact to the hand and wrist. The most common mechanism is a fall onto an outstretched wrist. Acute scapholunate ligament injuries typically present as dorsal, radial-sided wrist pain with associated decreased grip and pinch strength. Patients will often report difficulty with wrist extension. More specifically, patients will report that their symptoms are exacerbated with "push-off" activities, which require loading across an extended wrist. They may also report clicking or catching across the wrist due to abnormal translation of the scaphoid.

On physical exam, there may be a joint effusion with swelling seen over the dorsal aspect of the wrist. Wrist extension will typically cause increased pain. Palpation over the scapholunate interval, which is located distal to Lister's tubercle, elicits tenderness. The scaphoid shift test is a provocative test used to detect instability of the scapholunate ligament. Dorsally directed pressure is applied over the volar aspect of the scaphoid while the wrist is brought from ulnar deviation to radial deviation. Dorsal wrist pain while performing this maneuver reflects abnormal dorsal subluxation of the scaphoid due to loss of scapholunate ligament stabilization. A clunk can sometimes be appreciated when the dorsally directed pressure is released and reflects relocation of the scaphoid into the scaphoid fossa. In chronic injuries, the scaphoid shift test will no longer be positive as advanced arthritic changes stabilize the scaphoid, and wrist stiffness prevails. Patients may have tenderness at the radioscaphoid joint.

In cases of scaphoid fracture, patients typically report a remote history of a fall onto an outstretched wrist. SNAC presents with weakness with grip and pinch as well as joint stiffness, particularly with wrist extension and radial deviation. There may also be localized tenderness about the radioscaphoid articulation.

Differential Diagnosis and Suggested Diagnostic Testing

The diagnosis of acute scapholunate ligament injury is based on physical exam and imaging. Other causes of dorsal-sided wrist pain include wrist sprain, dorsal wrist ganglion cyst, extensor tenosynovitis, and intersection syndrome. Intersection syndrome is inflammation in the region where the extensor tendons cross, commonly localized 5 cm proximal to the wrist joint, and is associated with repetitive wrist extension.

Acute scapholunate ligament injury is initially evaluated with posteroanterior (PA) and lateral radiographs of the wrist. A clenched fist view is a stress view that may reveal diastasis between the scaphoid and lunate bones, which may not be appreciated on static views. Magnetic resonance imaging (MRI) can also be used to evaluate for scapholunate injuries but must be evaluated carefully due to the high sensitivity but low specificity for this type of pathology. Wrist arthroscopy is the gold standard to diagnose and appropriately grade the severity of a scapholunate ligament injury.

Advanced arthritic changes associated with chronic scapholunate injury are best evaluated on PA and lateral radiographs (Fig. 14.2). On PA radiographs, widening of greater than 3 mm is seen between the scaphoid and lunate. The severity of arthritic changes seen in SLAC is classified from Stage I to Stage III. In Stage I disease, there is narrowing of the joint space between the radial styloid and the scaphoid. In Stage II disease, arthritic changes have progressed to involve the entire scaphoid fossa, such that narrowing is seen between the scaphoid and the entire

Fig. 14.2 Plain radiograph of Stage III SLAC wrist with sclerosis and joint space narrowing of the radioscaphoid joint and lunocapitate articulation

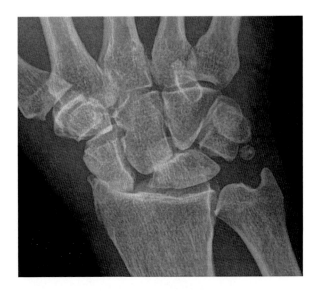

scaphoid fossa. Finally, in Stage III disease, sclerosis and joint space narrowing is also seen between the lunate and capitate and proximal migration of the capitate into the widened scapholunate interval ensues. There may also be localized tenderness about the radioscaphoid articulation.

In cases of SNAC wrist, it should be noted that radial-sided wrist pain can also be caused by deQuervain's tenosynovitis or adjacent base of thumb carpometacarpal osteoarthritis. SNAC can be diagnosed based on plain PA and lateral radiographs of the wrist. Radiographic changes seen in SNAC progress in a similar fashion as described for SLAC. In Stage I disease, there is joint space narrowing and sclerosis involving the radial styloid and scaphoid. In Stage II disease, degenerative changes are seen at the scaphocapitate articulation. Finally, in Stage III disease, periscaphoid degenerative changes are seen.

Non-operative Management

Treatment decisions for post-traumatic wrist arthritis are based mainly on symptom severity. Non-operative management is indicated as the first-line treatment in the majority of symptomatic patients. Non-operative management includes a trial of nonsteroidal anti-inflammatory (NSAID) medications, immobilization with a removable wrist brace or cast, and activity modification. A corticosteroid injection can also provide significant symptomatic relief.

Indications for Surgery

Surgical options may be considered in patients who continue to have debilitating symptoms despite an adequate trial of non-operative management.

Operative Management

The most appropriate surgical intervention for post-traumatic wrist osteoarthritis depends on the severity of arthritic changes. In early Stage I disease, open or arthroscopic approaches can be used to perform a radial styloidectomy to prevent impingement between the scaphoid and radial styloid. In select patients who have a symptomatic SNAC wrist, with minimal arthritic change, excision of the distal non-united scaphoid fragment can be considered.

In more advanced Stage II disease, there are two different techniques that eliminate the painful radioscaphoid articulation, while preserving motion through the wrist joint. A proximal row carpectomy involves excision of the entire proximal row of carpal bones. The capitate, originally part of the distal carpal row, comes to rest in the lunate fossa of the distal radius and wrist motion occurs through this new articulation. Alternatively, a scaphoid excision and four-corner fusion, or partial wrist fusion of the lunate, capitate, hamate, and triquetrum, can be performed. This procedure preserves motion through the wrist joint via the maintained articulation between the lunate and distal radius.

In Stage III disease, a total wrist fusion is typically recommended, often providing a stable and pain free joint. Total wrist joint replacement is rarely used to treat wrist osteoarthritis due to high implant failure rates over time and the need for activity restrictions following the procedure. Denervation of the wrist capsule via posterior interosseous nerve excision is often performed concurrently with the above procedures.

Expected Outcome and Predictors of Outcome

There are no studies that examine the long-term success of non-operative management of SNAC and SLAC wrists; however, non-operative management is typically more successful in the early stages of disease. With regard to surgical outcomes, proximal row carpectomy and scaphoid excision and four-corner fusion have similar functional outcomes. Patients generally report satisfactory pain relief, strength, and function following these procedures. Patients can expect to achieve postoperative wrist motion that is about 60% compared to that of the contralateral unaffected wrist. On average, patients achieve 80% grip strength compared to the contralateral unaffected wrist. After proximal row carpectomy, younger patients are at higher risk of developing secondary degenerative changes of the capitate, which may necessitate secondary procedures. Only a minority of patients who undergo proximal row carpectomy and scaphoid excision with four-corner fusion require secondary procedures for persistent pain or nonunion.

Total wrist fusion results in reliable pain relief and patient satisfaction at the expense of wrist motion. Patients often must adapt the way they perform certain activities that require manipulation of the hand in tight spaces and self-hygiene. With newer techniques, complications are rare, however include nonunion, extensor tendon adhesion, infection, poor wound healing, and painful hardware.

Wrist Osteoarthritis: Kienböck Disease

Kienböck disease is idiopathic necrosis of the lunate bone, characterized by fragmentation and progressive collapse of the lunate and subsequent degenerative changes of the wrist joints.

Summary of Epidemiology

Kienböck disease is most commonly seen in men between the ages of 20 and 40 years and is usually unilateral. The etiology is Kienböck disease remains poorly understood, but it is generally accepted that it is a multifactorial disease process. While some suggest that arterial insufficiency is to blame, others believe venous congestion plays a larger role. There is also evidence to suggest that certain anatomic variations of the wrist joint lead to increased force transmission across the radiolunate joint, which may lead to Kienböck disease.

Clinical Presentation

Patients typically present with non-activity-related dorsal wrist pain and limited wrist motion, without a clear history of trauma. Dorsal wrist swelling may be appreciated on exam. Patients typically do not seek medical attention in the early stages of disease; thus, the true prevalence and natural history of the disease remains unknown.

Differential Diagnosis and Suggested Diagnostic Testing

The differential diagnosis for dorsal wrist pain includes scapholunate ligament injury, dorsal wrist ganglion cyst, and extensor tenosynovitis. The unique feature of Kienböck disease is that pain is typically persistent both at rest and with activity.

Early Kienböck disease may be accompanied by normal radiographs. A subtle finding is relative shortening of the ulna compared to the distal radius, known as ulnar negative variance. In more advanced cases, lunate sclerosis, fragmentation, and eventual collapse can be seen. Normal plain films in a young adult with persistent non-activity-related wrist pain with ulnar negative variance warrants further evaluation with magnetic resonance imaging (MRI). MRI may reveal diffuse changes of the lunate, with low signal on T1-weighted images and increased signal on T2-weighted images.

Kienböck disease is staged using the Lichtman classification (Fig. 14.3). In Stage I disease, radiographs are relatively normal, and changes are only noted on MRI. In Stage II disease, sclerosis of the lunate can be seen, however without collapse. In Stage III, lunate collapse has occurred. Stage III disease is further divided into IIIA and IIIB, with IIIB disease associated with reduced carpal height due to proximal migration of the capitate and fixed flexion deformity of the scaphoid. In Stage IV disease, degenerative changes are seen in the radiocarpal and/or midcarpal joints.

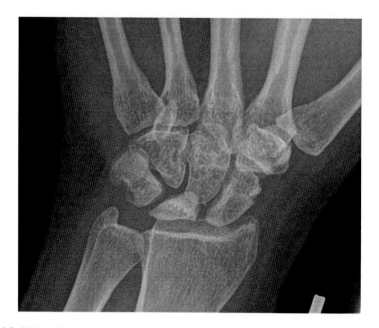

Fig. 14.3 Plain radiograph of Kienböck disease, noting sclerosis and collapse of lunate

Non-operative Management

Cast immobilization for 6–12 weeks is the initial treatment choice for the majority of patients and should begin at the time of initial diagnosis.

Indications for Surgery

Surgical treatment for Kienböck disease is indicated in patients who continue to have functionally limiting symptoms despite a period of cast immobilization.

Operative Management

In early disease (Stage II or IIIA) and in patients with ulnar negative variance, a radial shortening osteotomy can be performed in order to level the joint and "off-load" the lunate. A variety of vascularized bone grafting procedures have also been described in attempt to re-vascularize the lunate. Vascularized procedures are typically reserved for Stage II disease, when lunate avascularity is present but lunate collapse has not yet occurred. In late stages of disease (Stage IIIB and IV), namely, once carpal height has been lost and the capitate has migrated proximally, partial wrist fusions, proximal row carpectomy, and total wrist fusion are considered.

Expected Outcome and Predictors of Outcome

While some providers have reported success with non-operative management of Kienböck disease, many others have reported either no improvement in symptoms or progression of disease in most cases.

In early stages of disease, radial shortening procedures result in improved pain in over 90% of patients along with evidence of lunate revascularization in one third of patients. The majority of patients experience improved range of motion and grip strength following these joint-leveling procedures. In late stage disease, partial wrist fusion and proximal row carpectomy have been shown to have comparable results in terms of grip strength, pain relief, and wrist range of motion.

Thumb Carpometacarpal Arthritis

Summary of Epidemiology

Thumb carpometacarpal (CMC) joint osteoarthritis is the second most common arthritis of the hand. There is increasing prevalence of thumb CMC osteoarthritis with age over 40 years, especially in women. The overall prevalence of radiographic thumb CMC osteoarthritis in patients over 80 years of age has been reported to be over 90% in women and over 80% in men. Advanced destructive joint changes are more frequently seen in women compared to men.

Clinical Presentation

Patients present with insidious onset of pain at the base of the thumb and report difficulty with grip and pinch activities that impart stress across the joint. Classically, patients report trouble opening jars and turning doorknobs. On inspection, patients often have a prominent thumb carpometacarpal joint, which is reflective of dorsoradial subluxation of the metacarpal on the trapezium. In order to maintain a wide grip, compensatory hyperextension through the thumb metacarpophalangeal (MCP) joint is often seen. Pain is elicited with a grind test or axial compression across the thumb CMC joint.

Differential Diagnosis and Suggested Diagnostic Testing

Pain at the base of the thumb or radial side of the wrist can be caused by deQuervain's tenosynovitis, scaphoid fracture or scaphoid nonunion, radioscaphoid arthritis, or scaphotrapeziotrapezoid (STT) arthritis. STT arthritis often accompanies thumb CMC osteoarthritis and involves degenerative changes between the scaphoid, trapezium, and trapezoid.

Thumb CMC OA is evaluated using plain radiographs of the thumb, with the beam centered on the trapezium and the first metacarpal (Fig. 14.4). The radiographic stages of disease are graded based on the Eaton and Littler classification. In Stage I disease, radiographs remain unremarkable with preserved joint space. In Stage II and III disease, progressive joint space narrowing and osteophytes are seen at the thumb carpometacarpal joint. Stage IV disease is characterized by involvement of the adjacent STT joint.

Fig. 14.4 Plain
radiographs of thumb
carpometacarpal
osteoarthritis

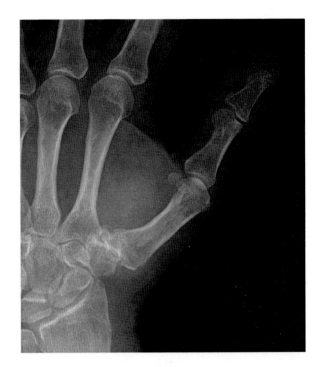

Non-operative Management

First-line treatment of thumb CMC osteoarthritis is non-operative management with anti-inflammatory medications, activity modification, and immobilization with a hand-based opponens splint, which encompasses the thumb metacarpophalangeal joint. The thumb interphalangeal joint can be left free if there is no osteoarthritis at this level, as this makes the splint better tolerated and allows the thumb to be more functional. These splints can be prefabricated or custom molded by an occupational therapist using thermoplastic material. Patients with persistent symptoms despite immobilization can consider corticosteroid injection. When corticosteroid injections are performed in patients with diabetes, patients must be made aware of the potential for temporary elevation of blood glucose levels, which may require supplementary treatment.

Indications for Surgery

Surgical treatment is elective and can be considered in patients who continue to be functionally limited despite non-operative management.

Operative Management

Multiple procedures for thumb CMC osteoarthritis have been described which include trapezium excision with or without tendon interposition and ligamentous reconstruction. All procedures have similar excellent results, and the surgeon's choice of procedure should depend on his or her comfort level. The use of non-biologic implants should be avoided. If the scaphotrapeziotrapezoid joint is also involved, which is quite common in advanced cases, removal of the proximal half of the trapezoid is additionally recommended. Thumb MCP joint hyperextension can be concurrently addressed with tightening of the volar capsule or MCP joint fusion.

In relatively younger patients with early stages of disease, some have advocated for arthroscopic partial excision of the trapezium. Joint replacement procedures are no longer performed as they were found to have unacceptably high failure rates.

Expected Outcome and Predictors of Outcome

Splint immobilization is an effective non-operative treatment modality, which has been show to dramatically improve symptoms within 6 months of use. Studies have reported that non-operative management can be successful in over 70% of patients, with better results seen in patients with earlier stage disease. Corticosteroid injection accompanied by splint immobilization has also been shown to have encouraging results, particularly in patients with earlier stages of thumb CMC osteoarthritis.

Surgical treatment of thumb CMC osteoarthritis is often successful. The majority of patients report improvement in pain, pinch strength, grip strength, and function. Over 80% of patients report complete pain relief or only mild pain with certain activities at 1 year postoperatively. Pain relief is maintained in the long-term in the majority of these patients. Although a variety of surgical techniques have been described, as noted above, no technique has demonstrated superiority over another.

Metacarpophalangeal Joint Arthritis

Summary of Epidemiology

Primary metacarpophalangeal (MCP) joint osteoarthritis is rare, and thus secondary causes, including trauma and systemic diseases such as inflammatory arthritis, hemochromatosis, and calcium pyrophosphate deposition disease (CPPD), must be considered. Moreover, it is notable that men more frequently develop MCP joint osteoarthritis than women, with a reported prevalence of 12% compared to 7% in women.

Clinical Presentation

Patients may present with pain, swelling, and limited motion across the MCP joint.

Differential Diagnosis and Suggested Diagnostic Testing

The differential diagnosis includes an underlying hemochromatosis, CPPD, and inflammatory arthritis. Proliferative synovitis is most commonly seen at the MCP joint in rheumatoid arthritis, as well as characteristic deformities of the joint such as volar subluxation and ulnar deviation. If these findings are noted, a rheumatologic work-up should be considered.

Non-operative Management

Activity modification and anti-inflammatory medications are the first-line treatment for MCP joint arthritis. Corticosteroid injections of the joint typically result in excellent relief and can be repeated every 9–12 months for several years if necessary. Medical treatment of any underlying primary disease processes is of utmost importance.

Indications for Surgery

Surgery is indicated for debilitating pain and stiffness despite non-operative treatment and optimization of the medical management of any associated systemic disease.

Operative Management

The operative procedure of choice in cases of MCP osteoarthritis is joint replacement using either silicone or pyrocarbon implants. Fusion of the MCP joint is avoided because it severely limits hand function.

Expected Outcomes and Predictors of Outcome

The majority of patients report pain relief, functional range of motion, and high satisfaction following joint replacement for MCP joint osteoarthritis. MCP joint range of motion is generally maintained postoperatively. MCP joint implants have demonstrated excellent durability, with over 80% survivorship after 10 years.

Proximal Interphalangeal and Distal Interphalangeal Joint Arthritis

Epidemiology

The distal interphalangeal (DIP) joint is the most common joint affected by primary osteoarthritis in the hand. The proximal interphalangeal (PIP) joint is the most common joint affected by post-traumatic osteoarthritis.

Clinical Presentation

DIP joint osteoarthritis is often asymptomatic. Symptomatic patients may report an aching pain across the DIP joint. Clinically, nodular deformities known as Heberden nodes can be observed at the DIP joint due to underlying osteophytes. Mucous cysts are also associated with DIP joint osteoarthritis, which can occasionally be painful or become secondarily infected. Mucous cysts may also lead to nail deformities due to pressure effects on the germinal matrix cells, which form the nail plate. At the PIP joint, nodular deformities from underlying osteophytes are referred to as Bouchard nodes. The natural history of PIP joint osteoarthritis is progressive loss of motion and pain secondary to joint contracture and collateral ligament fibrosis.

Differential Diagnosis and Suggested Diagnostic Testing

The diagnosis of interphalangeal joint OA can be made on plain radiographs of the hand (Fig. 14.5). The hallmark findings of osteoarthritis including joint space narrowing, osteophytes, subchondral sclerosis, and subchondral cysts can be seen.

The differential diagnosis of DIP joint and PIP joint arthritis is broad and includes inflammatory arthritis such as rheumatoid arthritis. It is important to remember that in rheumatoid arthritis, however, the DIP joints are often spared. PIP joints can be

Fig. 14.5 Plain radiographs of distal interphalangeal joint osteoarthritis of the index finger and long finger. There is evidence of joint space narrowing, osteophytes, subchondral sclerosis, and subchondral cystic change

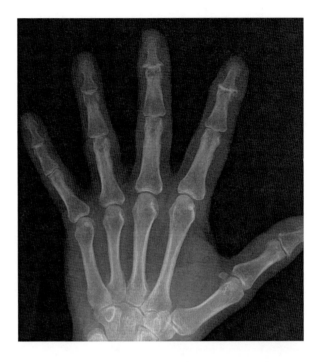

affected in rheumatoid arthritis; thus, it is important to examine whether there are accompanying deformities across the PIP joint that are characteristic of rheumatoid arthritis. For example, hyperextension of the PIP joint can occur due to attenuation of volar structures, while hyperflexion deformities of the PIP joint occur due to attenuation of the extensor mechanism. Seronegative spondyloarthropathies can also affect the interphalangeal joints. In psoriatic arthritis, more aggressive erosive changes are typically observed, namely, "pencil-in-cup" deformities at the DIP joint. Crystal-induced arthropathies, such as gout and calcium pyrophosphate disease present with a more acute onset of symptoms with considerable pain, swelling, and erythema. In addition, gout can be accompanied by soft tissue tophi.

Non-operative Management

Anti-inflammatory medications and activity modification are the initial treatment for patients with DIP or PIP joint osteoarthritis. Intermittent corticosteroid injections of the interphalangeal joints often provide good to moderate relief. However, injections should not be performed frequently as bone loss may occur resulting in increased deformity and ulnar drift, ultimately making reconstruction more difficult.

Indications for Surgery

Surgery is indicated for patients with pain despite the above non-operative measures.

Operative Management

DIP joint osteoarthritis can be addressed with fusion across the DIP joint. Fusion of the DIP joint in slight flexion typically enables the patient to maintain excellent function. A variety of methods can be used to achieve successful fusion, including wire fixation or headless compression screws. In the setting of symptomatic mucous cysts, cyst excision with removal of underlying osteophytes is performed. Occasionally, local soft tissue must be rotated in order to achieve adequate soft tissue closure following cyst excision.

PIP joint osteoarthritis is treated either with joint fusion or joint replacement. When the index or small finger joint is involved, joint fusion will reliably result in a painless and stable joint. In these cases, a stable index finger still allows for a strong pinch. When the long or ring fingers are affected, joint replacement can be considered to preserve motion across the PIP joint.

Expected Outcomes and Predictors of Outcome

DIP joint fusion results in reliable patient satisfaction and pain relief. Successful DIP fusion can be achieved using wire fixation or headless compression screws; however, nonunion rates have been reported to be as high as 30%. Recent studies examining outcomes of DIP fusion for degenerative arthritis using headless compression screws have reported lower rates of nonunion and overall complications, but there is no clear evidence that one method of fixation is superior to another.

Although PIP joint replacements and joint fusions have similar pain relief initially, the long-term results of joint replacements are quite variable, with a failure rate of over 30%. Subsequent revision surgeries are difficult due to bone loss and soft tissue changes. Following PIP joint replacement, it is important to counsel patients that there is typically no significant improvement in range of motion. In general, postoperative PIP joint range of motion is determined by preoperative range of motion. On average, patients achieve roughly 45 degrees of motion across the PIP joint.

Table 14.1 shows a summary of the clinical presentation, recommended diagnostic testing, and management of osteoarthritic conditions of the hand and wrist.

Table 14.1 A summary of the clinical presentation, recommended diagnostic testing, and management of osteoarthritic conditions of the hand and wrist

Clinical entity	Presentation	Diagnostic testing	Conservative management	Indications for surgery	Operative management
Wrist osteoarthritis: post-traumatic	Wrist pain, weak grip strength, limited wrist motion	Plain radiographs	Anti-inflammatory medications, wrist brace, activity modification	Pain and functional limitations despite conservative management	Determined by stage of disease: radial styloidectomy, proximal row carpectomy, scaphoid excision and four-corner fusion, or total wrist fusion
Wrist osteoarthritis: Kienböck disease	Wrist pain at rest, limited wrist motion	Plain radiographs; consider MRI if radiographs normal and high clinical suspicion	Cast immobilization	Pain and functional limitations despite cast immobilization	Determined by stage of disease; radial shortening osteotomy, vascularized bone grafting procedures, proximal row carpectomy, scaphoid excision and four-corner fusion, or total wrist fusion
Thumb carpometacarpal osteoarthritis	Insidious onset of pain at base of thumb, difficulty with pinch and grip	Plain radiographs	Anti-inflammatory medications, hand-based opponens splint, corticosteroid injection	Pain and functional limitations despite conservative management	Various procedures, including trapezium excision and ligamentous reconstruction

(continued)

Table 14.1 (continued)

Clinical entity	Presentation	Diagnostic testing	Conservative management	Indications for surgery	Operative management
MCP joint osteoarthritis	Pain, swelling, and limited range of motion across MCP joint	Plain radiographs, work-up for underlying systemic disease including hemochromatosis, CPPD, and rheumatoid arthritis	Anti-inflammatory medications, activity modification, corticosteroid injection, medical management of underlying systemic disease	Pain and functional limitations despite conservative management and optimal medical management	Joint replacement
Interphalangeal joint osteoarthritis (PIP and DIP joints)	Pain, swelling, and limited range of motion; Heberden nodes, Bouchard nodes, mucous cyst	Plain radiographs	Anti-inflammatory medications, activity modification, corticosteroid injection	Pain and functional limitations despite conservative management	DIP joint fusion, PIP joint fusion or joint replacement

CPPD calcium pyrophosphate deposition disease, *PIP* proximal interphalangeal joint, *DIP* distal interphalangeal joint, *MCP* metacarpophalangeal

Summary

Osteoarthritic conditions of the hand and wrist are common. Primary osteoarthritis in the hand can often be diagnosed with a thorough physical exam, clinical history, and plain radiographs. Surgery may be indicated for patients who have continued pain and functional limitations despite conservative management. While primary osteoarthritis in the wrist is uncommon, an understanding of the etiologies of secondary wrist arthritis as well as the functional demands of individual patients can help guide treatment.

Suggested Reading

Allan CH, Joshi A, Lichtman DM. Kienböck's disease: diagnosis and treatment. J Am Acad Orthop Surg. 2001;9(2). http://journals.lww.com/jaaos/Fulltext/2001/03000/Kienb_ck_s_Disease__Diagnosis_and_Treatment.6.aspx.

Berger AJ, Meals RA. Management of osteoarthrosis of the thumb joints. J Hand Surg Am. 2015;40(4):843–50. https://doi.org/10.1016/j.jhsa.2014.11.026.

Dickson DR, Badge R, Nuttall D, et al. Pyrocarbon metacarpophalangeal joint arthroplasty in non-inflammatory arthritis: minimum 5-year follow-up. J Hand Surg Am. 2015;40(10):1956–62. https://doi.org/10.1016/j.jhsa.2015.06.104.

Haugen IK, Englund M, Aliabadi P, et al. Prevalence, incidence and progression of hand osteoarthritis in the general population: the Framingham Osteoarthritis Study. Ann Rheum Dis. 2011;70(9):1581–6. https://doi.org/10.1136/ard.2011.150078.

Sodha S, Ring D, Zurakowski D, Jupiter JB. Prevalence of osteoarthrosis of the trapeziometacarpal joint. J Bone Joint Surg Am. 2005;87(12):2614–8. https://doi.org/10.2106/JBJS.E.00104.

Strauch RJ. Scapholunate advanced collapse and scaphoid nonunion advanced collapse arthritis—update on evaluation and treatment. J Hand Surg Am. 2011;36(4):729–35. https://doi.org/10.1016/j.jhsa.2011.01.018.

Villani F, Uribe-Echevarria B, Vaienti L. Distal interphalangeal joint arthrodesis for degenerative osteoarthritis with compression screw: results in 102 digits. J Hand Surg Am. 2012;37(7):1330–4. https://doi.org/10.1016/j.jhsa.2012.02.048.

Vitale MA, Fruth KM, Rizzo M, Moran SL, Kakar S. Prosthetic arthroplasty versus arthrodesis for osteoarthritis and posttraumatic arthritis of the index finger proximal interphalangeal joint. J Hand Surg Am. 2015;40(10):1937–48. https://doi.org/10.1016/j.jhsa.2015.05.021.

Weiss KE, Rodner CM. Osteoarthritis of the Wrist. J Hand Surg Am. 2007;32(5):725–46. https://doi.org/10.1016/j.jhsa.2007.02.003.

Part IX
Nerve Entrapment

Chapter 15
Upper Extremity Nerve Entrapment

Ariana N. Mora and Philip E. Blazar

Abbreviations

CTS   Carpal tunnel syndrome
CuTS   Cubital tunnel syndrome
MRI   Magnetic resonance imaging
NSAIDs   Nonsteroidal anti-inflammatory drugs

Introduction

Neurologic complaints involving one or both upper extremities are relatively common. The most frequent diagnoses for these complaints are carpal tunnel syndrome (CTS) and cubital tunnel syndrome (CuTS). These conditions present with similar symptoms of numbness, paresthesia, and sometimes pain but are distinct in their presentation and management.

Carpal Tunnel Syndrome

Summary of Epidemiology

Carpal tunnel syndrome (CTS) is the most common entrapment neuropathy. CTS is a mononeuropathy of the median nerve at the wrist, specifically in the carpal tunnel above the flexor tendons as they pass from the forearm to the hand. The prevalence of CTS has been studied in several populations and has been estimated to be approximately 4% in the United States. Classically, women account for approximately 75% of cases diagnosed, and the usual age of presentation, for both men and women, is around 50 years old.

A.N. Mora • P.E. Blazar (✉)
Department of Orthopedic Surgery: Hand and Upper Extremity, Brigham and Women's
Hospital, 75 Francis Street, Boston, MA 02115, USA
e-mail: amora1@partners.org; pblazar@partners.org

© Springer International Publishing AG 2018   253
J.N. Katz et al. (eds.), *Principles of Orthopedic Practice for Primary Care
Providers*, https://doi.org/10.1007/978-3-319-68661-5_15

A variety of risk factors have been identified, most common of which are female sex, pregnancy, or concomitant diagnosis of diabetes mellitus, obesity, and hypothyroidism. Specifically, the risk factors for CTS can be divided into systemic and anatomic factors. Systemic factors are more common and include diabetes mellitus and alcoholism resulting in neuropathy, fluid balance issues caused by pregnancy, myxedema, obesity, renal failure/hemodialysis, and metabolic issues arising from mucopolysaccharidosis or mucolipidosis. It is uncertain whether smoking affects the prevalence of CTS. Anatomic factors include paraplegia, position during sleep, deformity after fractures or other trauma, carpal bone anomalies, acromegaly, anomalous muscle bellies, hematoma resulting from anticoagulation therapy, lipoma and other neoplasms, hypertrophied synovium, infection, and increased adipose tissue volume in the carpal tunnel due to obesity.

Women who develop a first-time presentation of carpal tunnel syndrome during pregnancy are diagnosed with gestational CTS. Gestational CTS has not been well characterized in the literature. It is unclear as to what factors lead to the development CTS during their pregnancy—though some risk factors are the same as classical CTS, including diabetes mellitus and obesity. Interestingly, the majority of women who develop CTS during their pregnancy will have symptoms abate within 1–2 weeks postpartum, yet others will develop persistent CTS.

Over the past few decades, there has been a trend for CTS to be diagnosed in younger patients, a phenomenon that some have speculated is due to an increase in occupational repetitive motion activities. The link between CTS, occupational tasks, and repetitive activity is not clearly supported by the scientific literature. Most of the epidemiologic studies that have examined the correlation between CTS and repetitive motion have not found an association. However, exposure to some occupational factors, specifically vibration, has been consistently linked to compressive neuropathy, especially CTS. Some investigators have reported that occupational CTS is epidemiologically distinct, presenting at a younger age and at a nearly 1:1 sex ratio.

Clinical Presentation

The classic presentation of CTS is a gradual onset of numbness, paresthesia, and sometimes pain in the radial three and one half digits (Fig. 15.1).

The carpal tunnel is composed of a semicircular ring of carpal bones and an overlying, unyielding fibrous band, the transverse carpal ligament. Chronic compression and increases in pressure have been shown to reduce epineural blood flow and diminish axonal transport in peripheral nerves. For both unaffected patients and those with CTS, positioning the wrist in extreme flexion or extension further increases the pressure on the median nerve. The median nerve contributes motor fibers to the thenar muscles and sensory fibers to the thumb and the index and middle fingers, as well as to half of the ring finger.

Patients typically have subacute or chronic symptoms involving the median nerve distribution. However, a substantial number of patients will report symptoms

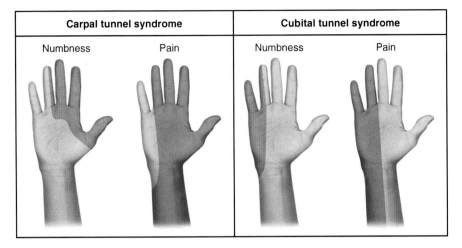

Fig. 15.1 Common symptom presentation of CTS and CuTS. *CTS* carpal tunnel syndrome, *CuTS* cubital tunnel syndrome

involving the entire hand. Development or worsening of symptoms at certain times or with particular activities is very characteristic and aids in diagnosis. While taking a patient's history, it is important to ask if the patient experiences numbness and pain in their hand while sleeping, driving, talking on the telephone, or reading. If so, carpal tunnel syndrome is very likely the cause.

Infrequently, patients will present with acute nerve compression secondary to swelling from trauma, spontaneous bleeding while on anticoagulation, or a rapidly progressing infection. In these scenarios, the acute process has likely caused complete intraneural ischemia and must be treated as a surgical emergency.

While many cases are idiopathic, it is important to check thoroughly for coexisting systemic disorders and local predisposing factors, which may have a substantial impact on the selection of appropriate treatment. Patients with bilateral symptoms are more likely to have metabolic or systemic risk factors. CTS may be the presenting complaint for a process with wide-reaching health implications; therefore, signs of secondary causes should always be sought, particularly in patients with bilateral symptoms.

The microvascular and anatomic changes in CTS create a spectrum of dysfunction, but patients generally can be grouped into one of three clinical stages:

(a) *Mild Stage CTS*: Characterized by intermittent paresthesia and frequent resolution of symptoms when predisposing activities are modified or ceased. In this stage, patients may respond well to nonsurgical treatment, but a moderate percentage still progress further.

(b) *Moderate Stage CTS*: Complaint of constant paresthesia/numbness. Pain and the severity of the paresthesia may be episodic. Conservative treatment is unlikely to be of long-term benefit to this population. This group shows the largest improvement in symptoms post-surgery.

256   A.N. Mora and P.E. Blazar

(c) *Severe Stage CTS*: Characterized by distinct sensory loss and thenar muscle atrophy. Chronic elevated pressure in the tunnel and reduced epineural blood flow are likely to lead to epineural fibrosis if untreated. A degree of persistent neurologic dysfunction despite treatment is likely after surgery, although the majority of patients will report significant symptom improvement, particularly in regard to pain relief.

The most sensitive and specific physical examination maneuver commonly employed is the carpal tunnel compression test, in which direct pressure is applied over the median nerve (Fig. 15.2). Other physical examination maneuvers that aid in the diagnosis of CTS are listed in the table below (Table 15.1). Other components of the peripheral nervous system in other limbs should be examined to exclude

Fig. 15.2 CTS compression test. Apply direct compression of the median nerve for 30 s to elicit paresthesia. *CTS* carpal tunnel syndrome

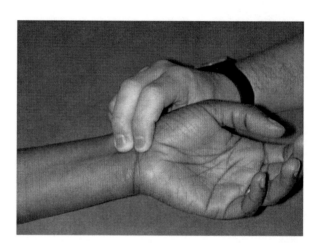

Table 15.1 Physical exam maneuvers that aid in the diagnosis of CTS

Test	Technique	Condition response	Positive result
Phalen's sign	Patient places arms on table, elbows extended, wrists in full flexion	Paresthesia in response to position	Numbness or tingling on radial sided digits within 60 s; probable CTS
Tinel's sign	Examiner lightly taps along median nerve at the wrist, proximal to distal	Site of nerve lesion	Tingling response in fingers at site of compression; probable CTS if response at the wrist
CTS compression test	Direct compression of median nerve by examiner	Paresthesia in response to pressure	Paresthesia within 30 s; probable CTS
Hand diagram	Patient marks sites of pain or altered sensation on an outline diagram of the hand	Patient's perception of site of nerve deficit	Diagram marked on palmar aspect; probable CTS

CTS carpal tunnel syndrome

systemic neuropathic predisposition. Examination of the median nerve more proximally, including at the cervical spine, should always be included because patients with proximal nerve entrapment are sometimes misdiagnosed and treated for CTS.

Differential Diagnosis and Suggested Diagnostic Testing

The differential diagnoses for CTS include various conditions that present with paresthesia, pain, or weakness involving the upper extremity:

(a) *Cervical radiculopathy* typically although not always presents with neck pain exacerbated with neck movement, reflex changes, and weakness of proximal arm muscles including elbow extension/flexion and arm pronation in addition to CTS symptoms.

(b) *Cervical spondylotic myelopathy* usually progresses to bilateral motor/sensory dysfunction in the hands not confined to the median nerve, unlike CTS.

(c) *Brachial plexopathy* is typically unilateral and accompanied with motor/sensory dysfunction in areas beyond the median nerve distribution.

(d) *Median neuropathy in the proximal forearm* is much less common than CTS. Symptoms overlap with CTS but include thumb flexion weakness and sensory loss over the thenar eminence, as these structures receive innervation from the median nerve proximal to the wrist.

(e) *Motor neuron disease* (e.g., *amyotrophic lateral sclerosis*) presents without pain, which is a hallmark of CTS.

(f) *Fibromyalgia* is characterized by chronic widespread pain and fatigue not isolated to the region affected by CTS.

Electrodiagnostic testing is often considered the diagnostic test of choice for CTS, but it remains operator dependent. As with any test, false-positive and false-negative rates are dependent on the threshold levels used by the particular practitioner. Systemic conditions (e.g., diabetes mellitus or aging) and laboratory conditions (e.g., limb temperature) can influence test results. The data are typically compared to population norms, but often information from the contralateral extremity or the ulnar nerve in the same wrist is more useful in diagnosis. The staging system for electrodiagnostic testing is similar to the clinical staging system, but it does not necessarily correlate. Electrodiagnostic tests will reliably detect cervical spine or more proximal upper extremity nerve compression only if the test examines the extremity proximal to the wrist.

Nerve conduction velocities and electromyography provide the only objective evidence of nerve dysfunction in CTS. Therefore, electrodiagnostic testing is especially useful for documentation in patients where there is an expected need for objective tools to monitor improvement, such as in the case of an active workers' compensation claim. Because patients frequently find the electrodiagnostic tests painful, recent literature suggests that electrodiagnostic tests may be substituted with ultrasound imaging in certain situations. Radiographs and magnetic resonance imaging (MRI) are rarely indicated, except in cases of limited wrist motion, trauma, or arthritis (radiographs) or for suspected soft tissue masses (MRI).

Nonoperative Management

The severity of the clinical stage of CTS usually dictates treatment choices. Any underlying systemic processes should be investigated and treated as appropriate. Mild stage CTS at first presentation is usually treated with splinting and/or activity modification. Nonsteroidal anti-inflammatory drugs (NSAIDs) have not been shown to be effective for CTS but are frequently effective for other hand conditions that also affect this population. However, if conservative management is unsuccessful, further activity restriction, corticosteroids, or surgery may be necessary.

(a) *Splinting*: The majority of patients are initially treated with wrist splinting in a straight position or in slight extension. Splinting protocols vary according to the severity of the patient's symptoms and the presence of exacerbating activities. Splinting only at night is typically sufficient for the vast majority of patients who have exclusively or predominantly nocturnal symptoms. Other patients may benefit from the additional use of splints during daytime activities that produce symptoms. In general, full-time splinting should be avoided to reduce the risk of atrophy and loss of motion. Disuse and atrophy are especially important to keep in mind for workers' compensation cases as this may delay or complicate the return to work.

(b) *Activity modification*: For patients with mild stage CTS who wish to avoid splinting or who are not appropriate candidates for it, some benefits can be achieved through activity modification. Limiting activities that exacerbate or produce symptoms is recommended; the patient may wish to consider adjusting his or her work schedule, taking frequent breaks from repetitive activities, or making ergonomic changes to the workstation. Activity modification is frequently unsuccessful and more restrictive modifications may be considered. The modification prescription will depend on a complex conversation in which patients may relate symptoms to occupational activities. Patients' options at this time may be limited to long-term work restrictions, surgical intervention, or continuing to manage the symptoms as above, as long as there are no signs of progressive neurologic dysfunction.

(c) *Diuretics and anti-inflammatories*: Patients with substantial peripheral edema may experience symptomatic improvement with diuretics. Frequently, NSAIDs are paired with diuretics. The use of NSAIDs has not been shown to be effective for idiopathic CTS in randomized trials; however, these agents are well tolerated if appropriately monitored. They are most beneficial for reducing inflammation in patients with multiple complaints or comorbidities. Anti-inflammatory medications are clearly indicated for those patients who have tenosynovitis from an inflammatory process.

(d) *Corticosteroids*: Injection with corticosteroids can be an effective treatment when the previous management strategies have not been successful. The response rate is best for patients who have experienced mild symptoms for less than 12 months. Injection is likely to reduce or eliminate symptoms in the majority of these patients; however, only a minority of these will have continued relief 1 year postinjection. Complications with carpal tunnel injection are uncommon, but injection into the nerve must be avoided. The goal is to introduce the steroid into the tenosynovium within the carpal tunnel but not directly into or immediately adjacent to the nerve. Any paresthesia in the median (or ulnar) distribution elicited during the procedure should prompt the physician to withdraw and redirect the needle. Complications from multiple injections at this site have not been reported; however, skin atrophy and tendon rupture from multiple corticosteroid injections at other sites have been documented. Therefore, multiple injections (more than two or three) are discouraged, except in the rare patient for whom surgery is medically contraindicated.

Indications for Surgery

Patients who present with moderate or severe stage CTS are managed in a more aggressive manner. Additionally, patients with mild stage CTS who have failed nonsurgical treatment may be considered surgical candidates. Moderate stage CTS patients typically have a limited or transient response to conservative treatment options. In these cases, surgical intervention is recommended to reduce the likelihood of permanent neurologic changes, and most patients report pain relief postoperatively. It should be noted, however, that even after surgery, many have some permanent neurologic dysfunction that can be seen through electrodiagnostic testing or subtle findings apparent during physical examination.

Patients presenting with severe stage CTS are best managed by surgical decompression of the carpal tunnel. In patients with CTS from coexisting systemic morbidities, it is unusual to see prompt diminution or resolution of symptoms with corrective measures (e.g., thyroid replacement therapy, improved control of blood glucose level). Thus, referral for consideration of surgery is appropriate even while actively addressing these comorbidities.

Clear indications for referral to a surgeon include:

(a) Patients who present with moderate or severe stage CTS, i.e., all patients with constant paresthesia. Those with limiting comorbidities also fall into this category. Carpal tunnel release can be performed expeditiously under local anesthesia with little physiologic stress; therefore, medical comorbidities are only considered to be an absolute contraindication for surgery in very extreme or unusual situations.

(b) Patients who have acute CTS as a result of trauma, suspected infection, or bleeding. Although rare, such patients should be referred emergently for surgical consultation and, if conclusively diagnosed, should be treated with emergent surgical decompression to avoid further neurologic injury.

(c) Patients with progressive neurologic dysfunction during nonsurgical treatment, such as progressive hand weakness noted in median nerve innervated muscles.

(d) A patient who fails nonsurgical treatment in the early stage of the disease is also an appropriate indication for referral. Patients must be counseled that decompression is an appropriate, but elective, procedure in these situations.

Operative Management

It remains controversial whether a particular surgical technique is optimal for treatment of CTS. Surgical division of the transverse carpal ligament has been shown to rapidly return pressure in the carpal tunnel in most patients with CTS to the same level as that in controls; however, standard surgical techniques have produced moderate rates of tenderness in the area of the palmar incision (Fig. 15.3). These symptoms almost always resolve, but improvement may take several months. Although temporary, this tenderness may slow rehabilitation and resumption of occupational and recreational activities.

Endoscopic techniques were developed to reduce this complication and to hasten rehabilitation. These techniques have been shown to decrease but not eliminate incisional pain. Although patients who undergo endoscopic surgery return to work slightly sooner, they may have very low but slightly elevated rates of neurovascular injury compared with patients treated with standard techniques.

Fig. 15.3 Postoperative incision for open carpal tunnel release

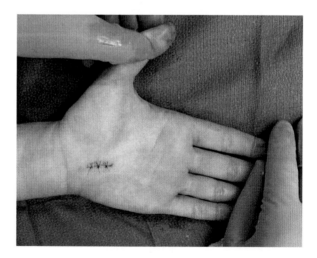

Expected Outcome and Predictors of Outcome

Studies of surgical treatment for CTS have typically focused on recovery of strength, resolution of paresthesia, and time to return to work. The persistence of symptoms after surgical release varies widely between studies and is highly dependent on patient selection; in well-selected case series with long-term follow-up, about 75% of patients report complete resolution of symptoms. Patients with intrinsic neurologic dysfunction and symptoms of more chronic and severe compression have generally experienced worse outcomes. Although many studies have documented that some patients will have persistent symptoms, reported satisfaction among patients is very high (over 90%) after surgical release. Little has been written on the outcomes of CTS in populations treated nonoperatively for extended time periods.

Additionally, studies suggest that patients with earlier surgical release have better outcomes. A study found that patients who underwent surgery within 3 years of diagnosis were twice as likely to have symptom resolution compared to those who underwent surgery more than 3 years after diagnosis. Other studies have suggested that after surgical release, patients with intermittent paresthesia (mild stage CTS) had better return of sensation than did those with constant paresthesia (moderate or severe stage CTS).

Cubital Tunnel Syndrome

Summary of Epidemiology

Cubital tunnel syndrome (CuTS) is the second most common upper extremity entrapment neuropathy after carpal tunnel syndrome (CTS). The prevalence of CuTS has not been studied as extensively as CTS; however, CuTS is estimated to have an annual incidence rate of 25 per 100,000, affecting men more than women, and has been associated with smoking and increased age. Besides the difference in gender prevalence in CTS, CuTS also differs from CTS in that BMI, diabetes, and hypertension are not predisposing factors for this syndrome.

Extrinsic compression of the ulnar nerve can be from acute trauma or prolonged pressure on the nerve caused by elbow flexion or leaning on the elbow, given that the ulnar nerve is situated tightly around the medial epicondyle in these positions. Trauma can lead to focal compression from osteophytes or scar tissue encroaching upon the nerve. Instability of the ulnar nerve can lead to repetitive subluxation or dislocation of the nerve during flexion, which in turn can lead to motor and sensory loss. Intrinsic factors around the elbow that can contribute to symptoms include arthritis, synovitis, mass lesions, and bone, muscle, or fibrous tissue anomalies.

Clinical Presentation

Patients with CuTS present with numbness and paresthesia in the volar aspect of the fourth and fifth digits of the hand and medial elbow pain, often with nocturnal symptoms. These symptoms worsen during sustained elbow flexion, leaning on elbow, or while performing activities that require repetitive lifting, gripping, pronation, or supination. While sensory complaints are more common, motor symptoms do occur, ranging from mild weakness of the intrinsic muscles of the hand to severe wasting of ulnar-innervated hand and forearm muscles, which is largely dependent on the duration of symptoms. Some patients will complain of difficulty performing tasks requiring fine dexterity and/or pinch such as using a key to open a door. Unlike CTS, this loss of dexterity in patients with CuTS is largely due to intrinsic hand muscle weakness and not sensory loss. This loss of intrinsic muscle strength can greatly affect grip strength.

The severity categories for CuTS are less defined than they are for CTS. Mild to moderate CuTS is characterized by intermittent or persistent sensory loss and weakness without wasting and without a causative structural lesion. When visible muscle atrophy accompanies symptoms of pain and paresthesia, CuTS should be classified as severe.

The ulnar nerve is positioned in the groove between the medial epicondyle and the olecranon process of the posterior elbow. It can be readily palpated to check for lesions, swelling, or nerve subluxation over the medial epicondyle. The examiner should inspect the elbow and forearm for deformity or atrophy. Visible muscle wasting, particularly of the intrinsic hand muscles, indicates a significant duration of ulnar nerve compression ranging from months to years. Examination maneuvers that assist in the diagnosis of CuTS are listed in the table below (Table 15.2).

Differential Diagnosis and Suggested Diagnostic Testing

The differential diagnoses of CuTS include various conditions that present with paresthesia, pain, or weakness involving the upper extremity:

(a) *Carpal tunnel syndrome* presents with numbness in the thumb, index, and middle fingers (palmar aspect) in addition to possible thenar muscle wasting.
(b) *Cervical radiculopathy* presents with neck pain exacerbated with neck movement, reflex changes, and weakness of proximal arm muscles including elbow extension/flexion and arm pronation in addition to CuTS symptoms.
(c) *Medial epicondylitis* is characterized by tenderness over the medial epicondyle; it is distinct from CuTS as it will not result in distal weakness, paresthesia, or numbness.

Table 15.2 Physical exam maneuvers that aid in the diagnosis of CuTS

Test	Technique	Condition response	Positive result
Tinel's sign	Percussion over ulnar nerve distally from ulnar groove to cubital tunnel	Site of nerve lesion	Tingling response in ulnar distribution of hand; likely CuTS
Elbow flexion test	Place index finger over ulnar groove throughout maximum elbow flexion	Ulnar nerve subluxation and presence of paresthesia	Ulnar nerve slips out of groove and patient reports paresthesia in ulnar distribution after 60 s of flexion; likely CuTS
Froment's sign	Patient actively adducts thumb to index finger	Thumb adductor muscle weakness (innervated by ulnar nerve)	Interphalangeal thumb joint flexes; in addition to positive sensory tests, could indicate more advanced CuTS
Abduction/adduction strength test	Cross index/ middle fingers; spread fingers (abduction), fingers together (adduction)	Finger abductor/ adductor muscle weakness (innervated by ulnar nerve)	Inability to cross fingers, weakness to resist antagonistic movement; in addition to positive sensory tests, could indicate more advanced CuTS

CuTS cubital tunnel syndrome

(d) *Thoracic outlet syndrome* includes neck and shoulder pain in addition to distal pain and numbness; patients will have normal nerve conduction studies at the elbow, and it rarely includes wasting in the hand.

(e) *Ulnar nerve entrapment at the wrist* will result in maintenance of strong wrist flexors and ulnar deviators, and sensation will remain intact over the dorsomedial hand and the dorsum of the little and ring fingers as these structures receive innervation from the ulnar nerve proximal to the wrist.

The clinical diagnosis of CuTS can be confirmed with electrodiagnostic testing. Electrodiagnostic studies can localize the lesion on the ulnar nerve, determine the severity, and provide objective evidence of the presence of CuTS. It should be noted that there are a high percentage of cases with mild CuTS, particularly among musicians, that present with clinically significant findings of CuTS however with negative electrodiagnostic tests. Many of these individuals have progressive symptoms and frequently elect to have surgery. Unlike electrodiagnostic tests for CTS, CuTS electrodiagnostic findings do not typically distinguish between mild and moderate categories; however, severe findings are usually noted as such. If elbow trauma has occurred, radiographs of the elbow should be ordered in addition to electrodiagnostic testing.

Nonoperative Management

The severity of paresthesia and pain due to CuTS usually dictates treatment choices. Mild to moderate CuTS at first presentation is usually treated with splinting and/or activity modification. Corticosteroid injections are not recommended. Nonoperative management is also recommended for those who are ineligible for surgical treatment.

(a) *Splinting:* The majority of patients are initially treated with nocturnal elbow splinting limiting flexion. Alternatively, and perhaps with better rates of compliance, patients can wrap the effected elbow with a pillow or towel instead of a traditional hard splint as this may be better tolerated during sleep.
(b) *Activity modification*: Patients should be instructed to avoid excessive or repetitive elbow flexion, putting pressure directly on the medial elbow during rest or activities, e.g., crossing arms, supporting significant weight on arm rests. Workplace modifications may also be necessary to limit repetitive lifting, elbow flexion, and direct pressure on the ulnar nerve.

Indications for Surgery

Those presenting with muscle atrophy and weakness in conjunction with sensory symptoms indicative of CuTS should be treated more aggressively and are recommended for surgery. Those who have had severe CuTS symptoms existing beyond 2 years will have variable improvement in sensory-related symptoms postoperatively, but surgery is beneficial to alleviate pain associated with CuTS. Surgery is also indicated in individuals with mild or moderate CuTS whose symptoms have progressed or those who have been unsuccessfully treated after 2–3 months of conservative management.

Operative Management

Typically CuTS is surgically treated with ulnar nerve decompression, which consists of cutting the flexor carpi ulnaris aponeurosis to decompress the ulnar nerve. However, in cases where the ulnar nerve subluxates upon flexion, ulnar nerve transposition is necessary. Ulnar nerve transposition is a more involved surgery that mobilizes and frees the ulnar nerve from the ulnar groove and repositions it anteriorly in the forearm. Ulnar nerve transposition requires a larger incision and can have higher rates of complications when compared to simple ulnar nerve decompression.

Expected Outcome and Predictors of Outcome

Patients with mild symptoms of intermittent ulnar sensory loss often improve with conservative treatment alone within 3–6 months. Many of these patients will never present to clinic. Those with more persistent sensory issues, ulnar nerve subluxation, or atrophy have less predictable outcomes. Duration of symptoms plays a significant role in both conservative and surgical treatment outcomes. The rate of surgical complications is very low, and these are usually minor issues such as erythema. If decompression surgery is performed, at times a revision surgery is still necessary to transpose the ulnar nerve. Overall, patient satisfaction achieved through surgical decompression is very high due to the improvements in sensory loss and pain, coupled with the short recovery time.

The syndromes discussed in this chapter are the two most common upper extremity entrapment neuropathies; thus, the primary care physician plays an important role in the initial care of these patients. A summary of carpal tunnel syndrome and cubital tunnel syndrome, including their presentation, diagnostic testing, conservative management, indications for referral and/or surgery, and operative management is provided below (Table 15.3).

Table 15.3 Summary of carpal tunnel syndrome and cubital tunnel syndrome

Clinical entity	Presentation	Diagnostic testing	Conservative management	Indications for surgery	Operative management
Carpal tunnel syndrome	Paresthesia in thumb, index, long, and half of ring finger; nocturnal hand pain	Electrodiagnostic testing for atypical clinical presentations and when surgery is indicated	Splinting, activity modification, diuretics (those with substantial peripheral edema), corticosteroid injections	Failed conservative treatment, muscle atrophy or weakness, constant paresthesia, CTS as a result of trauma	Division of the transverse carpal ligament (carpal tunnel release)
Cubital tunnel syndrome	Paresthesia in the ring finger or little finger, medial elbow pain, can have intrinsic muscle weakness with grasping	Electrodiagnostic testing for atypical clinical presentations and when surgery is indicated	Splinting and activity modification	Failed conservative treatment, muscle atrophy or weakness, constant paresthesia	Cubital tunnel release or ulnar nerve transposition

Suggested Reading

Blazar PE, Floyd WE 4th, Han CH, et al. Prognostic indicators for recurrent symptoms after a single corticosteroid injection for carpal tunnel syndrome. J Bone Joint Surg Am. 2015;97(19):1563–70.

Elhassan B, Steinmann SP. Entrapment neuropathy of the ulnar nerve. J Am Acad Orthop Surg. 2007;15(11):672–81.

Jain NB, Higgins LD, Losina E, et al. Epidemiology of musculoskeletal upper extremity ambulatory surgery in the United States. BMC Musculoskelet Disord. 2014;15:4.

Louie DL, Earp BE, Collins JE, et al. Outcomes of open carpal tunnel release at a minimum of ten years. J Bone Joint Surg Am. 2013;95(12):1067–73.

Part X
Knee

Chapter 16
Knee Osteoarthritis

Jeffrey N. Katz and Thomas S. Thornhill

Abbreviations

APM   Arthroscopic partial meniscectomy
COX   Cyclooxygenase
MRI   Magnetic resonance imaging
NSAID Nonsteroidal anti-inflammatory medication
OA   Osteoarthritis

Key Points
- Weight control and exercise are foundational management principles for knee OA
- Medications are directed at symptom control
- Total knee replacement is an effective, cost-effective intervention for advanced disease

Introduction

Osteoarthritis of the knee is characterized by pain, functional loss, and damage to cartilage, bone, meniscus, and other structures (Fig. 16.1).

J.N. Katz (✉) • T.S. Thornhill
Department of Orthopedic Surgery, Brigham and Women's Hospital, Harvard Medical School, 75 Francis Street, Boston, MA 02115, USA
e-mail: jnkatz@partners.org; tthornhill@partners.org

© Springer International Publishing AG 2018   269
J.N. Katz et al. (eds.), *Principles of Orthopedic Practice for Primary Care Providers*, https://doi.org/10.1007/978-3-319-68661-5_16

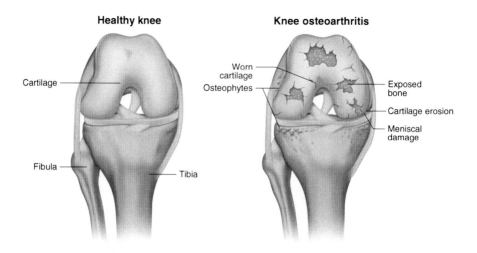

Fig. 16.1 A healthy knee and a knee with osteoarthritis, showing cartilage damage, osteophytes, and meniscal damage

Epidemiology

Osteoarthritis affects over 30 million Americans. The knee is among the mostly commonly involved joints, with symptomatic OA of the knee affecting over 14 million Americans and tens of millions more worldwide. OA is a costly condition. Over 600,000 persons in the US undergo total knee replacement, at a cost exceeding $12 billion. As with many chronic conditions, the indirect costs of lost productivity are even greater than the direct medical costs of osteoarthritis.

There are several important risk factors for knee osteoarthritis. The most powerful is age. While knee OA is uncommon in persons less than 40 years old, symptomatic radiographic knee OA occurs in over 15% of persons aged 65 or greater. With age, chondrocytes lose their capacity to produce the rich matrix of highly negatively charged macromolecules that enable cartilage to imbibe and retain fluid and bear load. Genetic factors also influence the loss of chondrocyte function. Obesity confers risk of OA both because of the excess biomechanical load borne by the knees of obese persons and due to metabolic factors associated with obesity. Prior injury is another powerful risk factor. Individuals who have sustained anterior cruciate ligament tears with concomitant meniscal tear by age 25, for example, face a lifetime risk of developing symptomatic, radiographic knee OA of around 30%. Long-standing occupational exposure to repetitive squatting confers risk, as does abnormal knee alignment (varus or excess valgus). Several medical conditions also may predispose to OA including hemochromatosis.

Clinical Presentation

History

The patient with osteoarthritis of the knee generally presents with gradual onset of knee pain with activity. Those with predominantly medial compartment disease typically perceive pain medially, and those with lateral compartment disease, laterally. It is possible, however, for patients with unicompartmental disease to feel pain on the contralateral side. Many patients will also have a global distribution of pain about the knee, reflecting concomitant involvement of the patella femoral and one or both tibiofemoral compartments. Pain rarely occurs at rest and is usually relieved by sitting or lying down. A complaint of stiffness is common and often associated with limited motion or an effusion. The quality of the pain varies; some patients describe it as sharp and others dull. Patients may notice intermittent swelling. Patients may also notice clicking, catching, popping, or a feeling that the knee is giving way. While these symptoms should alert the physician to the possible presence of a symptomatic meniscal tear, they may also arise from osteoarthritis per se (perhaps due to irregularities in the chondral surface of the osteoarthritic knee).

Patients may notice a gradual lack of knee flexion and extension. Stair climbing is frequently difficult for persons with knee OA, particularly those with involvement of the patellofemoral joint. Patients tend to seek care when they lose the capacity to perform valued activities, such as taking a walk with friends or climbing a flight of stairs in their house. Asking patients about their walking distance, the number of flights they can climb, and other functional activities that are relevant to their weekly routines is a useful way of assessing whether patients are improving or worsening. A number of patient reported outcome measures are available and are collected in clinical practice in some settings.

Physical Examination

Patients with knee OA often have an antalgic gait, in which they limp in attempt to place as little load across the knee as possible, for the shortest period of time. It is useful to observe knee alignment in the coronal plane. The normal alignment of the lower tibia compared to the thigh is about four degrees of valgus. Greater extent of valgus (tibia oriented excessively to toward the lateral side) overloads the lateral tibiofemoral compartment, while varus malalignment overloads the medial compartment. Patients with varus knees and more advanced OA may manifest a varus thrust with walking, in which the varus deformity is accentuated briefly as the patient pushes off in gait. Symptomatic patients tend to reduce weight bearing on the affected knee. As a result the examiner can often appreciate atrophy of the quadriceps (measured best 3 cm above the patella, as the vastus medialis obliquus is the most vulnerable muscle).

Tenderness is common over the medial or lateral joint line, depending on which compartment(s) are involved. Those with patellofemoral involvement often have pain with crepitus on manual compression of the patella against the femoral trochlea. Patients occasionally have palpable effusions; these are generally small and cool. Patients with effusions will sometimes have popliteal fullness on exam as well as pain, reflecting a popliteal cyst (Baker's cyst), which is a posterior outpouching of the synovium into the popliteal space. While range of motion tends to be preserved in early osteoarthritis, further in the course patients may develop limitations in flexion and extension.

Differential Diagnosis and Suggested Diagnostic Testing

Differential Diagnosis

The differential diagnosis of knee OA is broad. The chief challenge is not so much to determine whether the patient has knee OA but rather to discern whether knee OA is the principal source of the patient's symptoms or whether symptoms arise from one of several associated conditions. *Anserine bursitis* is a common source of pain in patients with knee OA. The anserine bursa is located at the insertion of the medial hamstring muscles into the tibia, just inferomedial to the tibial tubercle. Patients with *inflammatory arthritis* generally have warm effusions and often have involvement of other joints and prominent morning stiffness. *Infection* can generally be excluded on the basis of the more indolent presentation of osteoarthritis and the lack of warmth, substantial swelling, systemic symptoms, or monotonic worsening. A *strain of the medial collateral ligament* may mimic medial compartment osteoarthritis and can be identified by stressing the medial collateral ligament. *Patellofemoral dysfunction* due to malaligned patellar tracking tends to cause more diffuse anterior knee pain and can usually be provoked by patellofemoral compression. It is difficult to distinguish patellar dysfunction due to maltracking from patellofemoral OA; in fact, the two problems often overlap. (For more, see the chapter on patellofemoral syndromes in this text).

Meniscal tear is a frequent concomitant of knee osteoarthritis. Over 80% of patients with established osteoarthritis of the knee have meniscal tear on MRI. It is difficult to determine whether these tears are *symptomatic*. Popping, clicking, and catching sensations alert the physician to the possibility of meniscal tear, but these symptoms are nonspecific and may arise from osteoarthritis per se. The McMurray maneuver has modest diagnostic value. The examiner flexes and extends the knee using torque on the joint to stress the medial and then the lateral compartment. The test is designed to elicit a painful clicking sensation due to the direct irritation of the torn meniscus by loading and each tibiofemoral compartment through an arc of motion.

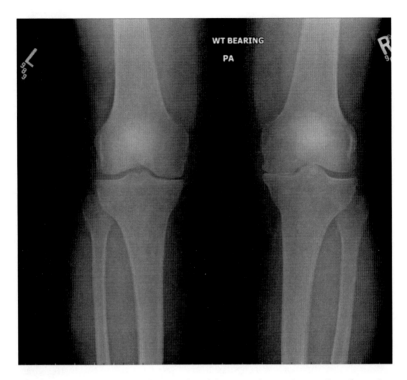

Fig. 16.2 Bilateral osteoarthritis with complete joint space loss and osteophyte formation medially on right; moderate to severe joint space loss on left

Diagnostic Testing

The diagnosis of knee OA can generally be made on the basis of characteristic history and physical examination findings, with no need for radiographs, advanced imaging, or blood tests. Radiographs obtained with the patient standing demonstrate the extent of joint space loss and osteophyte formation and are useful for assessing the severity of knee OA (Fig. 16.2). Flexed weight-bearing views are useful for assessing the extent of lateral compartment loss. Knee MRI is not necessary to diagnose knee OA but is sometimes used to evaluate for other problems that may mimic or accompany knee OA, such as meniscal tear. MRI should be ordered with caution in this setting, since over one third of all adults have meniscal tears and well over half of adults with knee OA have meniscal tears on MRI. MRI also provides detailed evaluation of OA features besides joint space loss and oteophytes, such as bone marrow lesions, synovitis, and effusion. Bone marrow lesions are subchondral areas of fluid signal on MRI. They are thought to arise from overload of subchondral bone (due, e.g., to destruction of the articular cartilage and/or meniscus, both of which bear load that is directly transmitted to subchondral bone when these tissues fail).

Nonoperative Management

Exercise and Core Lifestyle Changes

Substantial evidence documents that regular walking, knee strengthening, weight loss (for obese patients), and stretching to preserve a normal range of knee motion are all helpful in reducing pain and functional limitations in persons with knee OA. Consequently, the management of knee osteoarthritis should begin with patient education and engagement in self-care to initiate and sustain these lifestyle modifications. Physical activity and weight loss are notoriously difficult lifestyle changes for many patients. Programs and strategies are available to patients in the community to help persons with OA make these lifestyle commitments. Referral to a physical therapist is often useful so that patients can learn appropriate exercise techniques for strengthening, stretching, and improving neuromotor control of the lower extremity.

Medications

There is no validated and commercially available disease-modifying drug capable of arresting the process of joint destruction in persons with OA. In the absence of disease modification, treatment focuses on symptom relief and preservation of functional status. Acetaminophen is generally the first line of therapy. It is quite safe unless patients have liver dysfunction, but its analgesic effects are weak. Nonsteroidal inflammatory drugs (NSAIDs) are more potent but carry more toxicity, particularly in older patients and those with cardiac, renal, and gastrointestinal comorbidities. Thus, these drugs need to be used carefully, if at all, in patients with these comorbid conditions. Gastroprotective agents (e.g., proton pump inhibitors and H-2 blockers) reduce the frequency of gastrointestinal events in NSAID users. Several NSAIDs are also available in topical form (e.g., diclofenac). The topical formulations have similar efficacy to oral NSAIDs with less toxicity. Traditional NSAIDs such as ibuprofen and naproxen are predominantly cyclooxygenase 1 (COX-1) inhibitors. Predominant COX-2 inhibitors (such as celecoxib) do not inhibit platelets and thus are good options for patients with bleeding disorders or who are taking anticoagulants. The COX-2 inhibitors do increase risk of hypertension and cardiovascular events and thus should be used with care in patients with cardiovascular comorbidity.

Patients with pain that does not respond to any of these measures are often prescribed opiates. This prescribing practice is controversial. On the one hand, patients have limited options for addressing their pain. On the other, opiates carry risks of somnolence, respiratory suppression, falls, cardiac events, tolerance, addiction, and diversion of pills into the community. Physicians and their patients should discuss the risks and benefits of opiates carefully in this setting. Patients with chronic pain due to OA may benefit from duloxitene—an atypical antidepressant—or gabapentin, an antiepileptic that has been useful for neuropathic pain. Many physicians will suggest duloxitene or gabapentin for patients with features of centralized pain, such as amplification of pain severity and broadening of pain location.

Intra-articular Injections

Intra-articular corticosteroid injections have been shown to be safe and effective, though transient in their effect. Some patients benefit from a strategy of two or three injections annually. This is particularly useful for patients who wish to delay or avoid TKA. Injections of hyaluronate and related products—viscosupplementation—involve greater costs than steroid injections, but the effect appears to persist longer. The guidelines of various authoritative societies are mixed with respect to viscosupplementation.

Indications for Surgery

Patients with knee OA who have not responded to nonoperative therapy may wish to consider surgical options. High-quality randomized controlled trial data document that arthroscopic surgery is no better than a sham control or than a physical therapy program in reducing pain due to significant knee OA. Thus, there is no role for arthroscopic surgery in the management of knee osteoarthritis, per se.

On the other hand, if patients have suspected meniscal tear in association with their osteoarthritis, arthroscopy can be considered. This issue is covered in greater detail in the chapter on meniscal tear. Several large trials have been completed on the efficacy of arthroscopic partial meniscectomy in patients with knee OA. One trial documented a clear advantage for surgery; another showed that surgery is no more efficacious than a sham arthroscopic partial meniscectomy. In two other trials, surgery showed no advantage over a PT-based regimen in the intention to treat analyses but better outcomes in the as-treated analyses. Experts have generally interpreted this evidence as supporting a strategy of initial rigorous physical therapy with an emphasis on strengthening, with consideration of surgery for patients who have not responded and who recognize that the efficacy of surgery in this setting is somewhat uncertain.

For the patient with symptomatic unicompartmental osteoarthritis despite trials of nonoperative therapy, several surgical options can be considered including osteotomy, unicompartmental knee arthroplasty, and total knee arthroplasty. Osteotomy usually involves doing a tibial opening wedge for medial varus arthritis and a femoral lateral opening or medial closing for the patient with lateral compartment OA. For the patient with unilateral medial compartment OA, the osteotomy is designed to shift load bearing to the lateral compartments. Similarly, for the patient with lateral compartment OA, the osteotomy is designed to shift load medially. This procedure tends to be particularly well suited to younger patients (e.g., those in their 40s) with a good range of motion. If these patients were to receive a total knee arthroplasty, it would carry a high risk of failing in the patient's lifetime, requiring one or more revisions. Osteotomy is done infrequently in the US—just 1 for every 300 total knee arthroplasties. It is performed more frequently in Australia and Europe. Patients and referring physicians interested in considering osteotomy should inquire about surgeons who have expertise with this operation.

Unicompartmental knee arthroplasty (UKA) is another reasonable option for patients with unicompartmental knee OA. It is typically used in two settings. First, as with osteotomy, unicondylar arthroplasty has a role in younger, active patients because revision of a unicompartmental knee replacement involves less loss of bone than revision of a total knee arthroplasty. UKA patients report that their knee feels more normal than those with total knee replacements. In older patients with uni-compartmental involvement, UKA is sometimes used because the procedure involves less bone resection and reaming and therefore has a lower risk of cardio-vascular compromise due to fat embolism.

Total knee replacement (TKR) is performed on over 600,000 persons with advanced knee osteoarthritis annually in the US. The principal indications include evidence of advanced OA on radiographs, pain-related loss of functional activities that are important to patients, and absence of comorbidities that would make the procedure unsafe or the rehabilitation unsuccessful. Thus patients with unstable coronary disease, advanced heart failure, or advanced neuromuscular diseases are not appropriate candidates.

In TKR, the tibial plateaus are resected and a tibial plate is inserted. The femoral condyles are similarly sacrificed and femoral implants inserted (Fig. 16.3). In most implant systems, these components are made of metal alloys, and they are separated by a polyethylene liner that rests on the tibial plate. Many surgeons routinely also resurface the patella. Both UKR and TKR are technically demanding procedures, and poor surgical technique is the most common mode of implant failure. The incidence of complications and poor functional outcome is lower if the surgery is done by an experienced, high-volume surgeon in a high-volume center.

Expected Outcomes of Surgery

Approximately 80–85% of patients experience marked pain relief following TKA. The remainder has less complete pain relief, and a few patients actually feel worse or are frankly dissatisfied. There is considerable research focused on why 15–20% of patients continue to have persistence of pain after TKR. It appears that postoperative pain in these patients may be due to problems other than the index knee, such as contralateral knee or hip arthritis. Also, these patients may have psychological traits associated with persistence of pain, including catastrophizing and depression.

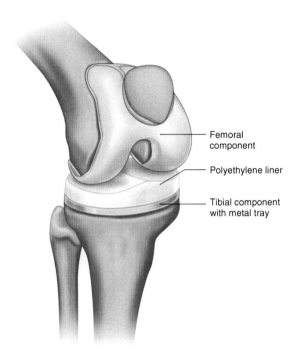

Femoral
component

Polyethylene liner

Tibial component
with metal tray

Fig. 16.3 Total knee replacement with femoral, tibial, and patellar components

Risks of complications depend upon the patient's general health. On average about 3–4% of patients have serious complications in the first 3 months after surgery including death, cardiac events, deep vein thrombosis or pulmonary embolus, pneumonia, or prosthetic infection. Over the longer term, infection remains a rare but worrisome risk and failure of the implant necessitating revision occurs at a rate of about 0.5% per year.

The outcomes of unicompartmental arthroplasty are similar to those of total knee arthroplasty. In most reports the risk of revision is somewhat higher for UKA than for TKA and the likelihood of symptomatic improvement similar. Osteotomy is less well studied but tends to have somewhat less complete pain relief than TKA. Patients undergoing osteotomy may ultimately develop OA on the weight-bearing side and at that point may progress to total knee replacement. The strategy guiding the use of osteotomy is to delay the need for TKA until the patient has reached his or her late 50s or 60s and faces a lower lifetime risk of TKA failure, which would necessitate revision.

Table 16.1 shows a summary of presentation and management of knee osteoarthritis.

Table 16.1. Summary of presentation and management of knee osteoarthritis

Presentation	Diagnostic testing	Conservative management	Indications for surgery	Operative management
Use-related pain and loss of valued activities	Diagnosis made by history and physical exam	Walking, quad strengthening, stretching	Persistent use-related pain and loss of valued activities despite conservative Rx	No role for arthroscopy in treating knee OA
Joint line tenderness	Radiographs to assess severity	Weight loss (if obese)		Role of arthroscopic surgery for OA with symptomatic meniscal tear evolving; requires careful discussion with physician
	MRI occasionally useful to exclude other entities	Analgesia (acetaminophen, NSAIDs, topical NSAIDs)	Patient understands and accepts short and long term risks	Osteotomy or unicondylar arthroplasty if unicompartmental OA
Occasional effusions		Intra-articular injection	Acceptable surgical risk	Total knee arthroplasty

OA osteoarthritis; *MRI* magnetic resonance imagining, *NSAIDs* nonsteroidal anti-inflammatory drugs

Suggested Reading

Deshpande BR, Katz JN, Solomon DH, et al. The number of persons with symptomatic knee osteoarthritis in the United States: impact of race/ethnicity, age, sex, and obesity. Arthritis Care Res. 2016;68(12):1743–50.

Katz JN, Brophy RH, Chaisson CE, et al. Surgery versus physical therapy for a meniscal tear and osteoarthritis. N Engl J Med. 2013;368:1–10.

Katz JN, Brownlee SA, Jones MH. The role of arthroscopy in the management of knee osteoarthritis. Best Pract Res Clin Rheumatol. 2014;28(1):143–56.

Konopka J, Gomoll AH, Thornhill TS, et al. The cost-effectiveness of surgical treatment of medial unicompartmental knee osteoarthritis in younger patients. J Bone Joint Surg Am. 2015;97:807–17.

Losina E, Weinstein AM, Reichmann WM, et al. Lifetime risk and age at diagnosis of symptomatic knee osteoarthritis in the US. Arthritis Care Res. 2013;65(5):703–11.

McAlindon TE, Bannuru RR, Sullivan MC, et al. OARSI guidelines for the non-surgical management of knee osteoarthritis. Osteoarthr Cartilage. 2014;22:363–88.

Moseley B, O'Malley K, Petersen NJ, et al. A controlled trial of arthroscopic surgery for osteoarthritis of the knee. N Engl J Med. 2002;347(2):81–8.

Sihvonen R, Paavola M, Malmivaara A, et al. Arthroscopic partial meniscectomy versus sham surgery for a degenerative meniscal tear. N Engl J Med. 2013;369:2515–24.

Skou ST, Roos EM, Simonsen O, et al. The effects of total knee replacement and non-surgical treatment on pain sensitization and clinical pain. Eur J Pain. 2016;20(10):1612–21.

Chapter 17
Cartilage Defects, Osteochondritis, and Osteonecrosis

Brian Mosier, Tom Minas, and Andreas H. Gomoll

Abbreviations

ACI	Autologous chondrocyte implantation
ACL	Anterior cruciate ligament
BMAC	Bone marrow aspirate concentrate
OAT	Osteochondral autograft transfer
OCD	Osteochondritis dissecans
PRP	Platelet rich plasma
SONK	Spontaneous osteonecrosis of the knee

Introduction

The spectrum of cartilage disease in the knee ranges from small isolated defects to end-stage osteoarthritis, each with differing treatment algorithms based on a multitude of patient and lesion characteristics. Chondral (cartilage) damage in the knee is a common finding during arthroscopy and can be due to a number of etiologies including acute or repetitive trauma, osteochondritis dissecans, and degenerative changes.

B. Mosier • A.H. Gomoll
Department of Orthopaedic Surgery, Brigham and Women's Hospital,
75 Francis Street, Boston, MA 02115, USA
e-mail: mosier619@gmail.com; agomoll@bwh.harvard.edu

T. Minas (✉)
Cartilage Repair Center, Brigham and Women's Hospital, Chestnut Hill, MA, USA
e-mail: tminas@bwh.harvard.edu

© Springer International Publishing AG 2018
J.N. Katz et al. (eds.), *Principles of Orthopedic Practice for Primary Care Providers*, https://doi.org/10.1007/978-3-319-68661-5_17

Fig. 17.1 Cartilage defect

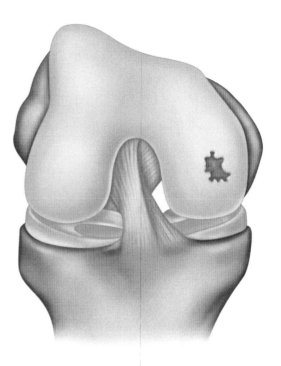

Chondral damage comes in many different forms. Typically the damaged portion of cartilage is classified according to its appearance, ranging from softening and swelling to partial-thickness fissures to full-thickness fissures and exposed subchondral bone. Full-thickness chondral defects, as discussed in this chapter, are focal injuries to the articular cartilage analogous to a pothole in the road (Fig. 17.1). They are classified according to their location and largest dimensions in order to guide treatment. Even though cartilage repair is generally indicated for the treatment of *focal* defects, it can be considered even in the case of *multiple* defects. However, there is no easy distinction between multiple isolated lesions versus early osteoarthritis. As a rule of thumb, patients considered for cartilage repair procedures should have a BMI less than 35, age less than 55 years, not smoke, and be able to comply with the prolonged rehabilitation that is necessary for many of the procedures.

In this chapter we discuss the management and treatments of cartilage disease, focusing on focal full-thickness cartilage defects (rather than established degenerative changes, which will be discussed in a different chapter). We also highlight two specific associated conditions, osteochondritis dissecans and osteonecrosis.

Cartilage Defects

Epidemiology

Symptomatic osteoarthritis of the knee affects over seven million persons in the US and accounts for tens of billions of dollars per year in direct and indirect medical expenses. The incidence of symptomatic osteoarthritis is increased in patients who have had a prior knee injury, especially injuries affecting the articular cartilage and/ or meniscus. The incidence of knee injuries is increasing, particularly ACL ruptures, patellar dislocations, and meniscal tears. These injuries are frequently associated with injuries to the articular surface and subchondral bone, which can compromise long-term outcomes and cartilage health. As discussed above, there is a high incidence of articular cartilage injury seen during arthroscopy; however, determining which defects require treatment—and with which modality—is key to successful outcomes.

Clinical Presentation

Patients seen in the office with symptomatic cartilage injuries have a wide variety of clinical presentations. Cartilage itself is an aneural structure; therefore, the pain resulting from a chondral injury is thought to be due to secondary damage of underlying subchondral bone or of surrounding soft tissues or to reactive synovitis from resultant debris. The patient may complain of mechanical symptoms such as catching or locking, which can result from a flap or delamination of the chondral surface. Both rapidly occurring hemarthrosis after injury and recurrent effusions are concerning and should raise suspicions of structural intra-articular damage, such as an ACL tear or intra-articular osteochondral fracture. The presence of such damage will require further investigation. In patients with a known injury, it is important to ascertain what treatments were rendered and what, if any, surgery was performed. If the patient had surgery, the intraoperative findings should be noted, as should the patient's response: did the patient experience at least transient pain relief? Lastly, it is important to gain a sense of the patient's activity level, functional demands, and goals for treatment; these factors (along with the patient's age) will guide treatment. In deciding on treatments, it is important to consider the modest healing capacity of cartilage, the complex nature of surgical treatment, and the lengthy rehabilitation protocols. The physician must engage the patient as an active member of the shared decision-making process in order to obtain the best possible functional outcome and highest patient satisfaction.

Differential Diagnosis

The diagnosis of cartilage defects is challenging given the vague and nonspecific symptoms that may be present and the clinical overlap that can occur with other pathologic entities such as meniscal tears. Symptomatic cartilage defects of the femoral condyles, similar to meniscal injuries, can result in joint line pain, mechanical symptoms of catching and clicking, and recurrent effusions. Cartilage defects within the patellofemoral compartment can present with pain associated with ascending or descending stairs, kneeling, squatting, and any other activity requiring prolonged or deep knee flexion. Patients with early osteoarthritis can present with all of the above, including pain with increased activity or impact.

Imaging

Painful mechanical symptoms, activity-related joint pain and recurrent swelling present a broad differential diagnosis. Therefore, patients with these complaints are often investigated with imaging modalities.

The initial work-up of a patient with knee pain concerning for cartilage injury should include weight-bearing radiographs. The typical series consists of an antero-posterior view, a Rosenberg flexed posteroanterior view, and lateral and merchant (patellar) views. While X-rays will not demonstrate specific cartilage lesions, they are useful to determine the amount of degenerative change that may be present due to osteoarthritis and can assess for prior evidence of injury or surgery. In patients who will be undergoing surgery, full-length alignment films should be performed to assess the mechanical axis of the lower extremity for malalignment that could require realignment osteotomy.

Magnetic resonance imaging (MRI) with high-resolution sequences is the imaging modality of choice to evaluate the chondral surfaces of the knee. Indications for MRI include evidence of joint line pain (by history and physical exam), swelling and/or mechanical symptoms. The development of cartilage-specific sequences such as proton density fat suppression (PDFS) has greatly improved our ability to accurately assess for the presence of cartilage defects. MRI also has the benefit of evaluating the joint for associated injuries to the ligaments or menisci and the presence of edema or cystic change in the subchondral bone, in order to help guide treatment as discussed further on in the chapter.

Computed tomography (CT), especially when obtained with arthrography, is a useful modality in patients unable to tolerate an MRI, or when associated bony pathology exists, such as in the case of osteochondritis dissecans (OCD) lesions (which are discussed later in this chapter). Advanced imaging with CT and MRI can also be a useful tool to evaluate biomechanical and anatomic factors such as trochlear dysplasia and patellar maltracking.

Nonoperative Management

The aim of conservative, nonoperative management should be symptom reduction followed by progression to strengthening and restoration of normal kinematics. Standard protocols of rest, ice, and anti-inflammatories are a mainstay of early treatment. Intra-articular corticosteroid injections can be a useful adjunct to decrease inflammation—especially in patients with acute flare–ups—even in the setting of advanced degenerative changes. Meanwhile viscosupplementation can alleviate symptoms in those with moderate osteoarthritis. More recent therapies such as platelet rich plasma (PRP), bone marrow aspirate concentrate (BMAC), and stem cell injections are being investigated; while some early results appear promising, further research is needed to delineate the efficacy of these approaches.

Other modalities that have been shown to help improve function in patients with cartilage injuries include bracing and physical therapy. Unloader braces, which shift the mechanical axis toward the unaffected weight-bearing portion of the joint, have demonstrated good results but are difficult to tolerate long term. Disadvantages of these braces include noncompliance, as some models may be too bulky for patients to tolerate—as well as the high cost. Physical therapy is another common treatment strategy, especially in patients with defects of the patellofemoral joint. Strengthening of the quadriceps has long been a tenet of physiotherapy programs aimed at reducing patellofemoral symptoms; however, as our understanding of lower extremity kinematics has improved, the focus of therapy has broadened to include hip and core musculature strengthening. These comprehensive programs have been shown to improve patellofemoral tracking and unload the joint to an extent that allows for relief of symptoms in a high percentage of patients.

Indications for Surgery

The decision for surgical intervention is generally based on the patient's response to conservative measures and the extent of structural damage, as well as the patient's age and physical demands. Cartilage repair or reconstruction is indicated for full-thickness symptomatic lesions in physiologically younger patients with recurrent pain and swelling during activities of daily living (ADLs). Contraindications for cartilage repair procedures include generalized tricompartmental arthritis, inflammatory arthritis, obesity, and nicotine use. Nicotine has been shown to negatively affect cartilage metabolism with decreased patient-reported outcomes and survival rates in multiple clinical studies. While there is no strict age limit for cartilage repair, age often functions as a surrogate for the extent of degenerative changes. Therefore, cartilage repair procedures are uncommon in patients older than 55.

Operative Management

Surgical management of cartilage defects is largely based on the size, depth, and location of the lesion. As the field of biologic reconstruction for cartilage injury evolves, techniques and indications for surgery continue to expand. Due to the limited innate ability of cartilage to heal, the use of traditional techniques in combination with emerging technologies including mesenchymal stem cells, platelet concentrates, and growth factors is a rapidly expanding point of interest. However, given the scope of this text, we will focus on providing an overview of the most commonly used surgical techniques in current clinical practice for the treatment of full-thickness cartilage lesions, as well as their observed outcomes.

Surgical Treatment for Small Cartilage Defects (<2 cm²)

Debridement/Chondroplasty

Chondroplasty is a widely performed arthroscopic procedure that is indicated for incidental findings during knee arthroscopy for pathology other than a cartilage defect (such as meniscal tear), small lesions in patients with lower functional demands, and in some instances, in-season athletes to carry them through the season until a more definitive intervention can be performed in the off-season. The goal of chondroplasty is thorough debridement of unstable flaps and loose tissue with the formation of a stable edge. Care should be taken to preserve the integrity of, and prevent undue damage to, the subchondral bone. With the correct indications and proper technique, chondroplasty can provide short-term symptomatic relief in up to 75% of patients in some series; however, there is limited evidence as to the extent and duration of benefit from this intervention. Postoperatively the patients can be weight bearing as tolerated and can resume activities once the postsurgical pain and swelling have subsided.

Marrow Stimulation

Microfracture is a marrow stimulation technique performed arthroscopically that was popularized over 20 years ago for the treatment of full-thickness cartilage defects. Similar to debridement and chondroplasty, microfracture is one of the most commonly performed procedures due to its low cost and familiarity among most orthopedic surgeons. The technique is indicated for cartilage defects of the femoral condyles and trochlea that are less 2 cm² and completely surrounded by a healthy rim of native cartilage tissue, in patients with moderate physical requirements. Marrow stimulation techniques, including microfracture, use awls or drills to create multiple perforations in the bed of the lesion, 2–3 mm apart, that penetrate the subchondral plate to allow for elution of marrow elements, resulting in the formation of a clot containing mesenchymal stem cells. Over time this clot matures into a fibro-cartilaginous tissue that fills the defect. This repair tissue lacks the intricate zonal organization and wear properties of native hyaline cartilage. Due to the inferior tissue created with marrow stimulation techniques, studies have demonstrated that outcomes are generally satisfactory in the first 2–3 years postoperatively but then begin to decline. Of note, a history of prior microfracture has been shown to worsen outcomes of certain subsequent revision procedures performed in the same compartment, such as autologous chondrocyte implantation (ACI); therefore, caution should be used while employing this technique as it can have a deleterious impact on future interventions.

Osteochondral Autograft Transfer (OAT)

OAT is primarily indicated for defects of the femoral condyles, less commonly for the patellofemoral joint. OAT is performed by creating a cylindrical recipient socket in the defect area that is filled with a corresponding cylindrical osteochondral plug taken from the intercondylar notch or the periphery of the trochlea of the same knee. The advantage of this technique is that it transfers mature hyaline cartilage to the defect along with a bony component that can address diseased subchondral bone. With proper technique and indications, the OAT technique has demonstrated good to excellent results in mid- to long-term follow-up. In randomized clinical trials, OAT has been shown to outperform microfracture in young active patients. Failure with OAT technique is seen if plugs are left prominent, extending past the native articular surface. This results in increased stresses to the transferred chondral surface and poor incorporation of the bony portion, resulting in resorption and cystic changes.

Surgical Treatment of Large Cartilage Defects (>2–4 cm^2)

Cell-Based Therapy

Autologous chondrocyte implantation (ACI) is one of the more common cell-based therapies used today for large symptomatic full-thickness lesions of the femoral condyles and the patellofemoral joint. Although it is only FDA approved for the femoral condyles, many surgeons use it to treat the patellofemoral joint as well, since the unique topography of the patellofemoral joint can be difficult to recreate with other techniques. ACI involves a two-stage process whereby an initial diagnostic arthroscopy is performed to document the size and location of the defect, as well as to obtain a cartilage biopsy from a lesser weight-bearing portion of the knee, usually the intercondylar notch. The cells are then sent off to a lab facility where they are expanded in culture and cryopreserved until implantation. The second stage is performed via an open procedure to debride the bed of the defect of fibrous tissue and create stable vertical walls. A collagen patch is then sewn in place to cover the

Fig. 17.2 Radiograph of spontaneous osteonecrosis of the knee (SONK)

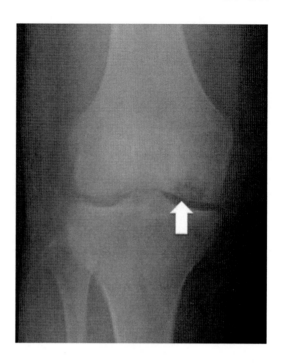

defect and create a closed space (Fig. 17.2). The suture line is sealed with fibrin glue, and the chondrocyte suspension is injected underneath the patch. The rehabilitation process for ACI is quite complex. For 6 weeks after implantation on a weight-bearing condyle, patients are made "touch down" weight bearing, meaning that they are permitted to put minimal weight on the affected extremity. Return to full weight bearing is permitted at 10–12 weeks and return to full sporting activities at a minimum of 1 year to allow for maturation of the reparative tissue. In experienced hands ACI has demonstrated good and excellent outcomes with pain relief and return to functional activities in 75% of patients. Complications of ACI vary with the most common being stiffness and hypertrophy of the transplanted surface; chondroplasty is required if mechanical symptoms persist, in approximately 5% of patients.

Osteochondral Allograft Transplantation

The use of osteochondral allograft transplantation has increased substantially since the early 2000s, when stricter procurement and storage regulations were brought upon tissue banks after a series of poor outcomes with the use of contaminated fresh allografts. Since these changes, the risk of disease transmission and infection has been considered minimal, with no documented cases of transmission of HIV or hepatitis for nearly 20 years. Indications for osteochondral allografting include large focal chondral and osteochondral defects after trauma, osteochondritis dissecans lesions, and salvage for prior failed cartilage restoration techniques. The technique is similar to osteochondral autograft transfer in that first a recipient socket is created. A corresponding osteochondral plug is then prepared from the same anatomical location on the size-, side- and compartment-matched allograft hemicondyle. The plug is thoroughly irrigated with pulsatile lavage to remove any residual donor bone marrow, reducing the antigenicity of the graft. The plug is then press-fit into the recipient socket in the correct orientation, avoiding high seating forces, which could injure or kill the chondrocytes.

Treatment of large cartilage defects with the use of osteochondral allografts has increased over the last decade, given the shorter rehabilitation than with cell-based techniques and the demonstration of good to excellent results in a number of cases series. Most series report pain relief in 85% of patients at 10 years. While long-term failure is controversial, a recent systematic review demonstrated a short-term complication rate of 2.4%. If failure occurs this is most commonly due to failure of incorporation of the bony portion of the graft. In cases of graft failure, revision osteochondral allograft transplantation is frequently an option.

Postoperative rehabilitation regimens vary based on surgeon preference and technique. If screws are used for graft fixation in a weight-bearing condyle, then weight bearing is limited until the screws are removed at 3–4 months. If the graft is satisfactorily press-fit and no fixation is used, then generally patients are allowed to be fully weight bearing by the 6-week mark.

Osteochondritis Dissecans (OCD) Lesions

OCD is best thought of as a disease of the subchondral bone with secondary effects on the overlying articular cartilage. Multiple classification and description schematics exist according to the patient's age, location of the lesion, and appearance—both on imaging studies and by surgical evaluation. The etiology of OCD and the exact mechanism by which these changes occur are still highly controversial; however, most believe that it is likely multifactorial in nature with histopathological studies failing to demonstrate osteonecrosis or an ischemic insult as the primary mechanism. One important distinction to note is that the name implies an inflammatory process; however, multiple studies have ruled this out. Currently, the most common theory indicates that genetics may play a role as well as repetitive microtrauma.

OCD lesions typically affect patients in their second decade of life with a higher incidence seen in males and with about one-quarter of patients demonstrating bilateral findings. The most common location for OCD lesions in the knee is on the lateral aspect of the medial femoral condyle. The treatment for OCD lesions is primarily based on the status of the physes and secondarily on symptoms and characteristics of the lesion. Patients with knee pain and/or swelling should be evaluated with radiographs and MRI to fully assess the lesion. Radiographs are helpful to determine bone age and mechanical alignment. Often the OCD lesion can be seen on X-ray as an area of increased lucency in comparison to the surrounding bone (Fig. 17.3). Through MRI and surgical evaluation, OCD lesions are typically

Fig. 17.3 Autologous
cartilage implantation

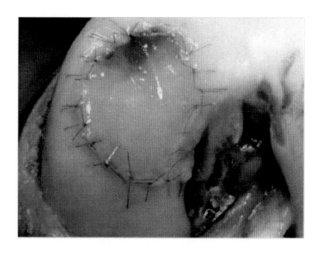

described by the appearance of the overlying articular cartilage with attention to softening and swelling, stable/partially detached flaps, or completely detached osteochondral loose bodies. MRI is useful for analyzing the integrity of the cartilage surface as well as the extent of pathology within the subchondral bone. Classifying the lesion by MRI can be a useful tool to help guide treatment. OCD lesions should be assessed on T2-weighted images and classified according to the extent of demarcation within the bony portion of the lesion, as well as the presence of fluid between the fragment and the underlying bone.

In patients with non-displaced OCD lesions and open growth plates, the treatment should be generally conservative with protected weight bearing, bracing, and modalities aimed at decreasing mechanical stress and inflammation within the joint. The majority of juveniles and most adolescents with open growth plates will heal non-displaced stable lesions. However, any lesion in adults is unlikely to heal. In young patients with non-displaced OCD lesions who fail conservative management, arthroscopic retrograde drilling of the defect with and without internal fixation is an established treatment alternative. In patients with unstable or displaced OCD lesions (as evidenced by fluid behind the fragment), surgery is usually indicated as the primary treatment given the low chance of success with conservative management. If there is intact articular cartilage, every attempt should be made to repair rather than remove the fragment in adolescents. Techniques vary but generally involve removal of diseased bone/cysts, autologous bone grafting, and fixation of the fragment. In juveniles with closed physes and adults with displaced OCD lesions, treatment depends on the amount of subchondral bone attached to the loose fragment. Fragments with a bony portion attached can be repaired by open reduction and internal fixation with bone grafting of the defect. Adult patients with completely displaced lesions usually require surgical intervention as these have been shown to progress toward symptomatic arthritis. Adult OCD lesions can be treated with a variety of methods; however, osteochondral allograft transplantation has grown in popularity with good to excellent results in approximately 75% of cases at 15 years follow-up.

Osteonecrosis of the Knee

Osteonecrosis of the knee has historically been divided into different types including primary or spontaneous osteonecrosis of the knee (SONK) and secondary osteonecrosis seen primarily in patients with high alcohol use, steroid treatment, or blood dyscrasias such as sickle cell anemia. Classically, SONK occurs more commonly in patients greater than 60 years old and most commonly affects the medial femoral condyle. More recently, SONK has been reclassified as a stress fracture frequently associated with posterior root medial meniscus tears rather than osteonecrosis. Yamamoto et al. published a case series of patients diagnosed with SONK and demonstrated that a subchondral insufficiency fracture was the primary event leading to localized osteonecrosis in the knee.

The Koshino classification is the most commonly used system, with stage one representing patients with clinical findings but normal radiologic studies. Stage two represents subchondral bone changes, while stage three demonstrates collapse on radiographs. Stage four represents degenerative disease with the classic signs of subchondral sclerosis and osteophyte formation.

Patients with secondary osteonecrosis of the knee are typically younger than those with SONK. The most common causes of secondary osteonecrosis of the knee are steroid and alcohol use. Just as in SONK, the femoral condyles are the most commonly affected; however, a substantial portion also develop osteonecrosis of the tibia or femoral diaphysis as well. The clinical presentation in patients with secondary osteonecrosis is usually insidious in onset. Symptomatic patients with secondary osteonecrosis very frequently require surgical intervention.

Patients with evidence of early osteonecrosis should initially be treated with protected weight bearing and other modalities, such as NSAIDs, aimed at reducing symptoms. Bisphosphonate treatment of early osteonecrosis has received substantial attention; however, a recent randomized placebo-controlled trial by Meier et al. demonstrated no benefit of bisphosphonates over traditional anti-inflammatories. Surgical management is reserved for patients with large lesions or those who fail to improve with conservative measures. In patients with intact articular surface, arthroscopic guided core decompression is a viable treatment option. In young patients with articular collapse, osteochondral allograft transplantation has been used with success. In older patients with collapse and evidence of osteoarthritis, treatment with unicompartmental or total knee arthroplasty has consistently demonstrated good results.

Summary

Cartilage repair is a viable treatment option for physiologically young patients with focal cartilage defects who failed conservative management. The field of biologic joint reconstruction continues to evolve rapidly and new treatment options including stem cell treatments are being explored. Current treatment options have been successful in delaying the need for joint replacement in young patients with intolerable symptoms.

Suggested Reading

Gomoll AH, Minas T. The quality of healing: articular cartilage. Wound Repair Regen. 2014;22(Suppl 1):30–8.

Henn RF 3rd, Gomoll AH. A review of the evaluation and management of cartilage defects in the knee. Phys Sportsmed. 2011;39(1):101–7.

Kanneganti P, Harris JD, Brophy RH. The effect of smoking on ligament and cartilage surgery in the knee: a systematic review. Am J Sports Med. 2012;40(12):2872–8.

Karim AR, Cherian JJ, Jauregui JJ, Pierce T, Mont MA. Osteonecrosis of the knee: review. Ann Transl Med. 2015;3(1):6. https://doi.org/10.3978/j.issn.2305-5839.2014.11.13.

Mall NA, Harris JD, Cole BJ. Clinical evaluation and preoperative planning of articular cartilage injuries of the knee. J Am Acad Orthop Surg. 2015;23(10):633–40.

Meier C, Kraenzlin C, Friederich NF, Wischer T, Grize L, Meier CR, Kraenzlin ME. Effect of ibandronate on spontaneous osteonecrosis of the knee: a randomized, double-blind, placebo-controlled trial. Osteoporos Int. 2014;25(1):359–66.

Minas T, Von Keudell A, Bryant T, Gomoll AH. The john insall award: a minimum of 10-year outcome study of autologous chondrocyte implantation. Clin Orthop Relat Res. 2014;472(1):41–51.

Schulz JF, Chambers HG. Juvenile osteochondritis dissecans of the knee: current concepts in diagnosis and management. Instr Course Lect. 2013;62:455–67.

Yamamoto T, Bullough PG. Spontaneous osteonecrosis of the knee: the result of subchondral insufficiency fracture. J Bone Joint Surg Am. 2000;82:858–66.

Chapter 18
Meniscal and Ligamentous Injuries of the Knee

Emily M. Brook and Elizabeth Matzkin

Abbreviations

ACL	Anterior cruciate ligament
BMI	Body mass index
LCL	Lateral collateral ligament
MCL	Medial collateral ligament
MRI	Magnetic resonance imaging
NSAID	Nonsteroidal anti-inflammatory drug
OA	Osteoarthritis
PCL	Posterior cruciate ligament

The Meniscus

The meniscus is a c-shaped fibrocartilaginous structure that lies between the femur and tibia on the medial and lateral aspects of the knee (Fig. 18.1). The meniscus serves as a cushion by absorbing the impact of weight-bearing forces, preventing bone-on-bone contact between the femoral condyle and tibial plateau. The meniscus is an important structure for both load bearing and stability of the knee joint.

Summary of Epidemiology

Meniscal injuries are a common source of knee pain and can occur in traumatic or nontraumatic settings. Traumatic meniscal tears most frequently occur in young and active individuals aged 15–45. Over a third of traumatic meniscal tears are related

E.M. Brook • E. Matzkin (✉)
Department of Orthopedic Surgery, Brigham and Women's Hospital,
75 Francis Street, Boston, MA 02115, USA
e-mail: ebrook@partners.org; ematzkin@partners.org

© Springer International Publishing AG 2018   291
J.N. Katz et al. (eds.), *Principles of Orthopedic Practice for Primary Care Providers*, https://doi.org/10.1007/978-3-319-68661-5_18

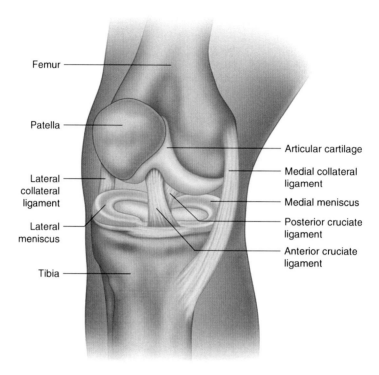

Fig. 18.1 The anatomy of the knee joint

to cutting and pivoting motions in sporting activities. Nontraumatic or degenerative meniscal tears most frequently present in older individuals, aged 45–70, and are often associated with osteoarthritis (OA). Individuals with a higher body mass index (BMI) have a greater occurrence of degenerative meniscal injury due to increased weight-bearing forces on the knee. In addition, medial meniscal tears are more common than lateral meniscal tears.

Clinical Presentation

Traumatic Meniscal Tears

Traumatic meniscal injuries are common injuries within the young and active population causing pain, loss of motion, and limitations in function. Common mechanisms of injury are noncontact decelerations including cutting and pivoting movements. These mechanisms of injury can be quite traumatic to the knee joint, and often there is a concomitant ligamentous injury. Traumatic meniscal tears commonly present with an effusion, pain, mechanical symptoms such as a locking or catching sensation, or a feeling of instability if a ligamentous injury is also involved. After an incident or event of the type described above, patients often have an immediate onset of pain that prevents them from continuing the activity or sport. Pain is localized to either the medial or lateral joint line, depending on the location of the tear. However, pain can be diffuse if a concurrent ligamentous injury is present. Individuals with a traumatic meniscal tear may report inability to fully flex or extend the knee because it is "stuck." A mechanical block with significant functional limitations may occur when the flipped edge of a torn meniscus catches between the femoral condyle and tibial plateau.

Degenerative Meniscal Tears

Degenerative meniscal tears can be difficult to diagnose because of vague or variable symptoms in addition to the presence of concomitant osteoarthritis in the knee. Not all degenerative meniscal tears are symptomatic, and patients typically do not report any history of specific trauma or injury to the knee. Patients often describe a gradual onset of pain and symptoms associated with an active lifestyle. An effusion may or may not be present at the time of clinical presentation, although many patients report a history of swelling after an increase in activity level or duration of exercise. Degenerative meniscal tears typically present with pain and point tenderness localized to the posterior aspect of the medial or lateral joint line, depending on the location of the tear. Mechanical symptoms such as catching and locking are not always present. Instead, the chief complaint may be activity limitation secondary to pain.

Physical Examination

Physical examination and evaluation of knee pain starts with a thorough patient history. It is important to gather information on whether the knee pain occurred in a traumatic versus nontraumatic setting and the specific mechanism of injury. A proper physical examination includes inspection, palpation, range of motion, and specific tests for the suspected meniscal injury. The clinician should inspect both the affected and unaffected knee for effusion and bruising or discoloration. Determine if there is any tenderness along the medial and lateral joint lines. This is the most sensitive test for a meniscal tear. Perform a ballottement test by placing one hand above the patella and the other hand below the patella and pushing inward with both hands to check for fluid in the knee, and compare it to the contralateral side.

The range of motion should be assessed with the patient supine on an examination Table. A normal finding for range of motion is 0 degrees of extension and 135 degrees of flexion.

The McMurray test should be performed as part of a standard physical examination of the knee. The McMurray test is performed with the patient lying supine and

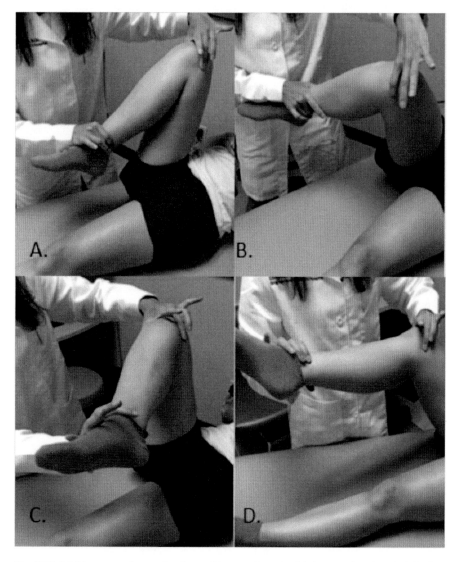

Fig. 18.2 McMurray test for meniscal tears. The examiner should place one hand on the joint line and the other hand around the ankle or heel (**a**). To test the medial meniscus, the examiner should rotate the lower leg externally (**b**). For the lateral meniscus, the examiner should rotate the lower leg internally (**c, d**)

the knee flexed to approximately 90° (Fig. 18.2). The examiner should have one hand over the joint line with the fingers placed on the medial joint line and the thumb placed on the lateral joint line. The other hand is placed at the heel of the foot (Fig. 18.2a). To test for a medial meniscal injury, the examiner should rotate the tibia externally, applying valgus stress to the knee, and twist the heel in an attempt to impinge any unstable torn edges of the meniscus (Fig. 18.2b). The presence of a lateral meniscal injury should be tested by rotating the tibia internally, applying varus stress to the knee, and twisting the heel in a similar fashion (Fig. 18.2c, d). A positive McMurray test is a "click" felt by the examiner along the joint line. However, a pseudo-positive test may not elicit a click, but rather pain with the motion. The sensitivity of the McMurray test is varied in the literature; one study reported a sensitivity of 50% on the medial side and 21% on the lateral side in 121 patients with meniscal injuries. Another study noted that a positive McMurray sign is indicative of good postoperative outcomes in patients with a meniscal lesion and concomitant osteoarthritis. Another examination for meniscal injury is the deep squat test. The examiner should have the patient bend into a deep squat where the knee is loaded and flexed past 90°. This allows the examiner to determine any pain coming from the meniscus as a deep squat may cause an impingement of the posterior horn of the meniscus against the femoral condyle. However, if the patient has an acute onset of injury and a large effusion, he or she may not be able to perform the deep squat test.

Suggested Imaging

All patients presenting with traumatic or persistent knee pain should have plain radiographs obtained. Anterior-posterior, lateral, sunrise, and bilateral weight-bearing views should be obtained to rule out presence of a fracture or bony pathology. Radiographs can be helpful in identifying osteoarthritis, which is associated with a degenerative meniscal tear.

Magnetic resonance imaging (MRI) is particularly useful in patients with minimal or no knee osteoarthritis. An MRI should be considered in the presence of an acute onset of knee pain or persistent pain that limits daily activities and has failed conservative treatment measures. A systematic review by Oei et al. (2003) of 29 articles indicated that MRI had a sensitivity of 93.3% for a medial meniscal tear and 79.3% for a lateral meniscal tear. The specificity was 88.4% and 95.7% for medial and lateral meniscal tears, respectively. MRI is highly effective in determining the specific type, size, and location of a meniscal tear, especially when planning surgical intervention.

Non-operative Management

Not all meniscal injuries require surgical intervention, and many degenerative meniscal tears that are not impinging significantly between the femur and tibia can be managed non-operatively. If a diagnosed meniscal injury is suspected, but it is not causing significant mechanical symptoms or limitations, non-operative management should be considered. It is important for the patient to understand that degenerative meniscal tears rarely extend to the vascular component of the meniscus and therefore have poor healing potential. Non-operative modalities such as physical therapy, regular use of ice and NSAIDS, and corticosteroid injections can help to alleviate the symptoms of a chronic degenerative meniscal tear. Physical therapy to maximize proximal musculature strength reduces the weight-bearing forces on the knee and can improve symptoms. An ice and NSAID regimen can help to alleviate swelling and provide pain relief. Symptomatic episodes with swelling and pain can be treated with an intra-articular corticosteroid injection, often allowing the patient to continue physical therapy or home exercise programs.

Outcomes of Conservative Treatment Measures

Traumatic Meniscal Tears

Traumatic meniscal tears tend to occur in patients under the age of 30 and often cannot be managed effectively with conservative treatments. These tears usually cause swelling and limitation not only of athletic activities but also of activities of daily living. In a bucket-handle meniscal tear, a flipped piece of meniscal tissue causes a mechanical block, preventing the patient from fully extending or flexing their knee. These tears generally do not respond to conservative measures and require prompt evaluation, reduction, and surgical repair.

Degenerative Meniscal Tears

Physical therapy or structured exercise programs can be successful in reducing symptoms and improving function from chronic degenerative meniscal tears. Several studies published in the last few years that compared surgical intervention versus non-operative strengthening exercises in patients with degenerative medial meniscal tears showed that both the operative and non-operative groups had significant pain relief and improved function at 2-year follow-up. Another study (Neogi et al. 2013) of patients with degenerative medial meniscal tears showed that a 6-week course of analgesics combined with a formal exercise program provided pain relief and improved function up to 6 months after initial diagnosis, but benefits began to decline. The study found that osteoarthritis continued to progress and was associated with worse outcomes in the long term. Current literature suggests an initial non-operative treatment protocol consisting of analgesics and a formal or home exercise program before considering surgical intervention in the treatment of chronic degenerative meniscal tears.

Indications for Surgical Intervention

Patients presenting with a traumatic meniscal injury with pain, mechanical symptoms, and an MRI confirming a torn edge of the meniscus may require surgical intervention. Bucket-handle-type meniscal injuries necessitate surgical intervention to reduce the flipped meniscus and restore range of motion. Bucket-handle tears are often amenable to suture repair, unlike the majority of other meniscal tears. These tears are commonly associated with a ligamentous injury, such as an anterior cruciate ligament (ACL) tear. Bucket-handle tears are best repaired surgically in a timely fashion to preserve as much meniscal tissue as possible.

For degenerative meniscal tears, surgery may be indicated if non-operative modalities such as physical therapy or corticosteroid injections have failed. Patients with degenerative meniscal tears who have persistent mechanical symptoms with no or minimal osteoarthritis may elect arthroscopic surgery in order to debride the unstable edge of the meniscus. Degenerative meniscal tears are often associated with some degree of OA. Therefore, it is important that patients understand that the symptoms of OA will not be alleviated with an arthroscopic surgery; however, any pain coming from a meniscal tear can be improved.

Operative Management

If surgery is indicated, patients will undergo an arthroscopic meniscal repair or meniscectomy. Arthroscopic surgery is performed through two small incisions—one anteromedial and one anterolateral—each measuring approximately 5 mm. An arthroscopic camera is first introduced into the knee joint in order to perform a diagnostic arthroscopy and assess the size and location of the meniscal tear (Fig. 18.3a, b). In addition, any degenerative changes to the cartilage or any ligamentous injury are also noted. The surgeon will evaluate the shape and size of the meniscal injury and determine if the meniscus can be repaired instead of debrided. An acute bucket-handle-type tear may be reparable. Arthroscopic meniscal repair involves the passing of a suture through the meniscus at the location of the tear to re-approximate the torn edges. Complex degenerative meniscal tears are irreparable and a partial meniscectomy is the appropriate intervention. In partial meniscectomy, an arthroscopic shaver is used to debride the torn and unstable edges, leaving behind the healthy and stable meniscal tissue.

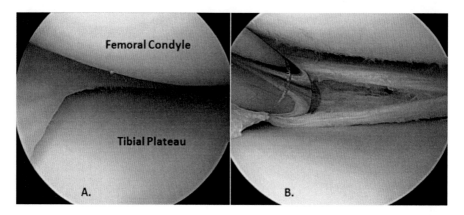

Fig. 18.3 Arthroscopic image of healthy meniscal tissue (**a**). Arthroscopic image of a meniscal tear occurring in a traumatic setting (**b**)

Expected Outcome

Surgical Intervention for Traumatic Meniscal Tears

Patients who have undergone a meniscal repair to treat a traumatic meniscal tear face a 4–6-month rehabilitation period before returning to sport or other recreational activity. A recent systematic review by Moulton et al. (2016) showed satisfactory healing of the meniscus and satisfactory patient-reported outcomes up to 71 months after a repair for a radial meniscal tear. It is thought that preserving meniscal tissue by using repair techniques instead of debridement provides better long-term outcomes in young patients since, with a repair, the meniscus can continue to maximize its anatomic function in weight-bearing. However, long-term data remains limited.

Expected Outcome for Degenerative Meniscal Tears

Conservative treatment measures provide adequate pain relief and improvement in function for most people with degenerative meniscal tears. However, patients who fail non-operative modalities may elect arthroscopic intervention to treat a symptomatic degenerative meniscal tear. The efficacy of an arthroscopic partial meniscectomy has been brought into question with a 2013 randomized, double-blind, and sham-controlled trial by Sihvonen et al. (2013) involving 146 patients with degenerative medial meniscal tears and no evidence on plain films of osteoarthritis. The study showed that at 12 months, there was no significant difference between the group who underwent a partial medial meniscectomy and the group who underwent a sham surgery. In contrast to these findings, however, a recent study by Gauffin et al. (2014) evaluated 150 patients aged 45–64 with degenerative medial meniscal tears and no evidence of osteoarthritis on radiographs. Patients who underwent arthroscopic partial medial meniscectomy had substantially more improvement in pain than those having non-operative therapy. Katz et al. (2013) randomized 351 symptomatic patients with a meniscal tear and concomitant mild-to-moderate osteoarthritis to a standardized physical therapy regimen or arthroscopic surgery with postoperative physical therapy. The investigators found no significant differences in the study groups in patient-reported outcomes at both 6 and 12 months after randomization. Of note, 30% of the patients who were randomized into the conservative treatment with physical therapy group elected to undergo surgery within 6 months of randomization. There are inconsistencies in the literature on the efficacy of surgical intervention for a degenerative meniscal tear, precluding definitive recommendations. The body of evidence does suggest that physical therapy should be the first line of treatment and that a partial meniscectomy remains a potential treatment for those with persistent pain and functional limitation despite a full complement of conservative treatments. It is important for patients to understand that the surgery will not alleviate symptoms from early concomitant osteoarthritis in the knee.

Ligamentous Injury

The knee is comprised of four major ligaments, each of which contributes to stability of the knee joint during movement. The anterior cruciate ligament (ACL) and posterior cruciate ligament (PCL) are located in the intercondylar notch. The ACL stabilizes anterior tibial translation, while the PCL stabilizes posterior tibial translation. The medial collateral ligament (MCL) is located on the medial aspect of the knee and connects the tibia and femur to prevent any medial translation of the tibia. The lateral collateral ligament (LCL) is located on the lateral aspect of the knee and prevents lateral translation of the tibia (Fig. 18.1). All four ligaments work together to stabilize all planes of motion during weight-bearing activities.

Summary of Epidemiology

Ligamentous injury is a common injury to the knee during more demanding activities such as cutting, pivoting, or twisting. The ACL and MCL are the most commonly injured ligaments in the knee. It is estimated that over 200,000 ACL injuries occur annually in the United States, the majority occurring in sports that involve cutting and pivoting movements such as soccer, basketball, skiing, and football. Injuries to the ACL are most prevalent in young and active patients aged 15–45. Females are 2–8 times as likely as their male counterparts to sustain ACL injury due to anatomical and biomechanical differences that place additional stress on the knee. MCL injuries also frequently occur in young and active patients who play sports that involve valgus stress, such as soccer, basketball, ice hockey, and football. MCL injuries such as sprains and partial tears are more prevalent than complete ruptures. PCL and LCL injuries can and do occur but are far less common than ACL and MCL injuries.

Clinical Presentation

Anterior Cruciate Ligament Injury

ACL injuries have become increasingly prevalent among the young and active population and cause pain, swelling, mechanical symptoms, and instability. The majority of ACL injuries occur during a sport or physical activity that involves quick changes of direction. Common sports or activities associated with a high incidence of ACL tears include soccer, basketball, football, skiing, and lacrosse. The mechanism of most ACL injuries is noncontact. Many patients will describe an attempted cut, pivot, or landing from a jump in which their knee subsequently "gave out." One of the hallmark descriptions of an ACL tear is a noncontact valgus stress, followed by an audible or felt "pop" in the knee. Some patients may describe a contact mechanism with hyperextension or player contact with the knee bending inward into valgus stress. Most patients have an immediate onset of pain and swelling and are not able to continue activity. Acute ACL injuries will often present to clinic with a large effusion, loss of motion, pain, and anterior instability. Some patients are not able to weight bear at all after an ACL injury, others are able to ambulate with difficulty, and some are able to ambulate but feel overt instability. The mechanism of injury for ACL tears, a rotational force, valgus stress, or hyperextension, can also be associated with injuries to the meniscus or MCL.

Medial Collateral Ligament Injuries

MCL injuries are another common knee injury and occur more frequently from a contact mechanism. A strong contact force to the outside of the knee that causes the knee to move inward into a valgus position puts stress on the MCL, causing a strain or tear. MCL injuries commonly result in a partial tear or strain rather than a full-thickness tear or avulsion from the attachment site. A strain may present with pain localized to the inner aspect of the knee with minimal swelling and no instability. Partial tears may present with moderate to severe pain, a sense of instability, and some swelling. Full-thickness tears often relate to severe pain, instability, loss of range of motion, and a large effusion.

Posterior Cruciate Ligament

PCL injuries are significantly less common than ACL injuries and may go unrecognized. Anatomically, the PCL is more robust and stronger than the ACL. The most common mechanism of injury for PCL tears is a strong force to the anterior aspect of the knee while the knee is flexed. For example, a flexed knee hitting the dashboard in a motor vehicle accident often results in a PCL injury. In more demanding activities such as sports, a force on the anterior aspect of the knee with hyperextension can also cause an avulsion injury to the PCL.

Lateral Collateral Ligament

Injuries to the LCL are significantly less common than MCL injuries. The mechanism of injury is a strong contact force on the inside of the knee that causes excessive varus stress on the LCL, causing it to strain or tear. Like injuries to the MCL, LCL injuries can range from a strain to a full-thickness tear. Presentation depends on the severity of the injury. Patients may present with a range of symptoms, from localized pain to the outermost aspect of the knee (in a strain or low-grade partial thickness tear) to loss of range of motion and functional limitations (in a full-thickness tear).

Physical Examination

Anterior and Posterior Cruciate Ligaments

A thorough patient history is essential in order to determine what structure has been injured. For ACL injury, a specific incident or event is usually associated with the onset of knee pain. Many patients feel or hear a "pop" in the knee followed by extreme pain, immediate swelling, and inability to continue physical activity.

Inspect both the affected and contralateral knee for bruising or discoloration and obvious swelling. Determine if fluid is present in the suprapatellar pouch or knee joint by performing a ballottement test. Check for point tenderness; an isolated ACL injury may have diffuse tenderness, while an ACL injury combined with a collateral ligament or meniscal injury may be point tender over the medial or lateral joint line. Test for range of motion on both the affected and contralateral knee to assess a baseline measurement (0–135°). Patients with a suspected ACL injury may have limitations in extension and flexion with moderate to severe pain.

The Lachman test is the most sensitive clinical examination test for ACL tears and measures the degree of anterior tibial translation. A proper Lachman is performed with the knee at approximately 30 degrees of flexion and slightly externally rotated. The examiner should place one hand around the patient's thigh approximately 3–5 cm above the patella and the other hand around the tibia with the thumb

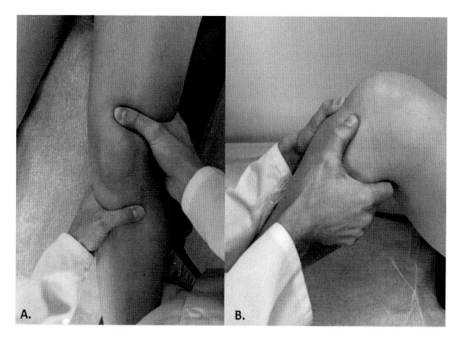

Fig. 18.4 Knee position and examiner hand placement for the Lachman (**a**). Knee position and hand placement for the anterior drawer and posterior drawer (**b**)

placed directly on the tibial tuberosity (Fig. 18.4a). The examiner should pull the tibia anteriorly while simultaneously pushing down on the thigh to assess anterior tibial translation. The Lachman test should first be performed on the contralateral knee to determine baseline tibial translation. A positive Lachman is characterized by increased anterior tibial translation on the injured knee and is highly predictive of a torn ACL.

Another specific test for instability of the knee is the anterior drawer, which similarly assesses anterior tibial translation. The anterior drawer is performed while the knee is flexed 90° with the examiner's thumbs on the anteromedial and anterolateral joint lines (Fig. 18.4b). The examiner should stress the tibia anteriorly while keeping the thumbs steady on the joint line to determine the amount of translation. The anterior drawer should also be assessed on the contralateral side for a baseline measurement. An anterior drawer resulting in increased anterior tibial translation is also predictive of an ACL tear. The posterior drawer test assesses posterior tibial translation and is sensitive to PCL injury. In a position similar to the anterior drawer test, the knee is flexed to about 90° with both thumbs placed on the anteromedial and anterolateral joint lines (Fig. 18.4b). The tibia is stressed posteriorly, while the examiner feels for any increase in translation compared to the contralateral side. Any increased posterior tibial translation is indicative of a PCL tear.

Medial and Lateral Collateral Ligaments

A thorough patient history should first be obtained. The description of the mechanism of injury is important to determine what ligament may be affected. MCL injuries are common with excessive valgus stress on the knee after contact to the outside of the knee. An LCL injury can be suspected if a patient describes a contact mechanism or varus force to the inside of the knee. Inspection, palpation, and range of motion should be performed for every suspected knee injury as described in the anterior and posterior cruciate ligament physical examination section.

The examiner should palpate for point tenderness on the medial or lateral joint line and apply pressure along the native location of the MCL or LCL, from femoral insertion to tibial insertion. Patients with injury to the MCL or LCL will feel pain and point tenderness along the ligament, not solely confined to the joint line. Point tenderness along the native MCL or LCL is a strong indication of injury.

The valgus stress test is useful for determining a partial or complete tear of the MCL. The patient should lie supine, with their knee flexed approximately 20–30°. The examiner should place their fingers over the joint line. A valgus stress is applied to the foot and ankle, and the amount of medial compartment opening or gapping is measured. The severity of an MCL injury (grades I–IV) can be determined by the amount of gapping upon valgus stress.

The varus stress test is used to determine the integrity of the LCL. The patient should lie supine with their knee flexed approximately 20–30°. The examiner should have their fingers over the joint line, and the distal femur stabilized. A varus stress is applied through the foot and ankle, and the amount of lateral compartment opening or gapping is measured. The severity of an LCL injury (grades I–IV) can be determined by the amount of gapping upon varus stress.

Diagnostic Imaging

Plain radiographs, including anterior-posterior, lateral, sunrise, and bilateral weight-bearing views, should be obtained to rule out evidence of fracture or bony pathology. For example, a Segond fracture is a small avulsion fracture of the lateral aspect of the tibia that is frequently associated with ACL injury. MRI is the gold standard for determining a ligamentous injury, as well as concurrent meniscal and cartilage injuries (Fig. 18.5a, b).

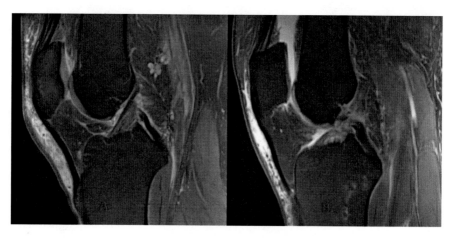

Fig. 18.5 MRI showing a healthy ACL (**a**) and a full-thickness ACL tear (**b**)

Non-operative Management

Anterior Cruciate Ligament

Patients with a torn ACL may be managed non-operatively or choose to have an ACL reconstruction. The majority of patients who participate in sports and are younger than the age of 35 opt for surgical reconstruction. However, ACL reconstruction is not for every patient. Patients with moderate to severe osteoarthritis are not candidates for ACL reconstruction as it can exacerbate arthritic pain. It is important to convey to the patient the function and purpose of the ACL and that a torn ACL will not impact forward or backward movements such as jogging or walking. Patients who are not as active and do not regularly participate in cutting and pivoting activities may have success with non-operative management. A formal course of physical therapy to reduce swelling and maximize proximal musculature strength often allows for the desired quality of life. Patients can also be fit for a functional ACL brace that provides added stability in cutting and pivoting activities such as tennis or skiing.

Outcomes of Non-operative Management for ACL Injury

Several studies have compared the outcomes of operative versus non-operative management for ACL injuries. Ericsson et al. (2013) compared physical performance and muscle strength between non-operative and operative treatments following an acute ACL tear and found no difference between the groups at 2- and 5-year follow-up. This study has provided evidence that non-operative treatment modalities can be an adequate treatment for ACL injury. Patients who are ACL deficient may be at risk for future instability episodes and subsequent injuries, causing a progression of osteoarthritis or further damage to the meniscus and cartilaginous structures of the knee. Sanders et al. (2016) showed that individuals who were treated non-operatively for an ACL injury had a significantly higher risk of secondary meniscal tear and osteoarthritis. However, it is ultimately the patient's preference in the decision to manage an ACL injury operatively or non-operatively. Younger, adolescent patients and those who wish to participate in heavy cutting and pivoting activities may wish to undergo a reconstruction for knee stabilization in physically demanding activities.

Medial and Lateral Collateral Ligament

The majority of collateral ligament injuries are strains and partial tears that should be managed non-operatively. Patients who have a strain or partial tear of the collateral ligament can undergo a formal course of physical therapy to reduce swelling, relieve symptoms, and increase proximal musculature strength. Formal physical therapy can alleviate symptoms and return the patient to activity after injury. Patients who have persistent instability when ambulating or participating in cutting or pivoting activities can be fit with a functional brace to provide added stability.

Non-operative management of ligamentous injuries can result in good outcomes with appropriate rehabilitation (physical therapy), use of a functional brace as indicated, and limitation of cutting and pivoting at-risk activities. The inherent laxity in non-operatively managed knees does increase the risk for additional injury, as recurrent episodes of instability can cause further damage to other ligaments, meniscus, or cartilage, as well as increasing the risk for early osteoarthritis.

Indications for Surgery

ACL or PCL reconstruction is indicated for young and active individuals who are unable to participate in their desired activities due to instability or pain in the knee with activities. ACL injuries are often indicated for surgical reconstruction in contrast to isolated PCL injuries, the majority of which are managed non-operatively. Knee dislocations resulting in multi-ligament injuries usually necessitate surgical intervention.

Patients with a full-thickness MCL or LCL tear who have recurrent feelings of instability or pain that limit their desired activity level may be candidates for an MCL or LCL reconstruction. While most MCL or LCL tears are treated non-operatively, full-thickness tears that do not improve with non-operative modalities should be considered for surgical reconstruction.

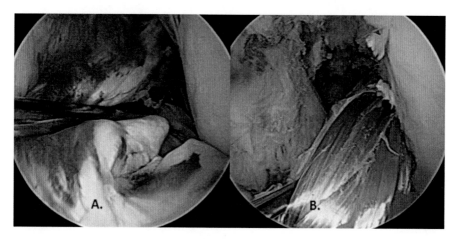

Fig. 18.6 Arthroscopic image of a ruptured ACL in the intercondylar notch (**a**). Arthroscopic image of a newly reconstructed ACL with hamstring autograft (**b**)

Operative Management

Anterior Cruciate Ligament Reconstruction

Arthroscopic ACL reconstruction is performed with small 5–10 mm incisions located on the anteromedial and anterolateral aspects of the anterior knee. An ACL can be reconstructed with the use of an autograft or allograft. Most commonly, autografts are used from the patellar tendon or hamstring tendons (semitendinosus and gracilis). An ACL reconstruction is performed first by debriding the torn fibers of the ACL and addressing any other concurrent meniscal or ligamentous injuries (Fig. 18.6a, b). After the graft has been prepared, a drill is used to create a tunnel for the graft on both the femoral and tibial sides. The reconstructed ACL graft is introduced into the joint and fixated with an interference screw or suture button on both the femoral and tibial sides. A PCL reconstruction follows a similar procedure. MCL and LCL reconstructions are fixated on the femoral and tibial sides with an interference screw, EndoButton, or suture button.

Expected Outcomes of Surgical Intervention

Patients undergoing a ligament reconstruction should expect a rehabilitation period of 6 months. The newly reconstructed ligament takes approximately 3 months to heal into the bone, and rehabilitation is controlled until that point. Patients are often managed in a hinged brace and may or may not utilize crutches for ambulation for the first 2–6 weeks. After 3 months, patients focus on regaining strength and function so that they may begin to resume their desired activities at 6 months.

Table 18.1 Meniscal and ligamentous injuries of the knee

Clinical entity	Presentation	Physical examination	Conservative management	Indications for surgery	Operative management
Traumatic or non-degenerative meniscal tear	– Knee effusion and pain – Traumatic mechanism – Mechanical symptoms such as locking and catching	– Range of motion – Joint line tenderness[a] – McMurray test – Ballottement test for fluid	– Ice and NSAID regimen – PT for proximal musculature strengthening	– Mechanical symptoms – Limitations in daily activities – Moderate to severe pain	– Arthroscopic surgical intervention – Depending on size and shape of the tear, meniscal repair vs. debridement
Degenerative meniscal tear	– Knee effusion and pain – Point tenderness over the medial or lateral joint line – Mechanical symptoms such as locking or catching	– Range of motion – Joint line tenderness[a] – McMurray test – Ballottement test for fluid – Deep squat test	– Ice and NSAID regimen – PT for proximal musculature strengthening – Corticosteroid injection(s)	– Failed conservative management – Mechanical symptoms – Limitations in daily activity	– Arthroscopic surgical intervention – Partial meniscectomy and debridement of the torn edges – Chondroplasty of cartilage surfaces if indicated

(continued)

Table 18.1 (continued)

Clinical entity	Presentation	Physical examination	Conservative management	Indications for surgery	Operative management
Anterior cruciate ligament tear	– Noncontact mechanism involving a rotation or hyperextension of the knee	– Range of motion	– Ice and NSAID regimen	– Recurrent feeling of instability daily activity	– Arthroscopic surgical intervention
		– Ballottement test for fluid	– PT for proximal musculature strengthening	– Unable to achieve desired activity level due to pain or symptoms	– ACL reconstruction with autograft or allograft
		– Lachman[a]			
	– Knee effusion	– Anterior drawer	– Functional brace to improve stability		– Address any other injuries
	– Moderate to severe pain				
	– Feeling of instability				
Posterior cruciate ligament tear	– Contact mechanism involving an excessive force pushing the anterior aspect of the knee posteriorly	– Range of motion	– Ice and NSAID regimen	– Recurrent feeling of instability with daily activities	– Arthroscopy surgical intervention
		– Ballottement test for fluid	– PT for proximal musculature strengthening	– Unable to achieve desired activity level due to pain or symptoms	– PCL reconstruction with autograft or allograft
	– Knee effusion	– Posterior drawer test[a]	– Functional brace to improve stability		– Address any other injuries
	– Moderate to severe pain				
	– Feeling of instability				

Medial collateral ligament tear	– Contact mechanism to the outside of the knee causing excessive valgus stress – Knee effusion – Pain localized to the medial aspect of the knee – Moderate to severe pain – Feeling of instability	– Point tenderness over native MCL – Ballottement test for fluid – Limited range of motion if complete or high-grade partial tear – Valgus stress test[a] – MRI to confirm diagnosis	– Ice and NSAID regimen – PT for proximal musculature strengthening – Functional brace to improve stability	– Complete tear of the MCL – Recurrent feeling of instability – Unable to achieve desired activity level due to pain or symptoms	– MCL reconstruction with autograft or allograft – Address any other injuries
Lateral collateral ligament tear	– Contact mechanism to the inside of the knee causing excessive varus stress – Knee effusion – Pain localized to the lateral aspect of the knee – Moderate to severe pain – Feeling of instability	– Point tenderness over the native LCL – Ballottement test for fluid – Limited range of motion – Varus stress test[a]	– Ice and NSAID regimen – PT for proximal musculature strengthening – Functional brace to improve stability	– Complete tear of the LCL – Recurrent feeling of instability – Unable to achieve desired activity level due to pain or symptoms	– LCL reconstruction with autograft or allograft – Address any other concurrent injuries

NSAID nonsteroidal anti-inflammatory drugs, *LCL* lateral collateral ligament
[a]Indicates most sensitive/specific test

ACL injuries have become far too common, especially in adolescent athletes, and youth prevention programs have been developed to reduce biomechanical risk factors. Fortunately, short-term outcomes from an ACL reconstruction are generally successful, with return to activity and relief of pain and instability symptoms after rehabilitation is complete. In the young athlete under 14 years of age, Chicorelli et al. (2016) found that 96% of athletes were able to return to sporting activity, and 85% were able to return to sport within 12 months postoperatively. Studies of NCAA Division I football players and NCAA Division I soccer athletes who underwent ACL reconstruction had return to play rates of around 85%. Rate of return to play is generally higher in recreational athletes.

Unfortunately, ACL reconstructions do not prevent the potential long-term consequences such as the early development of osteoarthritis 10–20 years after the procedure. A study of 135 patients with diagnosed ACL injuries (Barenius et al. 2014) found that the prevalence of osteoarthritis was three times higher in the group treated with a reconstruction at 14-year follow-up. The group also found that concomitant meniscal resection further increased the risk of OA. A systematic review by Oiestad et al. (2009) reported that osteoarthritis occurs in up to 13% of patients with an isolated ACL injury and reconstruction and in 21–48% of patients with concomitant injuries. The likelihood of osteoarthritis increases in patients with combined ACL and meniscal injuries, highlighting the importance of both structures in long-term knee function. Table 18.1 shows meniscal and ligamentous injuries of the knee.

Suggested Reading

Barenius B, Ponzer S, Shalabi A, et al. Increased risk of osteoarthritis after anterior cruciate ligament reconstruction: a 14-year follow-up study of a randomized control trial. Am J Sports Med. 2014;42(5):1049–57.

Calmbach WL, Hutchens M. Evaluation of patients presenting with knee pain: Part I. History, physical exam, radiographs, and laboratory tests. Am Fam Physician. 2003;68(5):907–12.

Chicorelli AM, Micheli LJ, Kelly M, Zurakowski D, MacDougall R. Return to sport after anterior cruciate ligament reconstruction in the skeletally immature athlete. Clin J Sport Med. 2016;26(4):266–71. https://doi.org/10.1097/JSM.0000000000000275. PMID:27359295

Ericsson YB, Roos EM, Frobell RB. Lower extremity performance following ACL rehabilitation in the KANON-trial: impact of reconstruction and predictive value at 2 and 5 years. Br J Sports Med. 2013;47(15):980–5.

Gauffin H, Tagesson S, Meunier A, et al. Knee arthroscopic surgery is beneficial to middle-aged patients with meniscal symptoms: a prospective, randomised, single-blinded study. Osteoarthr Cartil. 2014;22(11):1808–16.

Katz JM, Brophy RH, Chaisson CE, et al. Surgery versus physical therapy for a meniscal tear and osteoarthritis. N Engl J Med. 2013;368:1675–84.

Moulton SG, Bhatia S, Civitarese DM, et al. Surgical techniques and outcomes of repairing meniscal radial tears: a systematic review. Arthroscopy. 2016;32(9):1919–25. [Epub ahead of print]

Neogi DS, Kumar A, Rijal L, et al. Role of nonoperative treatment in managing degenerative tears of the medial meniscus posterior root. J Orthop Traumatol. 2013;14(3):193–9.

Oei EH, Nikken JJ, Verstijnen AC, Ginai AZ, Myriam Hunink MG. MR imaging of the menisci and cruciate ligaments: a systematic review. Radiology. 2003;226(3):837–48. Epub 2003 Jan 15. PMID:12601211

Oiestad BE, Engebretsen L, Storheim K, et al. Knee osteoarthritis after anterior cruciate ligament injury: a systematic review. Am J Sports Med. 2009;37(7):1434–43.

Paavola M, Malmivaara A, et al. Arthroscopic partial meniscectomy versus sham surgery for a degenerative meniscal tear. N Engl J Med. 2013;369:2515–24.

Sanders TL, Pareek A, Kremers HM, et al. Long-term follow-up of isolated ACL tears treated without ligament reconstruction. Knee Surg Sports Traumatol Arthrosc. 2017;25(2):493–500. [Epub ahead of print]

Sihvonen R, Paavola M, Malmivaara A, Itälä A, Joukainen A, Nurmi H, Kalske J, Järvinen TL, Finnish Degenerative Meniscal Lesion Study (FIDELITY) Group. Arthroscopic partial meniscectomy versus sham surgery for a degenerative meniscal tear. N Engl J Med. 2013;369(26):2515–24. https://doi.org/10.1056/NEJMoa1305189. PMID:24369076

Chapter 19
Anterior Knee Pain: Diagnosis and Treatment

Kaitlyn Whitlock, Brian Mosier, and Elizabeth Matzkin

Abbreviations

AMZ   Anteromedialization
CT   Computed tomography
MCL   Medial collateral ligament
MRI   Magnetic resonance imaging
NSAID   Nonsteroidal anti-inflammatory drug
PFPS   Patellofemoral pain syndrome
TT-TG   Tibial tubercle-trochlear groove distance

Introduction

Anterior knee pain is a common and challenging complaint. The differential diagnosis is broad, and making a diagnosis can be difficult due to vague physical manifestations and psychosocial contextual overlap, which may skew the patient's symptoms and perception of pain. There are numerous discrete entities that can contribute to anterior knee pain; therefore, a thorough history and focused physical examination is essential. This chapter outlines the most common causes of anterior knee pain including patellofemoral pain syndrome (PFPS), patellar tendinopathy, quadriceps tendinopathy, and pes anserine bursitis. The relevant structures are shown in Fig. 19.1.

K. Whitlock • B. Mosier • E. Matzkin (✉)
Department of Orthopaedic Surgery, Brigham and Women's Hospital,
75 Francis Street, Boston, MA 02115, USA
e-mail: kwhitlock@partners.org; mosier619@gmail.com; ematzkin@partners.org

© Springer International Publishing AG 2018   313
J.N. Katz et al. (eds.), *Principles of Orthopedic Practice for Primary Care
Providers*, https://doi.org/10.1007/978-3-319-68661-5_19

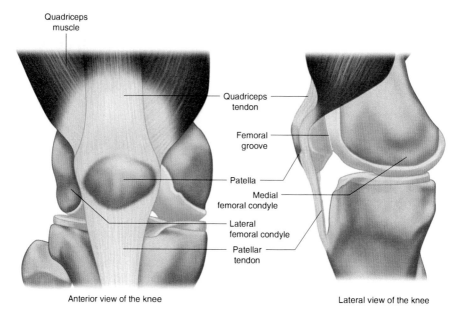

Quadriceps
muscle

Quadriceps
tendon

Femoral
groove

Patella

Medial
femoral condyle

Lateral
femoral condyle

Patellar
tendon

Anterior view of the knee

Lateral view of the knee

Fig. 19.1 Anatomy of the anterior aspect of the knee

Patellofemoral Pain Syndrome

Epidemiology

The etiology of anterior knee pain can be confusing as many terms are often used interchangeably to describe pain associated with patellofemoral symptoms. In general, patellofemoral symptoms reflect pain or instability, with some overlap between the two. Patellofemoral pain syndrome (PFPS) is generally classified as anterior or peri-patellar knee pain that occurs with activities that load the patellofemoral articulation, such as ascending or descending stairs. Patellar instability with true subluxation or dislocation is an entirely different entity with a completely separate treatment algorithm. PFPS is more common in females and often follows a change in levels of activity, such as an increase in running mileage or adding squats and lunges to a gym workout routine. Some studies have suggested that nearly 15–40% of patients presenting to the sports medicine physician have PFPS; however, there remains little consensus on its etiology or the factors responsible for causing pain.

Clinical Presentation

The patient presenting to the physician with PFPS will often complain of achy pain along the anterior aspect of the knee with associated pain in the peri-patellar region or directly behind the patella (Fig. 19.1). These symptoms are worsened by activities that require deep or prolonged knee flexion such as jumping, stair climbing, running, or sitting for an extended period of time. Patients may report vague pain with activity and occasional sharp or shooting pain around the anterior aspect of the knee or may complain that their knee feels like it will "buckle" or "give way."

True patellar instability indicates that the patella has come out of the trochlear groove. This is usually a traumatic event or can occur in someone with significant patellar laxity. In PFPS, a "buckling" or "giving way" sensation may be secondary to quadriceps inhibition and proximal muscle weakness. Patients may perceive instability; the evaluation needs to distinguish frank dislocation versus quadriceps inhibition/weakness pain resulting in knee "buckling" or "giving way." The patient may also complain of patellar crepitance or grinding without pain.

Important questions to ask include the onset of symptoms in relation to a change in exercise routine or trauma. Sharp, painful catching, locking, and recurrent effusions are red flags that should alert the physician that further diagnostic imaging and a referral to an orthopedist may be necessary. In particular, a knee effusion can suggest a full-thickness cartilage defect, causing symptoms. A prepatellar effusion would suggest prepatellar bursitis (septic or aseptic).

Physical examination may demonstrate pain on palpation of the peri-patellar tissues and retinaculum. Patellar mobilization in the medial-lateral and proximal-distal direction can be tested as well as an assessment of patellar tilt and tracking throughout the patient's range of motion. The examiner should note any direction of increased laxity, tightness, or apprehension on the part of the patient. The presence of a "J-sign," which is a lateral deviation of the patella as the knee is brought from flexion to terminal extension, can signal an imbalance between the medial (vastus medialis) and lateral (vastus lateralis) muscles.

Strength testing is a critical part of the clinical evaluation as muscular weakness and imbalance can lead to disrupted patellofemoral mechanics. The examiner should assess not only quadriceps strength but also hip flexor, hip abductor, as well as abdominal and lumbar core muscles. Weakness of the hip and core muscles can disrupt coronal plane mechanics leading to dynamic patellar mal-tracking.

Differential Diagnosis and Testing

Patellofemoral pain syndrome is a clinical diagnosis; there is no single imaging test or physical exam that establishes the diagnosis with certainty. As such, the clinician should rule out other causes of knee pain including patellar instability, patellar tendon or quadriceps tendon pathology, prepatellar bursitis, chondral pathology, meniscus tear, loose bodies, osteoarthritis, radicular pain, or a systemic cause that may portend a poor outcome if not treated. The clinician should be wary of a diagnosis other than PFPS in a patient with knee pain and persistent painful mechanical symptoms or evidence of an effusion (Table 19.1).

For most patients presenting with anterior knee pain, the best imaging studies to obtain initially are weight-bearing plain radiographs including an AP, PA flexion,

Table 19.1 Differential diagnosis of anterior knee pain

Diagnosis	Presentation	Diagnostic testing	Conservative management	Indications for surgery	Operative management
Patellofemoral Pain Syndrome	– Peri-patellar pain – Positive "J-sign" – Decreased strength of hip flexors/abductors/quadriceps	– Clinical diagnosis is often adequate – Plain radiographs to evaluate alignment and dysplasia – MRI to evaluate cartilage	– Physical therapy (strengthening hip/thigh musculature) – Ice and anti-inflammatories	– Persistent pain after conservative management	– Knee arthroscopy with debridement for cartilage abnormalities – Tibial tubercle osteotomy for patella maltracking
Patellar Tendonitis	– Tenderness over inferior pole of patella – Tenderness along patellar tendon – Positive "Bassett's sign"	– Clinical diagnosis is often adequate – MRI to confirm diagnosis	– Physical therapy (eccentric exercises, iontophoresis) – Ice and anti-inflammatories – activity modification	– Persistent pain after conservative management	– Tendon debridement with or without microfracture/drilling
Quadriceps Tendonitis	– Tenderness over superior pole of patella	– Clinical diagnosis is often adequate – MRI to confirm diagnosis	– Physical therapy (eccentric exercises) – Ice and anti-inflammatories – Activity modification	– Persistent pain after conservative management	– Tendon debridement with or without microfracture/drilling

Pes Anserine Bursitis	– Tenderness and local selling 5 cm below anterior-medial joint line	– Clinical diagnosis is often adequate	– Physical therapy – Ice and anti-inflammatories – Activity modification – Injection	– Persistent pain after conservative management	– Drainage/removal of bursa
Meniscus Tear	– Joint line tenderness (medial/lateral) – Effusion – Positive McMurray's (see Chap. 18) – Pain with deep squat	– MRI to confirm diagnosis	– Physical therapy – Ice and anti-inflammatories – Activity modification – Injection	– "Locked knee" – Persistent pain after conservative management	– Knee arthroscopy with partial meniscectomy or meniscal repair if indicated
Osteoarthritis	– Pain – Stiffness – Possible effusion	– Plain radiographs will show joint space narrowing/osteophytes/sclerosis/subchondral cysts	– Physical therapy – Weight loss – Ice and anti-inflammatories – Activity modification – Injection (corticosteroid) – Visco-supplementation	– Persistent pain after conservative management	– Total knee arthroplasty

(continued)

Table 19.1 (continued)

Diagnosis	Presentation	Diagnostic testing	Conservative management	Indications for surgery	Operative management
Fracture	– Tenderness – Possible effusion	– Presence on plain radiographs/MRI/CT scan	– Non-weight-bearing with crutches – Activity modification	– Displacement – Fracture not healing	– Open reduction, internal fixation
Patellar/Quadriceps Tendon Rupture	– Palpable defect – Effusion – Unable to perform straight leg raise	– Clinical diagnosis is often adequate – Plain radiographs will show patella alta/baja – MRI to confirm diagnosis	– Surgical intervention is indicated unless risks outweigh benefits	– Full thickness tendon rupture	– Patellar/quadriceps tendon repair
MCL sprain/tear	– Tenderness over MCL – Pain/laxity with valgus stress – Effusion	– Clinical diagnosis is often adequate – MRI to confirm diagnosis	– Physical therapy – Knee brace – Ice and anti-inflammatories – Activity modification	– Knee instability/laxity-full thickness tear	– MCL repair versus reconstruction

MRI magnetic resonance imaging, *CT* computed tomography, *MCL* medial collateral ligament

30° flexed lateral, and bilateral Merchant view. The weight-bearing AP and PA flexion views allow for the assessment of osteochondral lesions and arthritic change in the medial and lateral tibiofemoral compartments. The lateral X-ray can provide important information similar to the coronal views as well as an assessment of patellar height and the presence of trochlear dysplasia. Bilateral Merchant views allow for an evaluation of the patellofemoral joint including alignment, patellar tilt, and the presence of arthritis (Fig. 19.2).

Advanced imaging such as computed tomography (CT) and magnetic resonance imaging (MRI) is indicated in patients with PFPS who fail 3–6 months of conservative management. CT is useful for evaluating for any bony pathology as well as patellar height and the tibial tubercle-trochlear groove distance (TT-TG). The TT-TG is a measurement of the distance between the tibial tubercle and the deepest part of the trochlear groove. In patients with a TT-TG of 20 mm or greater, the tibial tubercle is too lateral, and the resultant vector of pull of the extensor mechanism results in mal-tracking of the patella. MRI can also be used to quantify TT-TG distance. Additionally, MRI is valuable for assessing the chondral surfaces and sub-chondral bone for cartilage abnormalities or evidence of arthritic changes. Both MRI and CT are good studies for analyzing trochlear morphology and dysplasia.

Non-operative Management

The majority of patients presenting with PFPS will improve with a comprehensive rehabilitation management strategy including nonsteroidal anti-inflammatories, ice, and physical therapy. Studies have demonstrated that 85% of patients improve with 8 weeks of appropriate physical therapy. The physician must be knowledgeable as to the correct protocols for PFPS rehabilitation as physical therapists differ considerably in the exercises they recommend. Initially, rehabilitation should consist of tactics aimed at reducing symptoms including activity modifications and modalities to improve flexibility and patellar tracking. The restoration of normal knee mechanics with capsular stretching and vastus medialis strengthening has long been the primary focus of rehab protocols in the treatment of patients with PFPS. As our knowledge of normal knee kinematics has evolved, the hip and core (abdominal/lumbar) musculature has emerged as another important aspect of treatment. Improving not only the strength but also the endurance of the hip and core muscles has been shown to better maintain the kinematics of the extensor mechanism.

Indications for Surgery and Operative Management

Surgical intervention for treatment of PFPS is rarely indicated, as most patients improve with conservative management. Accurate diagnosis is necessary for surgery to be successful. Cartilage injury on the underside of the patella or in the

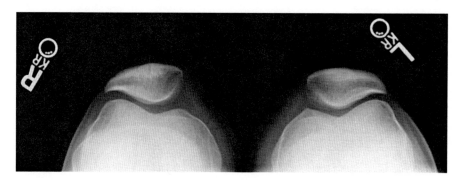

Fig. 19.2 Bilateral Merchant (sunrise) radiographic views of the knees

trochlear groove can often be treated with arthroscopic debridement. Should the patient fail or plateau after several months of dedicated rehab and exhibit evidence of mal-tracking, imaging studies should be performed to assess TT-TG distance and patellar height. Patients with evidence of lateral mal-tracking on exam with TT-TG distance greater than 20 mm are candidates for anteromedialization (AMZ) of the tibial tubercle combined with a possible proximal realignment procedure such as a lateral release or lengthening. In the past, many patients with lateral mal-tracking were treated with an isolated lateral release. This has fallen out of favor as many patients treated with a lateral release continued to have persistent pain and even developed iatrogenic medial instability. Current surgical treatment for lateral mal-tracking of the patella includes a tibial tubercle osteotomy, with or without a lateral release or lateral lengthening and vastus medialis advancement—depending on glide and tilt—performed through a single anterior incision. Using a saw, the tubercle is cut in the coronal plane in an oblique manner from an anteromedial to posterolateral direction. An oblique cut in this manner will allow for anteriorization with medialization of the tubercle. The cut tubercle is usually secured using two screws (Fig. 19.3). Typical medialization is approximately 10–15 mm with subsequent anteriorization of 10–15 mm depending on the angle of the osteotomy. This surgery requires a long postoperative rehabilitation. The patients are kept partial weight-bearing with crutches until there is healing at the osteotomy site which can take 6–8 weeks. Return to sports or athletic activities takes a minimum of 6 months.

Expected Outcomes

With some time and effort, 85–90% of patients with anterior knee pain secondary to PFPS will improve with conservative management. With better flexibility and strengthening of the hip and thigh musculature, improved load transfer and knee kinematics will result in enhanced functional capacity and a decrease in symptoms. In patients who have persistent pain and evidence of mal-tracking, an AMZ tibial tubercle osteotomy can provide significant symptomatic relief as this sufficiently

Fig. 19.3 Tibial tubercle transfer secured with two screws

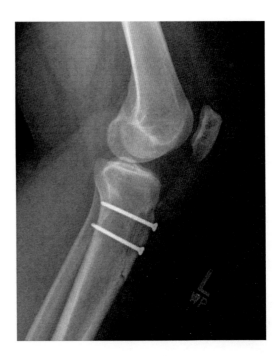

unloads the affected area and improves tracking. The use of an AMZ to treat chondromalacia of the lateral facet and inferior pole has also been met with good to excellent results in the majority of patients.

Patellar Tendinopathy

Epidemiology

Patellar tendinopathy is a common cause of anterior knee pain especially in the younger population. It is also referred to as "jumper's knee," since it is most common in athletes that participate in jumping sports, such as basketball and volleyball. However, patellar tendinopathy may be caused by any sport or activity that places repetitive load on the patellar tendon, such as football. It is most frequently diagnosed in athletes from ages 15 to 30 years and is more common in men than women. The onset of pain is usually insidious. The condition begins with microscopic injury to the tendon, with delayed healing because of repetitive loading or overuse.

Fig. 19.4 The anatomy of
the knee

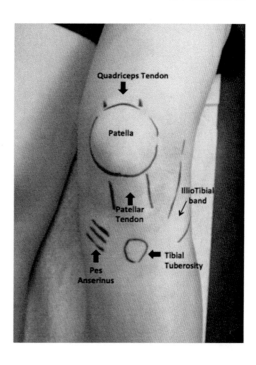

Clinical Presentation

Patients with patellar tendinopathy will localize the pain over the anterior aspect of
the knee, below the patella (Fig. 19.4). More specifically, the pain is most predominantly confined over its insertion at the inferior pole of the patella. Patients mainly
complain of pain and typically do not experience mechanical symptoms, such as
locking and catching or swelling. The pain is usually worse with activity (placing
increased load on the tendon) and can be very limiting to an athlete. Going down the
stairs or sitting for an extended period of time may exacerbate pain.

On physical examination, tenderness to palpation is common over the inferior
pole of the patella, although tenderness can occur anywhere along the patellar tendon down to its most distal attachment, the tibial tuberosity. Tenderness may be
elicited when the knee is either flexed or extended. "Bassett's sign" is a pattern
indicative of a patellar tendinopathy: increased pain from palpation is elicited when
the knee is extended/tendon is relaxed, with less pain when the knee is flexed. A
knee effusion is not common with tendinopathy. If a palpable defect is detected and
the patient cannot perform a straight leg raise, this indicates an extensor mechanism
disruption and needs immediate evaluation by an orthopedic surgeon. Operative and
non-operative treatment for patellar tendinopathy will be addressed together with
quadriceps tendinopathy in the Diagnostic Imaging section below.

Quadriceps Tendinopathy

Epidemiology

Similar to patellar tendinopathy, the pain is usually insidious in onset and affects males more than females. It is also very common in sports/activities that involve jumping and can lead to microscopic injury of the tendon. Quadriceps tendinopathy is significantly less common than patellar tendinopathy due to the richer vascularization, which promotes faster and more efficient healing.

Clinical Presentation

Quadriceps tendinopathy differs from patellar tendinopathy based on the location of pain. Though pain is also anterior, in quadriceps tendinopathy, the pain is localized over the attachment of the tendon at the superior pole of the patella (Fig. 19.4). Patients typically experience increased pain with going up and down the stairs and increased activity. Sitting for an extended period of time may also exacerbate pain. As in patellar tendinopathy, knee effusion and mechanical symptoms are not common.

The majority of patients will demonstrate tenderness to palpation just superior to the patella, without palpable defect. There is also frequently pain with resisted leg extension (strength testing of the quadriceps). Just as with the patellar tendon, immediate orthopedic evaluation is indicated for probable rupture if there is a defect where the tendon should be and the patient cannot perform a straight leg raise.

Diagnostic Imaging

Patellar and quadriceps tendinopathies are most often diagnosed based on history and clinical examination. When imaging is used, plain radiographs are a good first choice to determine if there is underlying pathology including degenerative change, calcification in the tendon, or patella mal-tracking. MRI is rarely indicated in these cases and is usually pursued only when conservative management has failed, and surgical intervention is the next option (Fig. 19.5).

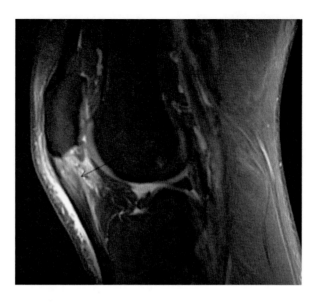

Fig. 19.5 MRI demonstrating chronic patellar tendinopathy

Non-operative Management for Patellar and Quadriceps Tendinopathies

Conservative management is the mainstay of treatment for both patellar and quadriceps tendinopathy, though it may take 3–6 months for some cases to fully resolve in. Physical therapy plays an important role in symptom reduction. More specifically, the eccentric exercises (introduced once the tendon is not considerably irritable) typically enhance rehabilitation and ultimate return to sport/exercise. Stretching and strengthening of the proximal musculature, including hamstrings, quadriceps, hip flexors, and abductors, also is an important aspect of treatment. Nonsteroidal anti-inflammatories (NSAIDs), ice, and activity modification are also beneficial. Surgical intervention is indicated rarely.

Operative Management of Patellar and Quadriceps Tendinopathies

Once it has been determined that conservative management has failed, usually after 6+ months with formal physical therapy, operative intervention is an option. At this point, an MRI may be obtained to definitively confirm the diagnosis and to determine if there are any other pathologies. The surgical procedures usually performed are first an arthroscopy (to evaluate the intra-articular structures including the tendon itself and the patella) and then an open patellar tendon/quadriceps tendon debridement with or without drilling/microfracture. The drilling of the patella (close to the tendon attachment) is performed to stimulate healing through increased vascularization to the area. Depending on the extent of debridement and quality of the tendon tissue itself, a patient may be put in a brace locked in extension for ambulation for the first 2–4 weeks postoperatively. Formal physical therapy will be beneficial in order for the patient to return to all activities anywhere between 3 and 6 months, depending on the extent of the surgery.

Expected Outcomes

Although patellar and quadriceps tendinopathies may linger for many months, the majority of cases will resolve with conservative measures as outlined above. It is important to determine that the patient is compliant with non-operative management before deciding that he/she has failed. Surgery is usually offered as a last option because there is more risk involved, and the vast majority should have resolution in symptoms if compliant with conservative treatments. If these patients still experience pain after surgery, it is usually secondary to noncompliance or secondary pathology.

Pes Anserine Bursitis

Epidemiology

The exact incidence of pes anserine bursitis is unknown, though it is fairly common among the adult population. Several studies have shown that overweight females are more at risk than male counterparts. Patients with diabetes mellitus also have been shown to be at increased risk of developing pes anserine bursitis. Approximately 5 centimeters (cm) below the anterior-medial joint line is the pes anserinus, where the semitendinosus, gracilis, and sartorius tendons attach. A bursa is located at this attachment site, below the tendons, and can become inflamed either by overuse or direct trauma, resulting in pes anserine bursitis.

Clinical Presentation

Clinically, patients with pes anserine bursitis will localize the pain over the anteromedial aspect of the proximal lower leg, about 5–6 cm below the medial joint line (Fig. 19.3). There will be tenderness to palpation over this area, and usually localized swelling will also be present. In some cases, resisted knee flexion may elicit pain to this area (strength testing of hamstring). Going up and down the stairs may intensify pain to the area as well. A knee effusion will not be present in isolated pes anserine bursitis.

Given the location of pain on the medial aspect of the knee, it is important that other causes of medial pain are excluded. Other diagnoses that can cause medial knee pain are medial meniscus tear, osteoarthritis, medial collateral ligament pathology, etc., discussed in separate chapters (Table 19.1).

Diagnostic Imaging

Pes anserine bursitis is diagnosed based on history and clinical examination. Plain radiographs will not make the diagnosis but are a good first choice in imaging in order to determine the amount of degenerative changes, whether there are any fractures, etc. MRI is rarely indicated but may be helpful in determining other pathologies of the medial aspect of the knee when the diagnosis is uncertain. Ultrasonography may aid in diagnosis, especially in cases where there is a significant amount of swelling, and can be used when administering an injection for diagnostic and therapeutic purposes.

Non-operative Management

Conservative therapy is the mainstay of treatment for pes anserine bursitis. Management options include ice, NSAIDs, activity modification, and physical therapy. Physical therapy is predominately focused on hamstring stretching and strengthening. Formal physical therapy may also include modalities meant to decrease inflammation and pain, such as topical corticosteroid treatment (iontophoresis with dexamethasone). An injection into the bursa with local anesthetic—with or without corticosteroid—may aid in diagnosis and improve symptoms. The injection serves as a diagnostic tool in that if pain completely resolves after the injection, it can be determined that it was the sole pain generator. Similarly, if the injection provides no relief, then other causes of pain must be considered, with the assumption that if a blind injection was performed, it was in the correct place (Table 19.1). Non-operative treatment should be successful in the majority of cases, and surgical removal of the bursa is reserved for cases that fail to resolve.

Operative Management

Surgical intervention is rarely ever indicated for pes anserine bursitis. This option may be presented to the patient if conservative management fails, usually after 6+ months of conservative treatment. The surgical procedure entails an incision over

the pes anserinus and drainage or removal of the bursa. If there is a bone prominence under the bursa, this will also be removed at the time of surgery. Once the soft
tissue is healed, patients will usually start a course of physical therapy until back to
all activities at about 2–3 months postoperatively.

Expected Outcomes

Nonsurgical management is the mainstay of treatment for pes anserine bursitis and
includes ice, NSAIDs, physical therapy, and local injection. Outcomes are typically
excellent. In the very rare occasion that conservative therapy fails, surgical intervention may be implemented. Surgical treatment is the last option given that it is associated with more risk. After surgery, symptoms are expected to resolve, and if not,
secondary pathology should be considered.

Suggested Reading

Calmbach W, Hutchens M. Evaluation of patients presenting with knee pain: Part I. Am Fam
    Physician. 2003a;68:907–12.
Calmbach W, Hutchens M. Evaluation of patients presenting with knee pain: Part II. Am Fam
    Physician. 2003b;68:917–22.
Clijsen R, Fuchs J, Taeymans J. Effectiveness of exercise therapy in treatment of patients
    with patellofemoral pain syndrome: systematic review and meta-analysis. Phys Ther.
    2014;94(12):1697–708.
Dejour D, Le Coultre B. Osteotomies in patella-femoral instabilities. Sports Med Arthrosc Rev.
    2007;15:39–46.
Helfenstein M, Kuromoto J. Anserine syndrome. Rev Bras Rheumatol. 2010;50(3):313–27.
Panni AS, Biedert RM, Maffuli N, et al. Overuse injuries of the extensor mechanism in athletes.
    Clin Sports Med. 2002;21:483–98.
Post WR. Anterior knee pain: diagnosis and treatment. J Am Acad Orthop Surg. 2005;13:534–43.
Wilson JD, Dougherty CP, Ireland ML. Core stability and its relationship to lower extremity func-
    tion and injury. J Am Acad Orthop Surg. 2005;13(5):316–25.

Part XI
Foot and Ankle

Chapter 20
Ankle Arthritis

Eric M. Bluman, Christopher P. Chiodo, and Jeremy T. Smith

Introduction

The tibiotalar joint, or ankle joint, is the major motion segment below the knee and plays a key role in locomotion. In addition to helping propel the body forward during ambulation, it also has an important role in shock absorption during walking and sporting activities.

The anatomy of the ankle joint is complex (Fig. 20.1). It is formed by the tibia, talus, and fibula. These three bones come together to form the bony mortise. The bony configuration alone does confer some stability to the joint. But the ligaments on the medial and lateral aspects of the joint are the most important components of the static stabilization system of the ankle. In addition to the static stabilizers, there are dynamic stabilizers (i.e., those requiring motion or applied tension), the most important of which are the peroneal tendons.

Although in a very simple sense the ankle can be thought of as a hinged joint, its motion is much more complex and involves sliding and some translation during normal joint motion.

E.M. Bluman (✉) • C.P. Chiodo • J.T. Smith
Department of Orthopedic Surgery, Brigham and Women's Hospital,
75 Francis Street, Boston, MA, USA
e-mail: emb43@cornell.edu; cchiodo@partners.org; jsmith42@partners.org

© Springer International Publishing AG 2018
J.N. Katz et al. (eds.), *Principles of Orthopedic Practice for Primary Care Providers*, https://doi.org/10.1007/978-3-319-68661-5_20

a   b

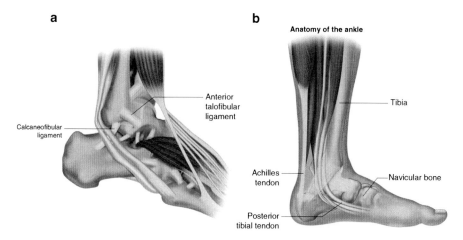

Fig. 20.1 Cartoon of (**a**) lateral and (**b**) medial ankle anatomy showing the static (joint morphology and ligaments) and dynamic (tendons) stabilizers of the joint

Summary of Epidemiology

Overall, the ankle is affected much less frequently by arthritis than the hip and knee joints. While almost 40% of individuals over 60 years of age have radiographic evidence of knee arthritis, in the same age cohort, approximately 5% of individuals have ankle arthritis.

It is not known why knee arthritis has higher prevalence than arthritis of the ankle. Biomechanical, histologic, and biochemical reasons have been postulated. The ankle joint is highly constrained when the dynamic and static stabilizers are considered in aggregate. This large degree of constraint has been suggested as one reason that arthritis is less likely to develop in the ankle. Ankle articular cartilage is thinner than that of other joints and better preserves its tensile stiffness and fracture stress with aging. The cartilage in the ankle has more resilience to biomechanical loading than that within the knee. In addition, there are metabolic differences between ankle and knee articular cartilage that may also help explain the relative rarity of primary ankle osteoarthritis. Biochemical assays have also shown that knee and ankle cartilage differ substantially. All of these factors may protect the ankle from developing primary osteoarthritis.

Unlike arthritis of the hip and knee joints, the majority (approximately 70%) of clinically important ankle arthritis is posttraumatic in nature. Those with significant end-stage ankle arthritis usually relate a history of ankle fracture, ankle dislocation, or a single or multiple severe sprains. Rarely, ankle arthritis develops without a history of significant ankle trauma (i.e., inflammatory or idiopathic pathologies).

Clinical Presentation

Patients with ankle arthritis typically complain of pain over the anterior aspect of the ankle. This pain may also feel as if it is deep within the joint. The pain usually develops over a long period of time and is not due to a single recent traumatic event.

Examination of patients may reveal limited joint motion as well as tenderness to palpation along the joint line. One needs to be careful that the ankle joint—and not the subtalar joint—is being tested. The ankle joint provides an arc of motion in the sagittal plane, while the subtalar joint provides the majority of motion in the coronal plane. Motion may be limited not only by mechanical blocks from osteophytes but also by contractures of the gastrocnemius and/or soleus musculotendinous units. There may be swelling, erythema, and/or an effusion about the ankle in these patients. In those who have developed arthritis from instability, the joint may show laxity in one or more planes.

Radiographic findings may include diminution of the tibiotalar joint space in a global sense or in a more limited distribution within the joint. Osteophytes can be present throughout the periphery of the joint but most often are seen over the anterior aspect of the joint. There can be subchondral sclerosis of bone and in some cases even cyst formation. Individuals who have developed arthritis of the ankle secondary to joint instability may show incongruity of the joint either on frontal views or lateral views. Some of the typical radiographic features of ankle arthritis are demonstrated in Fig. 20.2.

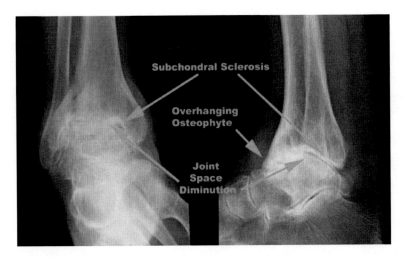

Fig. 20.2 Anteroposterior and lateral roentgenographic views of an ankle showing typical characteristics of ankle joint arthritis

Differential Diagnosis

The differential diagnosis for ankle arthritis includes ankle joint infections, inflammatory arthritis, osteochondral lesions of the talus, loose bodies within the joint, and ankle joint mechanically induced synovitis. In many of these cases, advanced imaging or lab work—including joint aspirates—can be very helpful in discerning among possibilities on the differential list.

A joint infection may cause swelling, pain, and erythema about the joint. There will likely be a significant limitation in motion, but this will be due to inflammation and pain of the synovium and not to a mechanical block. Patients with ankle infections generally do not want to move the ankle at all and may have fever, chills, nausea, or vomiting associated with the infection. If an ankle joint infection is suspected, an aspirate should be performed and sent for analysis to include Gram stain, culture, and antibiotic sensitivity determination.

Inflammatory arthritides may have similar signs and symptoms clinically and show similar joint space reduction radiographically. However, many patients with such pathologies will have polyarticular involvement.

Osteochondral lesions of the talus may cause complaints similar to those in ankle arthritis. However, clinical examination usually will demonstrate a localized point of maximal intensity on the talar dome, rather than the more global pain seen with tibiotalar arthritis. Osteochondral lesions are the localized softening of the talar bone and overlying articular cartilage. Loose bodies may cause locking and pain within the joint, but typically will do so intermittently, whenever the loose body impinges between the articular surfaces. This intermittent pain and locking are not typical of ankle arthritis. Mechanically induced ankle joint synovitis may have many of the clinical features of ankle arthritis but will not show joint space diminution, osteophytes, or bony changes on standard radiographs.

Nonoperative Management

Nonoperative management of ankle arthritis can provide substantial relief lasting years for many patients. Nonoperative treatment options include activity modification, cryotherapy, nonsteroidal anti-inflammatory drugs, shoe wear modification, bracing, and injections.

Activities that involve impact loading or require quick accelerations or decelerations tend to exacerbate ankle arthritis. If such activity can be minimized or limited, the patient will usually have a substantial decrease in pain.

Shoe wear modification can supplement activity modification to further reduce symptoms. Addition of a rocker bottom to the sole of a shoe can reduce the amount of ankle plantar flexion and dorsiflexion required for walking and, in doing so, greatly diminish the amount of pain experienced during ambulation. These modifications can be placed by a certified orthotist or in some cases by a cobbler. The

Fig. 20.3 Rocker bottom shoe that allows the patient to roll through the stance phase of gait so that there is less motion in the ankle joint

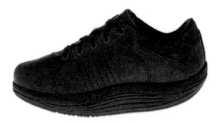

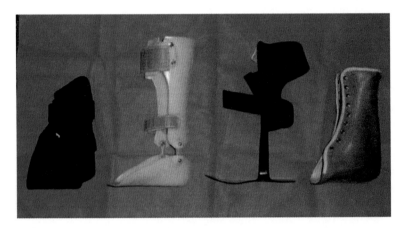

Fig. 20.4 Examples of fabric, custom molded plastic and carbon fiber ankle braces for use in patients with ankle arthritis. The appropriateness of each of these is dependent on a multitude of patient factors

modification is glued onto the bottom of a standard sneaker or shoe and provides a curved surface on the sole that allows the patient to roll through from the heel strike to toe off portions of gait (Fig. 20.3).

Bracing can also be an effective treatment for ankle arthritis. Effective ankle braces range from fabric ankle wraps to custom molded orthoses that provide rigid ankle and hindfoot stability. Each has the goal of limiting the amount of ankle motion. By closely applying a rigid or inelastic component to the ankle, bracing can prevent or significantly limit motion through the tibiotalar joint. Fabric ankle wraps have the advantage of being relatively cheap and easy to apply and remove. Custom molded orthotics, such as ankle foot orthoses, provide excellent fit and rigid stability for many patients. Some of these molded orthotics can be covered with soft leather to increase comfort. Carbon fiber ankle braces have the advantage of being lightweight, low profile, and very durable. They can fit easily into most shoes. Figure 20.4 shows examples of fabric, custom molded plastic and carbon fiber ankle braces.

Lastly, injections of corticosteroids can be placed intra-articularly to combat the pain and inflammation that the arthritis generates. These injections can be both diagnostic and therapeutic. The placement of a corticosteroid admixed with local anesthetic can provide immediate feedback in terms of pain relief. The steroid will usually take 48–72 h to reach a maximal effect. In some cases, injections can be used to manage ankle arthritis conservatively for extended periods of time. Frequency should be limited to no more than once every 3 months. This limit is meant to combat some of the adverse effects of corticosteroid on the cartilage as well as the soft tissues surrounding the ankle. For although the corticosteroid has a powerful anti-inflammatory effect, it can also cause some softening of structures containing collagen, including cartilage. It also may lead to thinning and bleaching of the skin at the injection site.

Although individual nonoperative treatments can have significant therapeutic effects in isolation, they can be combined for even greater effect.

Surgical Management

In general, patients should have exhausted nonoperative treatment options before considering operative treatment of their ankle arthritis. Surgical options include arthroscopic debridement of osteophytes and loose bodies, cheilectomy to remove osteophytes and increase ankle motion, distraction arthroplasty, ankle fusion, and total ankle arthroplasty.

Arthroscopic debridement of an arthritic ankle joint has the advantage of being a minimally invasive procedure with a short recovery time. However, in most cases, the effects obtained from such a procedure are short lived (i.e., weeks or months in duration) for those individuals with end-stage ankle arthritis. For those with milder cases of arthritis, there may be some beneficial effects that are more durable. Although debridement may be useful as a bridge procedure in select circumstances, it is generally not an effective method for end-stage arthritis.

Cheilectomy is a procedure in which osteophytes at the anterior margin of the ankle joint are removed. In certain cases, these osteophytes may be "kissing"; that is, they may physically abut each other on ankle dorsiflexion. This can cause either bony or soft tissue impingement. If the majority of pain is coming at the end of dorsiflexion range of motion, then a surgical procedure to remove these osteophytes can be very effective. This procedure does not treat the loss of articular cartilage directly. Here again, as with arthroscopic debridement, the procedure is less invasive than other large open procedures and has a fairly short recovery time. In certain individuals, it can be very effective, not only in the short run but also in the long run. Studies have shown that about 90% of patients undergoing cheilectomy for the proper indications will have improvement in their symptoms, with approximately 60% being pain-free at 2 years post-procedure.

Distraction arthroplasty is a technique used to regenerate painless articulating surfaces in the ankle joint. The procedure involves an arthroscopic debridement of the ankle joint followed by the application of an external fixator, which creates a distractive force across the ankle joint. Once the fixator is applied, the patient is allowed to be full weight bearing on the affected lower extremity. Allowing weight bearing—with the distractor on to remove shear forces from the articulating surfaces—maintains the beneficial effects of fluid pressure to the cartilage. Fluid pressure nourishes the cartilage, which obtains all of its metabolic needs through the joint fluid. This therapy has been shown to have durable effects. In fact, studies have shown that the results tend to improve with time after the frame has been removed. This therapy is not for everyone, as wearing a frame for 3–4 months is challenging for most. In addition, not all orthopedic surgeons are comfortable with putting on the type of circular fixators required. Some groups have reported that over 90% of patients will have improvement in their pain following ankle distraction arthroplasty.

For decades, fusion has been regarded as a very reliable definitive therapy for end-stage ankle arthritis. This procedure causes the tibia and talus to grow together and obliterates the ankle joint. In removing the joint, the arthritis is also eliminated. This therapy requires 6 weeks of non-weight bearing followed by 6 weeks of weight bearing in a cast. Following successful fusion, patients reliably experience a decrease in—and frequently the elimination of—pain in the ankle joint. This relief is durable. Once established, the fusion does not degrade and is able to sustain heavy loads placed upon it. The fusion does not require maintenance and does not need to be monitored after successful establishment. Ankle fusions can be performed in patients with many different comorbidities and levels of obesity.

As with any therapy, there are side effects to ankle fusion. These are usually not realized for years after the fusion is performed but can have a significant effect on patients in the long term. In addition to being a major motion segment for locomotion, the ankle joint also serves as a shock absorber. When this shock absorption is eliminated, the forces of locomotion are transmitted to other joints of the distal lower extremity, particularly the subtalar and transverse tarsal joints. Years after ankle fusion, these joints become arthritic and may eventually require fusion. When these additional joints are fused, the foot becomes extremely stiff and gait changes markedly. Activities such as walking long distance and hiking—relatively easy with an ankle fusion alone—become significantly more challenging. This is one major reason that ankle arthroplasty is generally reserved for those with end-stage ankle arthritis.

Total ankle arthroplasty (TAA) is a procedure that replaces the weight-bearing tibiotalar articulation of the ankle joint. Current designs use durable metal talar and tibial implants with a high molecular weight polyethylene component sandwiched between them. Unlike fusion, TAA maintains the tibiotalar articulation. The goal is to relieve arthritis pain while maintaining ankle motion and function. In addition to maintaining ankle function, TAA also aims to prevent the hindfoot arthritis that inevitably develops with ankle fusion.

Total ankle arthroplasty has been shown to be effective in properly selected patients in relieving the pain of ankle arthritis while maintaining ankle motion. Ankle replacement surgery—when performed properly and for the correct indications—has reliably provided pain relief. Historically, over 80% of patients undergoing total ankle arthroplasty had their pain levels reduced to three or less on a visual analog scale.

338 E.M. Bluman et al.

Table 20.1 Summary of diagnosis and treatment of ankle arthritis

Clinical entity	Presentation	Diagnostic testing	Conservative management	Indications for surgery	Operative management
Ankle arthritis	– TTP anterior ankle joint – Diminished ankle joint motion – Joint crepitus – Antalgic gait	– Standing Roentgenograms of ankle – Diagnostic injection (to rule out other sites of pathology)	– Bracing/splinting – Rocker bottom shoes – Steroid injection into joint	– Pain refractory to all conservative management	– Arthroscopic debridement – Distraction arthroplasty – Total ankle arthroplasty – Ankle fusion

Ankle arthroplasty, like any other joint arthroplasty, needs to be monitored intermittently once successfully established. As with other joint arthroplasty techniques, TAA has complications that can develop throughout the lifetime of the patient. These include osteolysis secondary to wear particle generation, arthrofibrosis, and infection. Long-term survival of total ankle arthroplasty implants at 10 years after implantation is 80–90%. Patients who have failure of their implants are able to be revised in some cases but, in other cases, require fusion after explant of the implant. Table 20.1 shows a summary of the diagnosis and treatment of ankle arthritis.

Suggested Reading

AOFAS. http://www.aofas.org/footcaremd/conditions/ailments-of-the-ankle/Pages/Arthritis.aspx.
Bluman EM, Chiodo CP. Tibiotalar arthrodesis. Semin Arthroplast. 2010;21:240–6.
Buckwalter J, Saltzman C. Ankle osteoarthritis: distinctive characteristics. AAOS Instr Course Lect. 1999;48:233–41.
Hayes BJ, Gonzalez T, Smith JT, Chiodo CP, Bluman EM. Ankle arthritis: you can't always replace it. J Am Acad Orthop Surg. 2016;24(2):e29–38.
Riskowski J, Dufour AB, Hannan MT. Arthritis, foot pain & shoe wear: current musculoskeletal research on feet. Curr Opin Rheumatol. 2011;23(2):148–55. https://doi.org/10.1097/BOR.0b013e3283422cf5.
Tellisi N, Fragomen AT, Kleinman D, O'Malley MJ, Rozbruch SR. Joint preservation of the osteoarthritic ankle using distraction arthroplasty. Foot Ankle Int. 2009;30(4):318–25.

Chapter 21
Soft Tissue Disorders of the Ankle

Jeremy T. Smith, Eric M. Bluman, and Christopher P. Chiodo

Abbreviations

AFO	Ankle foot orthosis
ATFL	Anterior talofibular ligament
CFL	Calcaneofibular ligament
ECSWT	Extracorporeal shock wave therapy
MRI	Magnetic resonance imaging
ORIF	Open reduction internal fixation
PT	Physical therapy
PTFL	Posterior talofibular ligament
PTT	Posterior tibial tendon
PTTD	Posterior tibial tendon dysfunction
RICE	Rest ice compression elevation

Achilles Tendon Disorders

The Achilles tendon is a confluence of the gastrocnemius and soleus muscles. These muscles, collectively referred to as the triceps surae, consolidate into the Achilles tendon—the largest and strongest tendon in the body. The Achilles then attaches broadly, with an approximately 2 × 2 cm attachment, to the posterior aspect of the calcaneus. During standing and throughout much of the gait cycle, the calf muscle-tendon unit is active and is either lengthening or shortening.

The blood supply to the Achilles comes from both proximal and distal directions. The proximal portion of the tendon receives its vasculature from intramuscular arterial branches. Distally, the tendon receives its blood supply from interosseous arterioles in the calcaneus. The result is that the central portion of the Achilles tendon, roughly 2–6 cm proximal to its insertion, is relatively poorly vascularized.

J.T. Smith (✉) • E.M. Bluman • C.P. Chiodo
Department of Orthopedic Surgery, Brigham and Women's Hospital,
75 Francis Street, Boston, MA, USA
e-mail: jsmith42@partners.org; emb43@cornell.edu; cchiodo@partners.org

© Springer International Publishing AG 2018   339
J.N. Katz et al. (eds.), *Principles of Orthopedic Practice for Primary Care Providers*, https://doi.org/10.1007/978-3-319-68661-5_21

Accordingly, much of the pathology that occurs in the Achilles tendon is at this vascular watershed.

Conditions affecting the Achilles muscle-tendon unit may involve the medial head of the gastrocnemius muscle, the non-insertional Achilles tendon (which involves the area of tendon typically 2–6 cm above the calcaneus), the insertional Achilles tendon, and the Achilles bursae. Two bursae sit adjacent to the Achilles insertion, one in front of the tendon insertion (retrocalcaneal bursa) and one behind (Achilles tendon bursa).

Achilles Tendinopathy

We advocate using three terms to describe Achilles tendon disorders: *tendinitis*, *tendinosis*, and *tendinopathy*. Tendinitis is an acute inflammatory pathologic process that involves inflammatory changes within either the substance of the tendon or the surrounding tendon layer, the peritenon. Tendinosis is a chronic degenerative process that occurs without inflammation of the peritenon. Tendinosis is characterized by degenerative lesions within the tendon substance with altered microscopic tendon structure. Macroscopically, a tendinotic tendon is thickened and lacks its healthy shiny appearance. Tendinopathy is a general term that includes tendinitis and tendinosis.

Achilles tendon disorders are often described by anatomic location, either at the calcaneal insertion (*insertional*) or within the substance of the tendon (*non-insertional*). The chronicity of the disorder is also often incorporated into its description with the use of the following terms: *acute* (<2 weeks of symptoms), *subacute* (2–6 weeks of symptoms), or *chronic* (>6 weeks).

Summary of Epidemiology

Tendinopathy of the Achilles tendon is most commonly caused by a combination of intrinsic and extrinsic factors. Intrinsic causes may include aging, foot or ankle deformity that contributes to added tendon stress, and a tight gastrocnemius muscle. Extrinsic factors include poor shoewear, hard surface conditions, and overuse which occurs at times with exercise. Achilles tendinitis develops frequently in athletes, often those who run or participate in sports that require frequent bursts of speed (e.g., soccer, basketball, tennis). Tendinitis therefore is seen more often in younger patients. Achilles tendinosis, in contrast, more often develops in older patients who have not begun any new or increasingly strenuous activity.

Clinical Presentation

Achilles tendinitis typically presents with an acute onset of pain in the Achilles that is exacerbated by activities that stress the tendon, including walking, stair climbing, running, and athletics. Additionally, worsened pain with the first steps in the morning is common. This start-up pain phenomenon is thought to be related to sleeping with the ankle plantar flexed, as most people do, which allows the tendon to tighten overnight and then stretch painfully with the first morning steps. Erythema or swelling may be present at the site of maximal discomfort. Upon examination, patients often have an antalgic gait in an attempt to limit motion at the ankle and stress to the tendon. The Achilles is focally tender, and while it may be somewhat swollen, there are not typically nodules within the substance of the tendon. Palpation should not reveal any gap in the tendon. The Thompson test—which evaluates the continuity of the tendon by squeezing the calf muscle and expecting a plantar flexion response of the ankle—should reveal a tendon that is intact and symmetric to the non-injured extremity. Ankle range of motion should be carefully assessed, as patients often have a tight gastrocnemius muscle; this may be part of the underlying cause of the tendinopathy.

In contrast to Achilles tendinitis, the onset of pain with Achilles tendinosis is often insidious. There is typically no acute event linked to the development of pain. Patients often report an area of swelling with a "knot" or "nodule" within the tendon. This nodule represents the area of greatest tendon degeneration. As with Achilles tendinitis, the tendon itself is often tender to palpation. The distinction between insertional and non-insertional tendinosis, or tendinitis, is based simply on the location of maximal tenderness on physical examination. However, whereas non-insertional tendinosis typically presents with a nodule within the tendon, insertional disease is often (but not always) accompanied by abnormal calcaneal bony morphology. A bony prominence at the posterosuperior calcaneus, just anterior to the tendon insertion, is called a Haglund's lesion (Fig. 21.1). This is distinct from insertional Achilles calcification, which can also contribute to pain at the tendon insertion. Insertional tendinopathy may be accompanied with retrocalcaneal or Achilles bursitis.

Fluoroquinolone antibiotics have been associated with disorders of the Achilles, including tendinopathy and rupture. This observation was first published in 1983 and has been documented in many studies since, including in vitro studies showing fluoroquinolone-related damage to collagen and tenocytes. As of yet, the exact mechanism of fluoroquinolone injury to tendons has not been fully established.

Differential Diagnosis and Suggested Diagnostic Testing

The diagnosis of Achilles tendinopathy is largely based on history and physical examination. Other causes of posterior leg pain include gastrocnemius strain, Achilles tendon rupture, plantaris rupture, chronic exertional compartment syndrome, calcaneal stress fracture, lumbar radiculopathy, and claudication.

Fig. 21.1 Lateral radiograph with Haglund's lesion (solid line) as well as insertional Achilles spur (dashed line)

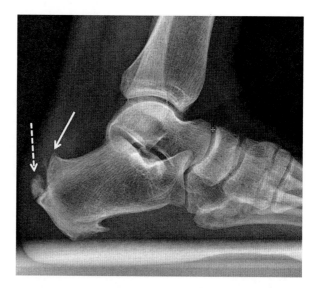

Fig. 21.2 Lateral radiograph showing a calcaneal stress fracture (solid line), seen as a sclerotic line through the calcaneus

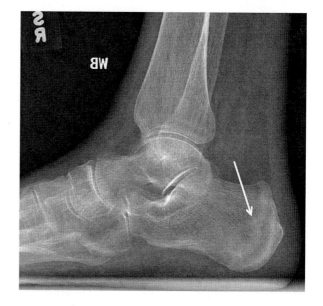

Plain radiographs of the ankle are useful in identifying abnormal calcaneal bony morphology. It is important to note that patients may have spurs on the calcaneus that are not associated with any pain or limitation. At times, a calcaneal stress fracture may be appreciated on plain radiograph as a sclerotic line through the calcaneus (Fig. 21.2). Advanced imaging, either MRI or ultrasound, is not often necessary but can be utilized to better clarify the extent of tendon involvement.

Non-operative Management

The majority of patients with Achilles tendinopathy can be successfully managed without surgery. For those presenting with tendinitis, particularly with the acute onset of severe pain, the use of a tall walking boot for a few weeks is often helpful. After that, and for those with tendinosis, treatment involves a carefully guided stretching and strengthening program with a physical therapist. Eccentric stretching, which occurs with firing of the muscle-tendon unit as it is being lengthened, has been shown to be an effective treatment. This program is accompanied by the use of a dorsiflexion night splint, which keeps the tendon stretched during sleep. Additional treatments may include activity modification, anti-inflammatory medications, and the use of a heel lift. For patients with pressure-related pain from shoes rubbing at the posterior heel, often called a "pump bump," the use of a gel heel sleeve to cover this area can be helpful. Corticosteroid injection into the tendon is *not* recommended as this is associated with Achilles rupture.

For those whose pain does not improve with those treatments just outlined— including boot immobilization, activity modification, and stretching and strengthening with physical therapy—additional nonsurgical treatments include the use of a custom ankle foot orthosis (AFO) or extracorporeal shock wave therapy (ECSWT). ECSWT, which uses a technology similar to lithotripsy, is performed as an in-office procedure and has shown promising results for patients with recalcitrant Achilles tendinopathy. The mechanism of its effect is not well understood, although theories include alteration in neural membranes or local vascularity.

Indications for Surgery

Surgical treatment may be indicated for patients with persistent pain and symptoms despite nonsurgical treatment. Most patients considered for surgery have had months of nonsurgical management and yet remain limited by pain in the Achilles tendon. Perioperative risk assessment is very important, and for certain patients, surgery is not appropriate due to systemic medical conditions, poor local physiology such as peripheral vascular disease, or an anticipated inability to comply with postoperative restricted weightbearing instructions.

Operative Management

Operative treatment for both insertional and non-insertional tendinopathy has traditionally involved open debridement of the diseased tendon and repair of the remaining tendon. This can at times require removal of a substantial portion of the Achilles, which may necessitate a transfer of one of the other flexor tendons to augment the remaining Achilles. For insertional tendinopathy, the Haglund's lesion and/or insertional spur are also removed. This involves surgically smoothing down the back of the calcaneus.

Less invasive surgical techniques include endoscopic Haglund's excision and retrocalcaneal bursa debridement for insertional disease and smaller incision release of adhesions surrounding non-insertional lesions. Gastrocnemius recession, which lengthens the Achilles muscle-tendon unit, has shown promise in offloading the Achilles.

Expected Outcome and Predictors of Outcome

Duration of symptoms prior to the onset of treatment has been associated with outcome. Those with symptoms for 6 months or longer are more likely to require surgical intervention. Additionally, insertional tendinopathy with a Haglund's lesion or insertional spur is less likely to respond favorably to nonsurgical treatment. For those who do require operative intervention, most studies report greater than 80% of patients with substantial pain relief.

Achilles Tendon Ruptures

Summary of Epidemiology

Rupture of the Achilles tendon occurs with an estimated incidence of 7 per 100,000 people annually in the USA. Ruptures occur with rapid loading of a tensed tendon. This condition is seen most commonly in men in the fourth or fifth decade of life, and injuries are often sports related. The majority of patients who sustain a rupture have microscopic and macroscopic alteration in the tendon integrity. Reports in the literature link Achilles rupture with fluoroquinolone use, certain endocrine abnormalities (hypothyroidism, renal disease), and systemic inflammatory arthritis (rheumatoid arthritis).

Achilles ruptures have a substantial societal cost, with many patients requiring an extensive time out of work. Most treatment programs require several months on crutches and then a gradual return to activities.

Clinical Presentation

Patients typically experience the immediate onset of pain and a pop or pull in the Achilles at the time of rupture. Many report feeling that someone kicked them in the Achilles and then turning around to see that no one was behind them. Patients may be able to ambulate by recruiting the deep flexors of the leg to push off, so ambulation does not exclude this diagnosis. On examination, the most consistent findings include a palpable gap in the Achilles, a lack of plantar flexion of the ankle when the calf is squeezed (abnormal Thompson test), and increased passive dorsiflexion of the ankle as compared to the non-injured extremity.

The diagnosis of Achilles rupture is missed initially in up to 25% of patients. This is likely because of patients' ability to compensate when walking and the difficulty of appreciating a gap in the swollen tendon. Treatment options and success rely upon early diagnosis, and thus making the diagnosis at time of presentation is critical.

Differential Diagnosis and Suggested Diagnostic Testing

Plantaris tendon rupture or gastrocnemius strain may also cause a pop or a pull at the back of the leg. These diagnoses can be distinguished from an Achilles rupture by palpation of a gap, a Thompson test, and assessment of passive ankle dorsiflexion. As with Achilles tendinopathy, the diagnosis of an Achilles tendon rupture is largely clinical. In many patients, radiographs are not necessary, although can be useful to ensure that there has not been a calcaneal avulsion fracture. MRI and ultrasound may be used to confirm the diagnosis, although are not required if the history and clinical examination is clear.

Non-operative Management

Achilles tendon ruptures can be treated both surgically and nonsurgically. Treatment goals include minimizing the risk of surgical wound healing problems or infection, restoring Achilles continuity and push-off strength, and minimizing the risk of re-rupture. Operative treatment carries inherent surgical risks. Nonsurgical treatment has historically led to decreased strength or unacceptably high rates of re-rupture. Over the past decade, though, significant strides have been made in approaches to both operative and non-operative treatments.

Traditional nonsurgical treatment of Achilles tendon ruptures involved cast immobilization of the ankle for 6–8 weeks. With this treatment, rates of re-rupture were reported to occur in roughly 20% of patients. Due to this high re-rupture rate, and based in part upon knowledge that tendons heal better when mobilized, current nonsurgical treatment protocols move the ankle early with a program called early functional rehabilitation. A randomized controlled trial published in 2010 randomized 144 patients to either operative or non-operative treatment using early functional rehabilitation and showed a re-rupture rate that was similar between both groups (3% in the surgical group versus 4% in the nonsurgical group). In this study, the nonsurgical group was treated with immobilization in a splint with the ankle in plantar flexion for 2 weeks, followed by gentle graduated range of motion while protected in a boot. It is critical to understand that nonsurgical treatment is not synonymous with nontreatment; the nonsurgical approach is a specific structured program.

Non-operative treatment of acute Achilles tendon ruptures is a viable and effective method of treatment. To date, it remains unclear whether operative or non-operative management is superior. Studies suggest that operative treatment carries an increased risk of surgical complications and yet provides benefits in push-off strength and an earlier return to work. The approach at our institution is to thoroughly present both treatment options, evaluate the patient's surgical risk profile, and work with the patient to determine the optimal treatment for him or her.

Indications for Surgery

Successful nonsurgical treatment of Achilles ruptures often requires early immobilization with the ankle plantar flexed. This is thought to start the tendon healing by bringing the tendon ends into closer proximity. It is thus thought by many that an initial delay in diagnosis by more than a few weeks is a relative indication for surgical treatment.

Patient comorbidities also guide the treatment decision for Achilles ruptures, as systemic or local factors can tilt the risk/benefit scale when deciding between operative and non-operative treatment. Surgical treatment should be approached cautiously in patients over age 65 and those with diabetes, immunosuppression, peripheral vascular disease, obesity, skin disorders involving the leg, and tobacco use.

Operative Management

The goal of operative treatment is to re-approximate the ends of the Achilles while minimizing the risk of surgical complications. Open surgical techniques typically approach the Achilles posteriorly and then suture the tendon ends together with tension that matches the contralateral extremity. With careful attention to detail, including gentle handling of the soft tissues, not using a tourniquet, and meticulous closure in layers, the risk of surgical wound complications can be lessened.

In an effort to further decrease the chances of wound healing complications, minimally invasive surgical techniques have been developed. Multiple techniques exist, but the general concept is that sutures are shuttled percutaneously through the tendon ends and then tied together through a small incision overlying the site of the rupture. Minimally invasive techniques have been shown to have very low surgical wound complication rates and, importantly, have functional outcomes that are similar to more traditional open surgical repair techniques.

Expected Outcome and Predictors of Outcome

Recovery from an Achilles tendon rupture takes many months. Patients are counseled that it can take up to one year to regain near-normal strength and that mild weakness in the injured extremity may persist. With appropriate treatment, either surgical or nonsurgical, good function can be achieved in the vast majority of patients.

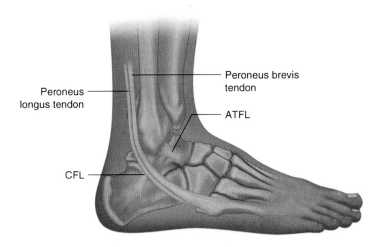

Fig. 21.3 Illustration of the lateral ankle, showing the lateral ankle ligaments, peroneus brevis tendon, and peroneus longus tendon

Peroneal Tendon Disorders

The peroneus brevis and peroneus longus muscle-tendon units run along the lateral aspect of the leg and cross the ankle posterolaterally, behind the fibula. The peroneus brevis tendon continues to its insertion at the base of the fifth metatarsal, and the peroneus longus crosses under the foot to attach at the plantar surface of the medial cuneiform and first metatarsal (Fig. 21.3). The peroneal tendons are adjacent to one another as they pass behind the fibula and then diverge at the peroneal tubercle, a bony prominence on the lateral wall of the calcaneus. The peroneus brevis tendon is thinner and more ribbon shaped than the longus and is more prone to injury.

Peroneal tendon injuries include tenosynovitis, tendon tears, and dislocation from their groove behind the fibula. Tears of the tendon are seen most commonly behind the fibula but can also occur at other sites such as the peroneal tubercle.

Peroneal Tendinitis/Tendon Tears

Summary of Epidemiology

Pathology of the peroneal tendons is uncommon without either a traumatic event (such as an ankle inversion injury), a pre-disposing mechanical abnormality, or a systemic inflammatory condition. Chronic ankle instability, resulting in frequent inversion ankle injuries, can also lead to injury of the peroneal tendons. Similarly, varus hindfoot alignment, which tilts the ankle and hindfoot inward and places stress on the structures at the lateral ankle and foot, can lead to peroneal tendinopathy.

Clinical Presentation

Tenosynovitis of the peroneal tendons typically presents with pain along the lateral and posterolateral aspects of the ankle. Patients often report activity-related pain with stair climbing and walking on irregular ground. This discomfort may be accompanied by swelling along the course of the tendons. Recent shoe wear changes or alternation in activity level is common. Peroneal tendon tears, which frequently accompany tenosynovitis, are typically longitudinal split tears, and therefore near-normal tendon strength is preserved.

Peroneal tendon subluxation, which occurs when the tendons dislocate laterally from behind the fibula, often occurs traumatically. Patients may be able to replicate the tendon instability by rotating the ankle in a large circle (circumduction). Tenderness just behind the fibula is common. With time, the pain from an acute injury may improve, but the tendons often remain unstable, which predisposes to tears. Clicking of the tendons may be due to subluxation from behind the fibula or intra-tendinous subluxation, in which one of the tendons clicks in and out of a tear of the adjacent tendon.

Physical examination should include assessment of gait, hindfoot and foot alignment (to assess for a varus hindfoot), site of maximal tenderness, peroneal tendon strength, ankle circumduction (to test for peroneal subluxation), and ankle stability.

Differential Diagnosis and Suggested Diagnostic Testing

Additional causes of posterolateral ankle pain and lateral hindfoot pain include injury to the fibula, calcaneus, or sural nerve, sinus tarsi syndrome, tumor, and radiculopathy. Plain radiographs are used to evaluate bony changes as well as to assess radiographic alignment, with particular attention to identifying any varus of the ankle or hindfoot. An enlarged peroneal tubercle may be appreciated by plain X-ray. Additional studies, such as MRI, can be very helpful in defining the extent of tendon involvement. In the setting of peroneal tendon instability, MRI enables measurement of the depth of the fibular groove. A shallow groove is associated with tendon subluxation and may necessitate surgery to deepen the groove. If the source of the patient's pain remains unclear, a diagnostic local anesthetic injection administered into the peroneal tendon sheath may help determine if the tendons are the source of the pain.

Non-operative Management

Peroneal tendon pain without tendon instability is most often treated with immobilization in a tall walking boot for 4–6 weeks. This period of rest is followed by a transitional soft ankle brace and physical therapy. Ice, anti-inflammatory medications, and activity modification may be helpful. For those with a high arch or varus hindfoot, orthotics can take pressure off the lateral hindfoot and peroneal tendons. As with Achilles tendon disorders, corticosteroid injections into the tendons are not recommended due to risk of rupture.

Peroneal subluxation or dislocation can also be treated nonsurgically, although this requires a 6-week period of cast immobilization with the ankle in plantar flexion. It is logistically difficult to ensure that the tendons remain reduced during this casting period, and tendon instability is successfully treated nonsurgically in only about 50% of cases.

Indications for Surgery

Surgery for peroneal tendinitis or tendon tears is considered for patients who have persistent symptoms despite extensive nonsurgical treatment. Surgery is more commonly recommended early for those with peroneal tendon instability.

Operative Management

The traditional approach for peroneal tendinitis or tendon tears is an open surgical procedure that exposes the tendons and enables debridement of inflamed tenosynovium and repair of tears as necessary. Some tears are amenable to repair, while others require removal of the torn portion of tendon. With extensive involvement, a tendon transfer may be necessary. Attention is also given to the underlying cause of the problem, which may be addressed simultaneously; this can include ligament repair for chronic ankle instability, correction of a varus hindfoot with osteotomies, or removal of an enlarged peroneal tubercle.

Recently developed arthroscopic techniques enable less invasive procedures and a quicker recovery. Tendoscopy allows for excellent visualization of the tendons and debridement of tissue from within the tendon sheath (Fig. 21.4).

Peroneal tendon subluxation is treated with an open repair of the peroneal retinaculum. Additionally, the tendons are exposed to address any associated tendon tears, and the fibular groove may be deepened with an osteotomy. This procedure, as is the case with most open peroneal tendon surgery, requires a period of 6 weeks of postoperative restricted weightbearing on crutches.

Expected Outcome and Predictors of Outcome

Due in part to the length of recovery required for healing after open peroneal tendon surgery, patients are counseled to expect a recovery period of at least three to 6 months. Clinical outcomes studies report good results with peroneal tendon procedures.

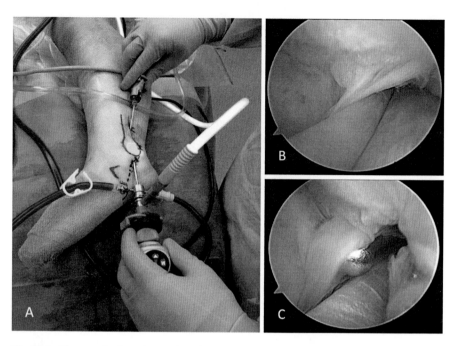

Fig. 21.4 Photograph of a patient undergoing peroneal tendoscopy (**a**). Arthroscopic photographs (**b**) show the peroneal tendons (stars), and a shaver device is utilized to remove scar tissue (**c**)

Posterior Tibial Tendon Disorders

The posterior tibialis muscle originates at the posterior aspect of the tibia, fibula, and interosseous membrane. The posterior tibial tendon (PTT) then passes behind the medial malleolus at the ankle and inserts broadly at the medial midfoot. The navicular is the primary site of attachment for the PTT. This muscle-tendon unit initiates push-off when walking and helps to maintain the arch of the foot.

Several anatomic features predispose the PTT to injury. As with the Achilles tendon, injury to the PTT often occurs at the site of poor tendon vascularity at the level of the medial malleolus. Secondly, the tendon has an excursion of only about two centimeters, meaning that the tendon travels a relatively small distance within its sheath as the muscle contracts and lengthens. Thus even minor injuries that lengthen the tendon impact its function.

Posterior Tibial Tendon Dysfunction

Summary of Epidemiology

Posterior tibial tendon dysfunction (PTTD) occurs most commonly in middle age and most often results from attritional wear of the tendon. Posterior tibial tendon pathology typically begins with inflammation without lengthening or loss of function of the tendon. With chronic inflammation, the tendon can then attenuate, lengthen, and then progressively deteriorate and weaken. As it deteriorates, it loses its ability to maintain the arch of the foot. As the foot begins to collapse, the hindfoot drifts laterally into valgus, and the midfoot begins to sag. Correspondingly, the Achilles tendon unit tightens as its working length shortens. This pathophysiologic process can then become cyclical, as the resultant shape of the foot puts added stress on the PTT and can lead to further injury.

The etiology of PTTD is often multifactorial. Causes may include repetitive microtrauma, anatomic predisposition to tendon injury (resultant from congenital pes planus alignment or an accessory navicular bone), systemic inflammatory conditions such as seronegative spondyloarthropathy, vascular insufficiency, and obesity. Posterior tibial tendinitis also occurs in younger patients, although more commonly after traumatic events such as an ankle eversion sprain, fracture, or repetitive sports-related injury.

Clinical Presentation

Posterior tibial tendon dysfunction is classified into four stages of increasing severity and often progresses through the stages if untreated. The first stage of PTTD is tendinitis without deformity. This typically causes pain and localized swelling along the course of the PTT. Examination should always include a standing analysis of alignment, which, in stage I disease, will reveal a neutrally aligned hindfoot. Patients may have difficulty initiating a single leg heel rise due to pain along the PTT. Stage II PTTD occurs when the hindfoot has drifted into valgus (Fig. 21.5), and yet the deformity remains flexible. The tendon is often tender and swollen. With manipulation, the alignment of the foot may be corrected, which distinguishes Stage II from Stage III. The rigid deformity in Stage III disease often is caused by hindfoot arthritic changes. As the deformity progresses, the site of pain may shift as well. If the posterior tibial tendon completely tears, this may alleviate pain at the medial ankle as the inflamed tendon has now released. Pain may occur laterally due to impingement of the calcaneus against the lateral soft tissues and the fibula. As the condition worsens, the long-standing valgus deformity can lead to injury to the deltoid ligament, which is the primary medial ankle ligamentous support. As this occurs, the ankle joint can drift into valgus alignment, which is Stage IV PTTD.

Fig. 21.5 Photograph of a patient with a left valgus hindfoot. On the uninvolved right side, the hindfoot alignment is neutral

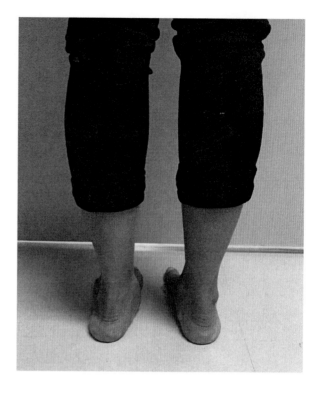

Differential Diagnosis and Suggested Diagnostic Testing

Additional causes of medial ankle pain include bony injury such as stress fracture of the medial malleolus or navicular, tendinitis of the flexors to the toes, and tarsal tunnel syndrome.

Examination should begin with a barefoot standing examination to assess alignment. Localized swelling along the PTT may be appreciated and range of motion testing will often reveal a contracture of the gastrocnemius muscle. A single leg heel rise assesses the competence of the posterior tibial tendon. Plain radiography of the foot and ankle is indicated to evaluate the source of the pain and to assess alignment. To evaluate alignment, it is critical that the radiographs be *weightbearing*. MRI is a useful study to assess the degree of injury to the PTT, although is not required if the diagnosis is clear.

Non-operative Management

Many patients with PTTD can be effectively managed without surgery. The approach to treating this disorder is to rest the tendon, train the tendon with physical therapy, and then protect the tendon with an orthotic. Immobilization is accomplished with a tall walking boot. Patients with milder symptoms or who are unsteady on their feet—and therefore not safe in a boot—may be treated with a smaller ankle brace. The duration of immobilization is typically 4–6 weeks, and then patients transition from the boot into orthotics that support the medial hindfoot. Over-the-counter orthotics, although much cheaper, are often not sufficient to adequately off-load the PTT, and therefore many patients require custom molded orthotics. If orthotics are not sufficient, larger braces such as an ankle-foot orthosis may be considered. Physical therapy begins after boot immobilization and concentrates on training the tendon and stretching the tight gastrocnemius muscle. Corticosteroid injection is not recommended as it can further attenuate the PTT.

Indications for Surgery

Surgery may be considered for patients who have persistent or worsening symptoms despite the treatments outlined above. The specifics of surgery depend upon the stage of disease, age, and functional level. Larger reconstructive procedures often require 6-week non-weightbearing after surgery, and thus patients must be able to manage this challenging restriction.

Operative Management

The classification scheme outlined previously guides treatment. Stage I disease (inflammation without deformity) is typically treated with tenosynovectomy. This can be done either in an open fashion or tendoscopically. Stage II PTTD (flexible deformity) is most commonly managed with a combination of procedures that reshape the foot while removing the painful tendon. Often this involves lengthening the tight gastrocnemius muscle, removing the diseased PTT, transferring another tendon into its place (most commonly the flexor to the lesser toes), and correcting the bony alignment with osteotomies. Since stage II disease is flexible and joints of the hindfoot are typically non-arthritic, the joints are preserved. In stage III PTTD (fixed deformity), corrective osteotomies and tendon transfers are not powerful enough, and thus treatment often involves fusions of the joints of the hindfoot. When the ankle is involved in stage IV disease (valgus ankle deformity), procedures typically address both the hindfoot and ankle deformity. This may preserve the ankle joint as with a deltoid ligament reconstruction or sacrifice the ankle with an ankle replacement or fusion.

Expected Outcome and Predictors of Outcome

As PTTD progresses, the surgical treatment increases in complexity. While surgical intervention for all stages of disease has been shown to be successful, the more complex procedures carry increasing risk, and it is therefore optimal to interrupt the disease progression early. Pain relief along the medial ankle is a good indicator of successful non-operative treatment, so if a pain-free state can be achieved with the use of an orthotic, for example, then progressive deterioration of the tendon is unlikely to occur.

Ankle Ligament Injuries

Ankle Sprains

Summary of Epidemiology

Ankle sprains are the most common musculoskeletal injury, and it has been estimated that one ankle sprain occurs every second in the USA. The majority (85%) of these injuries involve the lateral ankle ligaments, with the remaining injuries occurring either to the medial ankle ligaments or the syndesmotic ligaments. Ankle sprains have been reported to account for 30% of all sports-related injuries and are more common in contact sports such as basketball and soccer. Up to 30% of ankle sprains can lead to chronic symptoms. These resultant problems may include chronic ankle instability, osteochondral lesions, ankle impingement syndromes, and peroneal tendinopathy.

Lateral ankle sprains most commonly cause injury to the anterior talofibular ligament (ATFL), the calcaneofibular ligament (CFL), and/or the posterior talofibular ligament (PTFL) (Fig. 21.6). Medial ankle sprains cause injury to the deltoid ligament. And the syndesmotic ligament complex, which maintains stability between the tibia and the fibula, is the site of injury in a *high ankle sprain*.

Fig. 21.6 Lateral ankle illustration showing anterior talofibular (ATFL) and calcaneofibular ligament (CFL)

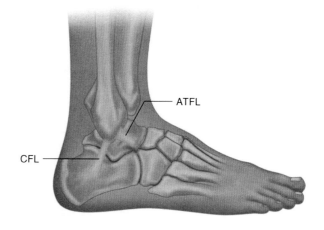

Clinical Presentation

The majority of patients presenting with an ankle sprain report a twisting injury to the ankle. Lateral ligament injuries often occur from supination (rolling inward), medial ligament injuries from pronation (rolling outward), and syndesmotic ligament injuries from external rotation while the foot is planted and fixed to the ground. Patients report the immediate onset of pain and swelling and may hear or feel a pop. Many patients have difficulty weightbearing after the injury.

The site of maximal tenderness often indicates which ligament(s) were injured. Medial ankle pain may accompany a lateral ligament injury, as the talus abuts the medial tibia during an inversion injury. With syndesmotic sprains, discomfort may radiate up the syndesmosis along the anterolateral leg. In the acute setting, specific tests to assess ligamentous instability are not feasible due to patient discomfort. As the acute pain subsides, an anterior drawer test is used to assess the degree of anterior shift of the talus relative to the tibia. Alignment should be evaluated as well, best done by examining the foot and ankle with the patient standing. Varus alignment of the hindfoot predisposes the ankle to rolling inward.

Ankle sprains are graded depending upon the severity of the injury. Grade I ankle sprains occur with minimal ligament injury, minimal swelling and tenderness, and minimal pain with weightbearing. Grade II injuries occur when the ligaments have been stretched but remain in continuity. These patients have moderate swelling, tenderness, and pain with weightbearing. Grade III sprains occur with complete rupture of the ligaments and cause significant pain and swelling.

Differential Diagnosis and Suggested Diagnostic Testing

In addition to lateral ligament sprain, supination injuries may cause ankle fracture, lateral process talus fracture, anterior process calcaneus fracture, peroneal tendon injury, osteochondral lesion of the talus, and stretch injury to the superficial peroneal nerve. For this reason, we routinely obtain weightbearing radiographs of the ankle to ensure that there is no bony injury or malalignment through the ankle joint. Pronation injuries similarly can cause medial ligament, bone, and/or tendon injury.

Acute surgical intervention is rare when the ankle joint remains properly aligned, whereas surgery is often necessary in cases with altered alignment. While disruption of normal alignment is very uncommon with lateral or medial ankle sprains—in part since the talus is nestled within the confines of the lateral and medial malleoli—syndesmotic injuries more commonly cause disruption of the ankle alignment. With high-grade injury to the syndesmotic ligaments, the fibula may shift laterally, allowing the talus to follow. This is detrimental to the long-term function of the ankle due to abnormal loading of the thin cartilage of the ankle joint and the development of post-traumatic arthritis. It is for this reason that we stress the importance of weight-bearing ankle radiographs to assess alignment, with imaging of the contralateral, presumably normal, ankle for comparison as needed.

Additional imaging is not typically necessary when radiographs demonstrate a well-aligned ankle. If symptoms persist a few months after an ankle sprain, MRI may be indicated. Additionally, stress radiographs can quantify laxity at the tibiofibular or tibiotalar joints.

Non-operative Management

Ankle sprains are treated with rest, ice, compression, and elevation (RICE). The severity of the ligament injury guides treatment. In minor injuries where weight-bearing, walking, or even sporting activities can be performed immediately following the injury, the use of a soft ankle brace and ankle strengthening exercises may be sufficient. These exercises concentrate on range of motion, proprioception, and peroneal strengthening. With more significant injuries, immobilization in either a restrictive ankle brace or a walking boot may be necessary. For many patients, a few weeks of immobilization is followed by physical therapy. Activity can then be gradually resumed, although care should be taken not to sustain a reinjury when playing cutting sports or when on irregular ground. Patients are instructed to wear a soft supportive ankle brace for up to 6 months following an ankle sprain. Similarly, patients are instructed to avoid high heels as this can increase the likelihood of recurrent injury.

Medial ankle sprains and high ankle sprains take considerably longer to recover from than lateral ankle sprains. In these injuries, boot immobilization for 1 month is followed by physical therapy.

Indications for Surgery

Weightbearing ankle radiographs after an acute ankle sprain evaluate the alignment of the ankle joint. If there is no malalignment of the ankle, which is the case in the vast majority of patients, then surgery is rarely indicated. If malalignment of the ankle has developed as a result of the injury, which occurs most commonly at the level of the syndesmosis, then acute surgical intervention is often recommended to reduce and stabilize the ankle.

Surgical treatment after ankle sprains is more commonly performed as a result of persistent symptoms months after the injury. Indications for surgery typically include a failure of nonsurgical treatment and objective pathologic findings, such as documented mechanical ankle instability or an osteochondral lesion seen on MRI.

Operative Management

Ligament reconstruction procedures can address lateral or medial ankle instability. These procedures utilize either native local tissue or reroute tendons, or use allograft tendon to provide stability to the joint. More than 50 lateral ligament reconstruction

Table 21.1 Ten common soft tissue disorders of the ankle with associated typical presentation, diagnostic testing, and treatment

Clinical entity	Presentation	Diagnostic testing	Conservative management	Indications for surgery	Operative management
Achilles tendinosis	– TTP midportion of Achilles, posterior heel – Achilles pain with active plantar flexion (single leg raise)	– Thompson test to rule out rupture – radiograph to evaluate for Haglund's lesion or insertional spur – ultrasound or MRI for confirmation of tendinosis	– PT: Eccentric strengthening, ankle/foot intrinsic strengthening – heel lift – dorsiflexion night splint	– pain refractory to conservative management	– tendon debridement – gastrocnemius recession
Achilles tendon rupture	– acute onset pain and weakness in calf – may hear or feel a pop	– Thompson test – plantar flexion strength – passive ankle dorsiflexion	– nonsurgical treatment can be effective treatment but must follow specific protocol	– healthy patient who elects for operative intervention	– tendon repair using either open or minimally invasive technique
Gastrocnemius strain	– acute onset of pain in upper calf – may hear of feel a pop	– Thompson test to rule out Achilles rupture – vpalpation for site of maximal tenderness	– immobilization in tall walking boot – PT: Strengthening and stretching to begin when pain improved	– very uncommon to treat surgically	– Na

(continued)

Table 21.1 (continued)

Clinical entity	Presentation	Diagnostic testing	Conservative management	Indications for surgery	Operative management
Peroneal tendinopathy	– pain at posterolateral ankle – may have clicking or tendon instability	– identify site of maximal tenderness – assess hindfoot alignment – test ankle ligament stability – circumduction testing for peroneal instability – MRI	– immobilization in tall walking boot – PT: Strengthening and range of motion	– persistent symptoms despite nonsurgical care – peroneal tendon instability	– open tendon exploration and repair – Tendoscopy
Posterior tibial tendon dysfunction	– pain at medial ankle – deformity may be present	– standing evaluation of alignment – plain weightbearing X-rays – MRI	– immobilization in tall walking boot – PT: Stretching of calf and training of tendon – orthotic to offload tendon	– persistent symptoms despite nonsurgical care	– depends upon stage of disease – may include tenosynovectomy, deformity correction, hindfoot fusions
Ankle sprain	– acute onset pain after twisting injury – swelling and ecchymosis present	– Weightbearing plain ankle X-rays palpation for site of maximal tenderness	– boot immobilization followed by PT and return to activities	– altered ankle alignment on X-rays (rare) – chronic associated injury with persistent symptoms	– ORIF if altered alignment (rare) – ligament reconstruction for chronic symptoms – ankle arthroscopy
Ankle instability	– recurrent ankle sprains	– Weightbearing plain ankle X-rays – MRI	– PT: Strengthening, proprioception, peroneal strengthening	– persistent limiting symptoms despite PT	– ligament reconstruction – ankle arthroscopy

Condition	History/Symptoms	Diagnosis	Nonsurgical treatment	Surgical indication	Surgical treatment
Ankle impingement syndrome	– pain along ankle joint line – may follow injury	– identify site of maximal tenderness – plain X-rays – MRI	– immobilization in tall walking boot – Pt – intra-articular corticosteroid injection	– persistent pain or mechanical symptoms of locking or catching	– ankle arthroscopy
Tarsal tunnel syndrome	– pain at posteromedial ankle – sensory changes at plantar foot	– tenderness along tibial nerve – replicated symptoms with tibial nerve testing (Tinel's sign)	– immobilization in tall walking boot – orthotic if associated valgus hindfoot – anti-inflammatory medication – local corticosteroid injection	– persistent symptoms despite nonsurgical care	– tarsal tunnel release
Flexor hallucis longus tenosynovitis	– pain at posterior ankle – pain exacerbated with great toe flexion	– Weightbearing plain ankle X-rays – MRI	– immobilization in tall walking boot – Pt	– persistent pain despite nonsurgical care	– FHL tenosynovectomy (open or arthroscopic)

TTP tender to palpation, *PT* physical therapy, *MRI* magnetic resonance imaging, *FHL* flexor hallucis longus, *NA* not available

procedures have been described. The most commonly used is the modified Bröstrom procedure, which involves tightening the lateral ankle ligaments while also incorporating part of the extensor retinaculum into the repair. All ligament reconstruction procedures require a lengthy recovery.

Associated injuries may require operative treatment as well. Osteochondral lesions may be treated with open or arthroscopic cartilage procedures that stimulate healing or replace injured cartilage. Ankle arthroscopy can be effective in treating loose bodies or ankle impingement syndromes, which cause pain with ankle range of motion due to chronically inflamed tissue within the ankle joint. And peroneal tendon injuries, as mentioned previously, may require operative intervention.

Expected Outcome and Predictors of Outcome

The majority (more than 80%) of patients with ankle sprains are effectively treated without surgery. In those requiring surgery, studies report that roughly 80% of patients experience substantial pain relief and a sense of ankle stability. Surgical treatment is less effective, and should be utilized infrequently, in patients with pain after an ankle sprain yet without objective findings on clinical examination or imaging. Surgical outcomes also become less predictable in cases of revision surgery.

Table 21.1 shows ten common soft tissue disorders of the ankle with associated typical presentation, diagnostic testing, and treatment.

Suggested Reading

Alfredson H, et al. Heavy-load eccentric calf muscle training for the treatment of chronic Achilles tendinosis. Am J Sports Med. 1998;26(3):360–6.

Alvarez RG, et al. Stage I and II posterior tibial tendon dysfunction treated by a structured non-operative management protocol: an orthosis and exercise program. Foot Ankle Int. 2006;27(1):2–8.

Baumhauer JF, O'Brien T. Surgical considerations in the treatment of ankle instability. J Athl Train. 2002;37(4):458–62.

Beals TC, et al. Posterior tibial tendon insufficiency: diagnosis and treatment. J Am Acad Orthop Surg. 1999;7:112–8.

Guss D et al. Acute Achilles tendon rupture: a critical analysis review. J Bone Joint Surg Rev. 2015;3(4).

Philbin TM, et al. Peroneal tendon injuries. J Am Acad Orthop Surg. 2009;17(5):306–17.

Willits K, et al. Operative versus non-operative treatment of acute Achilles tendon ruptures: a multi-center randomized trial using accelerated functional rehabilitation. J Bone Joint Surg Am. 2010;92(17):2767–75.

Chapter 22
Midfoot Arthritis and Disorders of the Hallux

Christopher P. Chiodo, Jeremy T. Smith, and Eric M. Bluman

Abbreviations

CT   Computed tomography
MP   Metatarsal-phalangeal

Hallux Rigidus and Hallux Valgus

The hallux, or great toe, has an important role in normal foot function. Biomechanically, it contributes to foot strength, stability, and balance. It is comprised of two bones, the proximal and distal phalanges (Fig. 22.1). These bones are relatively large when compared to the bones of the other toes. The base of the proximal phalanx articulates with the head of the first metatarsal at the first metatarsal-phalangeal (MP) joint. The two most common conditions that affect the great toe are hallux rigidus and hallux valgus.

Hallux Rigidus

Osteoarthritis of the first MP joint is referred to as hallux rigidus, which is Latin for "stiff big toe." Many patients with hallux rigidus are minimally symptomatic. In these instances, the disease results only in decreased motion that often goes unnoticed by the patient. The frequent absence of pain in the face of radiographic changes and reduced motion make stiffness typical of this disease, as reflected in the name

C.P. Chiodo (✉) • J.T. Smith • E.M. Bluman
Department of Orthopedic Surgery, Brigham and Women's Hospital,
1153 Centre Street, Boston, MA 02130, USA
e-mail: cchiodo@partners.org; jsmith42@partners.org; ebluman@partners.org

© Springer International Publishing AG 2018   361
J.N. Katz et al. (eds.), *Principles of Orthopedic Practice for Primary Care Providers*, https://doi.org/10.1007/978-3-319-68661-5_22

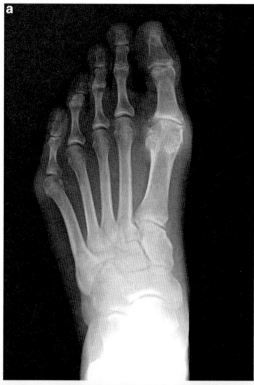

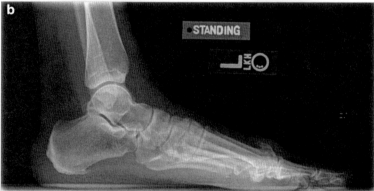

Fig. 22.1 Anteroposterior (**a**) and lateral (**b**) radiographs of a patient with hallux rigidus. Note the dorsal osteophyte formation as well as the loss of joint space at the metatarsal/phalangeal joint

Fig. 22.2 Line drawing of a moderate hallux valgus deformity before (**a**) and after (**b**) surgical correction using a proximal osteotomy stabilized with screw fixation. Note the preoperative lateral deviation of the hallux as well as the medial angulation of the first metatarsal

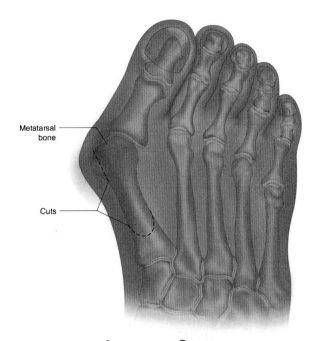

Metatarsal bone

Cuts

A   Pre-op

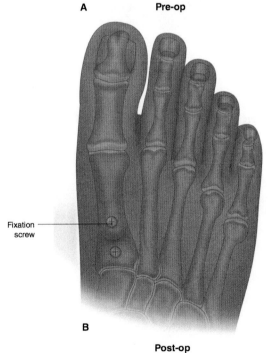

Fixation screw

B

Post-op

"hallux rigidus." As the disease progresses, large osteophytes form on the dorsal aspect of the MP joint (Fig. 22.2). These may cause pain by irritating adjacent soft tissue structures or by impinging with terminal dorsiflexion of the joint.

Summary of Epidemiology

Hallux rigidus generally affects middle-aged and elderly individuals. In a minority of cases, it may be caused by trauma or inflammatory disease. In most cases, however, the etiology is unknown. Some have speculated that it may be secondary to subtle dorsiflexion malalignment of the first metatarsal, contracture of the flexor hallucis brevis tendon, or chondral injury.

Clinical Presentation

Patients with hallux rigidus typically complain of pain on the dorsal aspect of the joint, centrally within the joint, or both. This contrasts with medial pain, which is more typical of a bunion, or plantar pain, which usually indicates sesamoid pathology. Two pertinent factors in the patient's history are (1) pain that is exacerbated by the joint rubbing against shoes and (2) pain that occurs when the affected foot pushes off. These indicate that the dorsal osteophytes are the primary pain generator. If, on the other hand, symptoms persist throughout the gait cycle or in the absence of shoes rubbing on the joint (e.g., going barefoot), then it is more likely that the underlying arthritis of the MP joint is the main pain generator.

Differential Diagnosis and Suggested Diagnostic Testing

The differential diagnosis for central and dorsal MP joint pain includes gout, stress fracture, and osteochondral injury. Gout will typically present more acutely and with a greater degree of inflammation. Meanwhile, pain and tenderness from a stress fracture will typically be localized more proximally at the metatarsal neck. Finally, an osteochondral injury will usually not be associated with dorsal spur formation.

Weight-bearing radiographs should be obtained in all patients with suspected hallux rigidus. Dorsal osteophyte formation and joint space narrowing will be apparent in most cases. Beyond radiographs, advanced imaging is usually not indicated. One exception would be the use of magnetic resonance imaging to rule out a stress fracture or sesamoid pathology. Similarly, laboratory studies are generally not needed, unless ruling out gout or infection. In these instances, however, joint aspiration is more specific and accurate.

Non-operative Management

There are several non-operative treatment options available. Shoewear modification, specifically choosing shoes with a deep toe box, makes room for the dorsal osteophytes that are typically present. Wider shoes may also helpful in this regard. Unfortunately, some patients report that while wider and deeper shoes provide relief for the hallux, such shoes are ill fitting in other regions of the foot. This may lead to excessive motion, shear, and blister formation.

Shoes with a stiff sole may also be helpful. The stiff sole will decrease dorsiflexion through the MP joint, effectively "stress shielding" it. Both custom-made and commercially available rocker bottom shoes may also stress shield the joint by creating a biomechanical "rocker" that decreases motion at the joint.

Finally, shoe stretching may also help. Stretching the toe box in the region of the osteophytes may minimize or eliminate spur pain. There are several available devices that accomplish this; however, in our experience a "ball-and-ring" shoe stretcher is the most effective. In contrast to other shoe stretching devices, this device stretches the shoe material locally, over the enlarged joint. As such, it avoids problems with shear and improper shoe fitting elsewhere in the foot that may occur when using other devices.

With regard to custom orthoses, these devices are often expensive, not covered by insurance, and ineffective in the treatment of hallux rigidus. Their poor efficacy is due to the fact that, with hallux rigidus, the dorsal spurs normally crowd the shoe. Placing a custom orthosis in the shoe only further exacerbates this crowding.

Instead of orthotics, many providers have begun using carbon fiber inserts to treat hallux rigidus. These are non-custom devices that are very thin and as such do not "overstuff" the shoe. However, they are relatively stiff and thus still stress shield the MP joint. When prescribing these devices, the phrase "Morton's extension" is used to specify that the device extends to the tip of the hallux.

Finally, cortisone injections are another reasonable non-operative treatment option for hallux rigidus. The accuracy of these procedures likely increases when performed under fluoroscopic or ultrasound guidance. Repeated injections, however, may have a harmful effect on the remaining cartilage. As such, only one or two injections are considered prior to surgery. In one clinical study, two-thirds of patients with mild disease who underwent injection combined with gentle manipulation were able to avoid surgery.

The clinical literature with regard to the non-operative treatment of hallux rigidus is sparse. Nevertheless, in the authors' experience, many—if not most—patients with hallux rigidus will enjoy sufficient relief and avoid surgery with one or more of the measures listed above.

Indications for Surgery

Patients with hallux rigidus are considered appropriate surgical candidates if they have regular pain that has been present for at least three months, is refractory to non-operative measures, and interferes with activities of daily living. This functional criterion includes the ability to wear reasonable shoes.

Operative Management

The surgical management of hallux rigidus may be divided into joint-sparing and joint-sacrificing procedures. Traditionally, joint-sparing procedures are reserved for patients in whom there is some cartilage remaining or in whom pain is caused primarily by irritation or impingement of the dorsal osteophytes, rather than by the osteoarthritic process within the joint. Such patients will typically complain of shoe pain and pain as the affected foot pushes off during the gait cycle. The most commonly performed joint-sparing procedure for hallux rigidus is a cheilectomy, in which the offending dorsal osteophytes are resected. Less commonly, distal metatarsal and proximal phalangeal osteotomies have been described to "decompress" the joint.

Arthrodesis is indicated when there is pain throughout the gait cycle and not just at terminal push-off. With arthrodesis, the first metatarsal and proximal phalanx are surgically fused. The joint is eradicated and the bones are fixed together with a plate and/or screws. Of note, the hallux is positioned in slight valgus to facilitate shoe-wear. It is also fused in slight dorsiflexion. With this adjustment, the tip of the toe will not touch the ground. This positioning creates a plantar rocker to allow for more efficient ambulation, and patients should be reassured that this is planned and advantageous.

Expected Outcome and Predictors of Outcome

Most patients undergoing treatment for hallux rigidus are able to return to the activity level they enjoyed prior to the onset of symptoms. In one recent study examining arthrodesis, high levels of function in both everyday life and recreational activities were noted postoperatively. For instance, 92% of patients could hike, 75% of patients could return to jogging, and 80% of patients could resume golfing. Nearly all patients could return to work.

Hallux Valgus

A hallux valgus deformity, or bunion, is characterized by lateral deviation of the great toe. This leads to an angular deformity at the MP joint and the development of a secondary bony prominence (Fig. 22.2). While in some patients the medial eminence of the distal first metatarsal may be slightly enlarged, it is important to note that the abnormal physical appearance of the hallux is due primarily to angular deformity.

Summary of Epidemiology

Bunions are one of the most common conditions treated by foot and ankle specialists. They affect over 30% of adults, occur primarily in shoe-wearing societies, and are more prevalent in females compared to males. The narrow toe box of many shoes, especially women's shoes, applies a laterally directed force on the hallux. This may contribute to the development of a bunion or irritate an existing deformity due to rubbing of the shoe. Other factors that have been implicated in the etiology of bunions include joint instability, muscle imbalance, hindfoot pronation, skeletal abnormalities, and hereditary predisposition. Symptomatic bunions occur in patients of all ages, although the prevalence is higher in middle-aged and elderly individuals.

Clinical Presentation

Many patients with mild bunion deformities have little to no pain. Patients who do have symptoms typically will note pain localized to the medial aspect of the first MP joint. This is an important clinical finding, as dorsal or plantar pain should alert the clinician to another pathology, such as hallux rigidus or sesamoid pain. Symptoms are typically aggravated by shoes, and especially fashionable shoes with a narrow toe box. Pain may also be exacerbated by repetitive joint motion from prolonged walking, running, and sports. It may occasionally radiate proximally due to irritation of the dorsal medial cutaneous nerve as it courses over the MP joint.

Differential Diagnosis and Suggested Diagnostic Testing

Two radiographic parameters are particularly important when assessing hallux valgus. The first is the hallux valgus angle, formed by the intersection of the long axes of the hallux and first metatarsal. This is useful in grading deformities as mild (15–30°), moderate (30–40°), or severe (>40°). Meanwhile, the intermetatarsal angle measures the divergence between the first and second metatarsals. This angle is useful in determining the type of procedure that will be necessary if surgical correction is performed.

Non-operative Management

The non-operative management of hallux valgus includes shoe stretching as well as local pads and braces. As with hallux rigidus, a ball-and-ring shoe stretcher is able to focally stretch the toe box over the deformity while preserving the contour of the remaining shoe. Numerous braces, pads, and spacers are available commercially. Soft, low profile devices are tolerated best. One appealing option is a forefoot neoprene sleeve with a seam along the medial side of the device. This both cushions the bony prominence and also draws the hallux into more anatomic alignment.

Custom orthoses are usually not effective in the treatment of hallux valgus. The one exception is in the case of advanced hindfoot pronation that results in increased pressure on the medial hallux.

Indications for Surgery

Patients are considered appropriate surgical candidates if they have substantial, chronic pain that is not alleviated by reasonable shoewear or shoe stretching. It is important to note that cosmesis and the desire to wear high heels or fashionable shoes are generally not considered indications for surgery. Patients who inquire about bunion surgery should be carefully counseled that cosmesis is not considered an indication for surgery. Patients must also be cognizant of—and be able to comply with—a non-weight-bearing period of up to six weeks postoperatively, depending on the nature of the procedure performed.

Operative Management

Numerous procedures have been described for the treatment of hallux valgus. More mild deformities may be addressed with a "modified McBride" procedure, in which the contracted lateral structures of the MP joint are released while, medially, the metatarsal eminence is shaved and the joint capsule is tightened. This realigns the hallux at the MP joint and to some degree may correct the elevated intermetatarsal angle. Alternatively, a "chevron" osteotomy of the distal first metatarsal may also be performed to shift the metatarsal head laterally.

When the intermetatarsal angle is substantially elevated (e.g., greater than 14°), a proximal procedure may also be necessary. Most surgeons will perform some type of metatarsal osteotomy to address the malalignment of this bone. Other options include arthrodesis of the first TMT joint or even suture-button fixation.

Advanced arthritis or instability of either the first MP or TMT joint is an indication for surgical arthrodesis (fusion). With this, the deformity is corrected through the joint, which is then fused in more anatomic alignment.

Expected Outcome and Predictors of Outcome

Approximately 90% of patients undergoing surgery for hallux valgus are satisfied and have lasting relief. One common complication of surgery, however, is recurrent deformity. This occurs in less than 15% of patients and is likely due to residual soft tissue contractures as well as changes in the bony anatomy on the plantar aspect of the metatarsal. In our experience, though, pain relief and patient satisfaction usually persist despite recurrent deformity. Another complication associated with hallux valgus correction is decreased motion at the first MP joint. This is particularly noticeable for patients who attempt to wear high heels postoperatively. Finally, residual sesamoid malalignment on postoperative X-rays has been associated with recurrent deformity. This is likely due to the persistent eccentric pull of the flexor hallucis brevis tendon, within which the sesamoids are located.

Midfoot Arthritis

The midfoot is composed of the navicular, cuboid, and cuneiform bones. It connects the hindfoot to the metatarsals and allows for efficient force transmission and propulsion, which are critical for ambulation. Osteoarthritis often affects the joints of the midfoot, and, as with other foot arthritides, can be quite debilitating.

Summary of Epidemiology

Symptomatic midfoot arthritis affects both middle-aged and elderly individuals, and is present in approximately 10% of individuals over 50 years of age. There may be a slightly higher prevalence in females, and both obesity and occupation have been cited as risk factors. While usually idiopathic, in some cases the condition may be secondary to a prior midfoot sprain or Lisfranc fracture dislocation.

Clinical Presentation

Patients typically complain of insidious aching pain localized to the midfoot. There is usually "start-up" pain, which occurs when standing after sitting for a long period of time or when first arising in the morning. A tight shoe counter may irritate dorsal osteophytes. Deformity may also be noted, specifically, abduction of the forefoot. This, in turn, may compromise the medial longitudinal arch and lead to the development of an acquired flatfoot.

Differential Diagnosis and Suggested Diagnostic Testing

Two important items in the differential diagnosis for midfoot arthritis are tendon pathology and stress reaction. The posterior tibial tendon is the main dynamic stabilizer of the medial longitudinal arch. It inserts primarily on the medial pole of the navicular. Associated pain and swelling are usually more medial and extend proximally into the hindfoot and medial ankle. Meanwhile, a navicular stress fracture can present with symptoms similar to midfoot arthritis. The pain associated with this diagnosis, however, usually has a more acute onset and is of greater intensity. A period of strict non-weight-bearing is integral to healing navicular stress fractures and, as such, provider awareness is critical.

Weight-bearing X-rays of the foot are usually sufficient to establish the diagnosis of midfoot arthritis. Computed tomography (CT) is helpful in further specifying which joints are involved and the extent of disease present. CT is also important for surgical planning. Magnetic resonance imaging is helpful in differentiating midfoot arthritis from stress fractures and tendinopathy and should be considered if the diagnosis is in question.

Non-operative Management

The non-operative treatment of midfoot arthritis includes nonsteroidal anti-inflammatory medications, shoe modification, inserts, and cortisone injections. As with hallux rigidus, the use of a rocker bottom shoe and carbon fiber baseplate decreases bending moments at the joints of the midfoot. In the absence of significant dorsal spur formation, this often provides substantial relief. Cortisone injections also play a valuable role in the treatment of midfoot arthritis. Some patients have long-term relief with a single cortisone injection into the diseased joint(s), while others require serial injections every 4–6 months. Of note, the joints of the midfoot are small and often occluded by dorsal osteophytes. As such, the accuracy and efficacy of injections are significantly enhanced by either fluoroscopic or ultrasound guidance.

Indications for Surgery

Surgery is indicated for those patients who have chronic, recalcitrant pain that interferes with daily living. Those patients who require arthrodesis must also be willing and able to comply with a postoperative protocol that may entail up to three months of protected weight-bearing. Contraindications for fusion include active infection as well as insufficient perfusion and soft tissue coverage. Finally, many orthopedists insist on smoking cessation given the negative impact smoking has on fusion rates.

Operative Management

The surgical management of midfoot arthritis generally entails either exostectomy or arthrodesis. An exostectomy—i.e., removal of painful osteophytes—is indicated when patients have pain that is felt to be caused by irritation of the soft tissue structures that overlie a prominent osteophyte. Patients must understand that with an exostectomy, the arthritic joint is still present and could potentially result in persistent pain. Arthrodesis better addresses this concern and is indicated for patients who have pain both with and without shoes, and in whom the primary pain generator is felt to be the arthritic joint itself.

Expected Outcome and Predictors of Outcome

Most patients with mild disease respond to non-operative measures as delineated above. For more advanced disease in which fusion is indicated, modern success rates have ranged from 92 to 100%. Risk factors for nonunion include diabetes, smoking, poor nutrition, compromised bone stock, and a history of trauma with advanced soft tissue stripping. A low vitamin D level may also predispose to nonunion.

Suggested Reading

Brodsky JW, Passmore RN, Pollo FE, Shabat S. Functional outcome of arthrodesis of the first metatarsophalangeal joint using parallel screw fixation. Foot Ankle Int. 2005;26(2):140–6.

Deland JT, Williams BR. Surgical management of hallux rigidus. J Am Acad Orthop Surg. 2012;20(6):347–58.

Easley ME, Trnka HJ. Current concepts review: hallux valgus part II: operative treatment. Foot Ankle Int. 2007;28(6):748–58. Review

Nemec SA, Habbu RA, Anderson JG, Bohay DR. Outcomes following midfoot arthrodesis for primary arthritis. Foot Ankle Int. 2011;32(4):355–61.

Suh JS, Amendola A, Lee KB, Wasserman L, Saltzman CL. Dorsal modified calcaneal plate for extensive midfoot arthrodesis. Foot Ankle Int. 2005;26(7):503–9. PubMed PMID: 16045838

Thomas MJ, Peat G, Rathod T, Marshall M, Moore A, Menz HB, Roddy E. The epidemiology of symptomatic midfoot osteoarthritis in community-dwelling older adults: cross-sectional findings from the Clinical Assessment Study of the Foot. Arthritis Res Ther. 2015;17:178.

Verhoeven N, Vandeputte G. Midfoot arthritis: diagnosis and treatment. Foot Ankle Surg. 2012;18(4):255–62.

Yee G, Lau J. Current concepts review: hallux rigidus. Foot Ankle Int. 2008;29(6):637–46.

Chapter 23
Foot and Ankle Plantar Fasciitis

James P. Ioli

Abbreviations

ABI	Ankle-brachial index
BMI	Body mass index
CBC	Complete blood count
CRP	C-reactive protein
CT	Computed tomography
ECSWT	Extracorporeal shock wave therapy
EMG	Electromyography
ESR	Erythrocyte sedimentation rate
HLA-B27	Human leukocyte antigen B27
MRI	Magnetic resonance imaging
NSAID	Nonsteroidal anti-inflammatory drugs
OTC	Over the counter
PT	Physical therapy
PVR	Pulse volume recording
RICE	Rest, Ice, Compression, Elevation
S1	Sacral one
US	Ultrasound

Summary of Epidemiology

Plantar fasciitis accounts for about one million patient visits per year in the USA. It affects 10% of the general population and makes up 10% of runner-related injuries. It is estimated that between \$192 and \$376 million is spent annually on treatments for this condition. It usually affects adults of all ages and peaks between 40 and 60 years of age. Adult women present twice as often as men, while in younger

J.P. Ioli (✉)
Department of Orthopedics, Brigham and Women's Hospital, Harvard Medical School,
75 Francis Street, Boston, MA 02115, USA
e-mail: jpioli@bwh.harvard.edu

© Springer International Publishing AG 2018   373
J.N. Katz et al. (eds.), *Principles of Orthopedic Practice for Primary Care Providers*, https://doi.org/10.1007/978-3-319-68661-5_23

Fig. 23.1 Plantar fasciitis

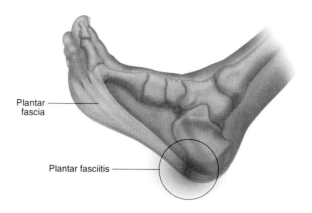

Plantar
fascia

Plantar fasciitis

patients men and women are affected equally. There is no association with race or ethnicity. One-third of the patients experience plantar fasciitis bilaterally.

Clinical Presentation

The fascia is a long, thick, ligament-like structure that is located on the plantar aspect of the foot (Fig. 23.1). It extends from the medial and lateral calcaneal tubercles distally toward the toes. The fascia consists of medial, central, and lateral bands. The plantar medial heel attachment is the most common area of pain and discomfort. The pain is usually acute when the patient first steps out of bed or first moves after a period of inactivity. The heel pain usually subsides after a few minutes of activity. At times, the pain will worsen as the day progresses. Some patients may also complain of burning, tingling, and sharp pain in the heel. The discomfort can also be felt in the medial arch. Factors that can influence or trigger the onset of pain are foot structure (pes cavus, pes planus); overpronation (an excessive inward roll and collapse of the medial arch and foot); tightness and/or weakness of the gastrocnemius, soleus, or Achilles tendon; weight; occupations such as factory workers, teachers, and postal workers; worn-out or poorly fitting shoes; and sudden increase in activity. Some studies report that plantar fasciitis can linger for 12–18 months. It is possible for the condition to resolve spontaneously, and 80% of cases resolve in 1 year. About 5% of patients for whom conservative therapy is ineffective choose surgery in an attempt to resolve their symptoms. Some patients are concerned when they see a plantar heel spur on a radiograph. Advise them not to be concerned. Many people have heel spurs and have no heel pain.

Differential Diagnosis and Suggested Diagnostic Testing

When investigating the origin of heel pain, one should think of the musculoskeletal, vascular, dermatological, and neurological systems. As mentioned previously, the musculoskeletal system is usually the primary cause of heel pain (plantar fasciitis). If the pain worsens and does not respond to treatment, it is important to rule out a stress fracture, bone cyst, apophysitis (pain in the growth plate of the heel, known as Sever's disease), and inflammatory arthropathy. Conditions of the vascular system, such as peripheral arterial disease and vascular insufficiency, can also cause heel pain. Plantar verrucae, porokeratoses, ulcers, and foreign bodies fall into the dermatological system. Neurological causes of heel pain can be tarsal tunnel syndrome, medial or lateral plantar nerve neuritis, entrapment, or neuroma. S1 radiculopathy should also be considered. A proper and thorough physical exam will aid in the assessment of all four systems.

Recalcitrant heel pain requires further diagnostic assessment, which may include some of the following studies: X-rays to look for bony lesions; MRI to rule out soft tissue or bony lesions; electromyography (EMG) to detect tarsal tunnel syndrome; three-phase bone scan for stress fracture or bone infection; computed tomography (CT) for subtalar arthritis, calcaneal cysts, and stress fractures; Ankle-Brachial Index/Pulse Volume Recording (ABI/PVR) to rule out peripheral arterial disease; ultrasound to rule out soft tissue pathology; or bone scan. If there is a suspicion of an inflammatory arthropathy, laboratory studies may include a complete metabolic panel, a complete blood count (CBC), erythrocyte sedimentation rate (ESR), C-reactive protein (CRP), a rheumatoid factor, and HLA-B27 (to evaluate for spondyloarthropathy).

Nonoperative Management

If a patient presents to your office and complains of symptoms, which you determine to be consistent with plantar fasciitis, consider furnishing a handout with information about plantar fasciitis, including an explanation of its origin and general treatment regimens. Pictures and/or drawings of the anatomy and of stretching and strengthening exercises are extremely helpful to patients, so that they can develop insight into the problem (Fig. 23.2). Initial recommendations would also include an evaluation for new supportive shoes and over-the-counter orthotics; custom orthotics may be considered if there is no or minimal progress after 3 months of treatment. OTC and custom orthotics are used to provide support and a better alignment of the foot in order to decrease the mechanical forces that aggravate the condition. Initially, a home exercise program is usually recommended. It has been shown that plantar fascia and intrinsic foot muscle stretching techniques have reduced pain associated with the plantar fascia. As illustrated later in this article, a towel stretch, plantar

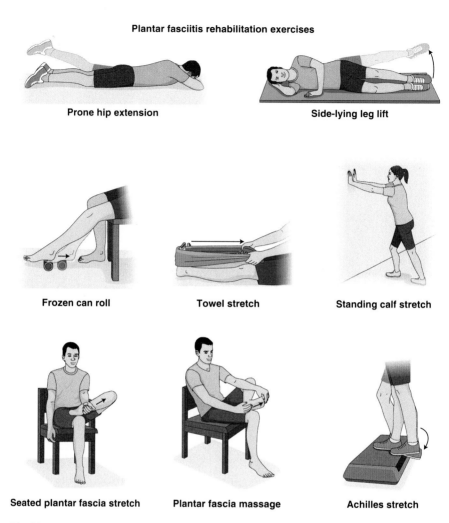

Fig. 23.2 Plantar fasciitis exercises

fascial stretching and massage, and Achilles stretches are all helpful in decreasing pain and discomfort. If this fails, then physical therapy would be recommended. There is no evidence that a formal PT program is better than the home exercise program. Evidence of the effectiveness of nonsteroidal anti-inflammatory agents is inconsistent and of limited quality. A night splint is usually prescribed if the patient complains of pain on the first step out of bed. Keeping the foot and ankle in a neutral 90° position, the night splint prevents ankle plantar flexion (and associated tightening of the heel cord) during sleep. There is evidence that the night splint helps; however, patients may complain of foot discomfort and interrupted sleep.

Typically, a follow-up appointment is scheduled for 6–8 weeks following the initial visit in which plantar fasciitis was diagnosed. When the patient returns, the initial treatment regimen is reassessed. If there has been improvement with formal physical therapy, the prescription is usually renewed. A physical therapy program that focuses on lower extremity stretching and strengthening can be beneficial and provide reinforcement for present and future patient compliance. It is also important to review the home exercise program—which supplements the formal PT program—use of the night splint, and OTC NSAIDs. The new shoes and inserts should also be evaluated. If the pain has worsened, then review the differential diagnosis. If there is moderate pain, a prescription for NSAIDs can be considered. If there is severe pain from plantar fasciitis, then immobilization in a removable, below-the-knee walking boot would be recommended at that visit. It is important to both inform and remind the patient about activities that can aggravate or exacerbate the condition. It is especially important to advise patients, particularly those who run or participate in strenuous athletic activities, to avoid such activities while treatment is in progress. Encourage the patient to cross-train and to limit long periods of standing and walking barefoot on hard surfaces. If the patient has a high BMI, a frank discussion about nutrition and weight loss is paramount.

If, at the time of the patient's next appointment (generally within 6–8 weeks), the patient still complains of plantar fasciitis pain, a steroid injection could be considered. The patient should be advised that there can be a weakening or possible rupture of the plantar fascia, especially from multiple steroid injections. Many primary care providers will have little experience with plantar fascial injections; it would be reasonable to refer these patients to foot specialists (e.g., podiatrists or foot and ankle surgeons) for an injection.

Extracorporeal shock wave therapy may be another conservative option for recalcitrant plantar fasciitis. A recent study of the effectiveness of ECSWT demonstrated success rates between 50 and 65% as compared with 34.5% with placebo. This study involved 250 subjects in a prospective, multicenter, double-blind, randomized, and placebo-controlled US Food and Drug Administration trial. If, after 12 months of conservative treatment, the patient is still in severe pain, surgery may be an option.

Indications for Surgery

Surgery is only an option if all conservative treatment has failed and the patient is in severe pain.

Operative Management

Fasciotomy: Part or all of the fascia is sectioned. This can be accomplished by an endoscopic or open procedure.

Table 23.1 Plantar fasciitis

Clinical entity	Presentation	Diagnostic testing	Conservative management	Indications for surgery	Operative management
Plantar fasciitis	– pain in heel after stepping down out of bed or after a period of inactivity – tender to palpation plantar medial heel – nature of pain: Sharp, achy, burning	– physical exam – X-ray – MRI or ultrasound for recalcitrant cases – laboratory studies	– weight loss – new shoes with support – OTC heel cups, orthotics – RICE (rest, ice, compression, elevation) – OTC/Rx ibuprofen, naproxen – night splints – physical therapy – stretching and strengthening of plantar fascia and gastrocnemius soleus before and after activity – respite from sport or activity that aggravated the condition – steroid injection – limit prolonged standing and walking barefoot on hard surfaces – cross-training – extracorporeal shock wave therapy	– pain refractory to all conservative management	– plantar fascia release – percutaneous partial fasciotomy – cryosurgery – bipolar radiofrequency microdebridement – Strayer procedure

MRI Magnetic resonance imaging, *OTC* over the counter, *RICE* rest, ice, compression, elevation

Other: Certain other procedures have initially appeared promising in small studies, including percutaneous partial fasciotomy, cryosurgery, bipolar radiofrequency microdebridement, and Strayer procedure (a gastrocnemius recession procedure to increase ankle dorsiflexion). If these treatments prove to be successful in larger studies, they will likely become more common.

Expected Outcome and Predictors of Outcome

The reported success rate for fasciotomy ranges from 70 to 90%. Postoperatively, most patients begin weight bearing to tolerance after 24 h. After suture removal at 10 days, an athletic shoe can be worn as tolerated. Post-op course for open plantar fasciotomy can vary. One study showed that those patients who wore a below-knee walking cast for 2 weeks required less time to obtain 80% pain relief, needed less time to return to full activities, and had fewer complications. Both open and endoscopic fasciotomies have been associated with instability complications such as lateral foot pain (calcaneal-cuboid and metatarsal-cuboid joints), overload, and medial foot pain. A decrease in the longitudinal arch, numbness in the heel, medial arch pain, and strain are potential complications.

Table 23.1 is a summary of the presentation, diagnostic testing, and conservative and operative management of plantar fasciitis.

Suggested Reading

Goff JD, Crawford R. Diagnosis and treatment of plantar fasciitis. Am Fam Physician. 2011;84(6):676–82.

Gollwitzer H, Saxena A, DiDomenico LA, Galli L, Bouhe RT, Caminear DS, Fullem B, Vester JC, Horn C, Banke IJ, Burgkart R, Gerdesmeyer L. Clinically relevant effectiveness of focused extracorporeal shock wave therapy in the treatment of chronic plantar fasciitis: a randomized, controlled multicenter study. J Bone Joint Surg Am. 2015;97(9):701–8.

Martin RL, Irrgang JJ, Conti SF. Outcome study of subjects with insertional plantar fasciitis. Foot Ankle Int. 1998;19(12):803–11.

Riddle DL, Schappert SM. Volume of ambulatory care visits and patterns of care for patients diagnosed with plantar fasciitis: a national study of medical doctors. Foot Ankle Int. 2004;25(5):303–10.

Riddle DL, Pulisic M, Pidcoe P, Johnson RE. Risk factors for Plantar fasciitis: a matched case-control study. J Bone Joint Surg Am. 2003;85-A(5):872–7.

Singh D, Angel J, Bentley G, Trevino SG. Fortnightly review. Plantar fasciitis. BMJ. 1997;315(7101):172–5.

Tong KB, Furia J. Economic burden of plantar fasciitis treatment in the United States. Am J Orthop (Belle Mead NJ). 2010;39(5):227–31.

Wolgin M, Cook C, Graham C, Mauldin D. Conservative treatment of plantar heel pain: long-term follow-up. Foot Ankle Int. 1994;15(3):97–102.

Part XII
Bone Stress Injuries

Chapter 24
Bone Stress Injuries

Adam S. Tenforde

Abbreviations

BSI Bone stress injury
DXA Dual energy X-ray absorptiometry
MRI Magnetic resonance imaging

Summary of Epidemiology

Bone stress injury (BSI) is a common form of overuse injury in athletes and active individuals who present to sports medicine clinics. The injury is the result of cumulative microtrauma to the bone that exceeds the capacity for remodeling, resulting in development of injury. A BSI exists on a continuum of injury with early changes seen on imaging that include bone marrow edema. If the bone is continually loaded, advanced injury may include presence of fracture line on imaging, commonly referred to a stress fracture. Land-based sports such as running can cause repetitive overload to the skeleton and place athletes at elevated risk for this form of injury. Biological factors including the female athlete triad (Triad), biomechanical influences, and bone anatomy may each contribute to increased susceptibility to BSI.

Clinical Presentation

Chief Complaint

The most common symptom for an athlete with BSI is focal pain with weight bearing. In general, an athlete with BSI will typically provide a history of pain that occurs with sport activity. As the injury advances, a BSI may cause pain outside sport including

A.S. Tenforde (✉)
Department of Orthopedics and Physical Medicine and Rehabilitation, Brigham and Women's Hospital, Spaulding Rehabilitation Hospital, 1575 Cambridge Street, Cambridge, MA 02138, USA
e-mail: atenforde@partners.org

© Springer International Publishing AG 2018
J.N. Katz et al. (eds.), *Principles of Orthopedic Practice for Primary Care Providers*, https://doi.org/10.1007/978-3-319-68661-5_24

during weight bearing and at rest. When a medical provider is obtaining the history, it is important to identify risk factors that may have contributed to the injury. This includes changes in frequency, volume, or intensity of training or preparing for a sports competition/event. In all female athletes, the female athlete triad (Triad) risk assessment score and screening should be performed. Additionally, relevant history includes medical conditions that predispose to BSI or impaired bone health (including thyroid disease, rheumatological conditions, and osteopenia/osteoporosis), family history of fracture or osteopenia/osteoporosis, and review for culprit medications (including steroids, proton pump inhibitors, and antiepileptic drugs). Given that impaired nutrition can contribute to BSI, dietary patterns including restrictive eating, disordered eating behaviors, symptoms of malabsorption, food allergies, and amount of calcium and vitamin D intake from food and supplements should be characterized.

Sex-Specific Considerations

In female athletes, medical professionals should screen for presence of the Triad. The Triad is defined as the interrelationship of energy availability, menstrual function, and bone mineral density in female athletes (Nattiv et al. 2007; De Souza et al. 2014). An increased number of Triad risk factors are associated with elevated risk for BSI (Barrack et al. 2014). Each component of the Triad may fall on a spectrum of health to disease (Nattiv et al. 2007; De Souza et al. 2014).

Energy Availability

Energy availability is calculated as the difference of energy intake to estimated energy expenditure standardized to kilogram of metabolically active fat-free mass per day (Ihle and Loucks 1994). With body weight constant, energy availability is reduced with lower caloric intake, increased exercise energy expenditure, or a combination of both. Low energy availability has been defined as 30 kcal per kg of fat-free mass per day. Low energy availability has been shown to alter both metabolic and reproductive hormones. Resulting reductions in sex hormones including estradiol may manifest as changes in menstrual periods (increased interval of time between menstrual periods, lighter periods, and cession of menses) and are an important early marker for inadequate energy availability. Low energy availability may occur inadvertently due to mismatch of energy intake to energy expenditure. Active female athletes may have low energy availability without disordered eating or an eating disorder.

Menstrual Function

Menstrual function is initially determined by obtaining a menstrual history. Key components include age of first menstrual period (menarche) and least number of periods over 12 months. In the absence of pregnancy, females should have ten or more periods per year. Note that females using hormonal therapy including oral contraception pills may experience withdrawal bleeding. However, withdrawal bleeding is not the same as having normal menstrual periods and should not be equated to sufficient menstrual health. Female athletes on hormonal therapy should be asked why the medication was prescribed. Menstrual function is a good initial measure of hormonal function in a female patient. The cyclic patterns of estradiol and progesterone associated with menstrual periods influence bone turnover and bone mass accrual.

Bone Mineral Density

Both energy availability and menstrual function influence skeletal health, including bone mineral density. In setting of adequate energy availability, menstrual function is preserved, and hormones including estradiol promote bone health. In the setting of inadequate energy availability, reduced estradiol and nutritional deficiencies result in reduced bone mass and an increase risk for BSI.

Screening for the Triad

The Female Athlete Triad Coalition has developed a series of screening questions that should be asked at time of annual pre-participation evaluation in athletes (Box 24.1) (De Souza et al. 2014). However, these questions can also be incorporated into clinical evaluation for a female athlete with suspected BSI. In those screening positive for risk factors for the Triad, a risk assessment score can be generated to guide management and return to play. The risk assessment score can be used to categorize athletes at low, moderate, or high risk (Figs. 24.1 and 24.2). The questions cover menstrual health, including age of menarche and number of periods over the past 12 months. Late menarche is defined as first menstrual period at age 15 or older. Oligomenorrhea is defined as 6–9 periods over 12 months, and amenorrhea is fewer than six periods in 12 months or absence of menses for 3 months. Regarding nutrition, a diagnosis of eating disorder or disordered eating is important to elicit. Additionally, other markers may include reduced body mass index (defined as less than 18.5 kg/m^2 in female athletes), concerns about weight, or restrictive dietary patterns or attitudes. Bone health is more challenging to assess without direct measure of bone density using dual-energy X-ray absorptiometry (DXA); screening questions include history of prior stress fractures or stress reactions or diagnosis of low bone mineral density.

Box 24.1 Triad Consensus Panel Screening Questions[1]

Have you ever had a menstrual period?

How old were you when you had your first menstrual period?

When was your most recent menstrual period?

How many periods have you had in the past 12 months?

Are you presently taking any female hormones (oestrogen, progesterone, birth control pills)?

Do you worry about your weight?

Are you trying to or has anyone recommended that you gain or lose weight?

Are you on a special diet or do you avoid certain types of foods or food groups?

Have you ever had an eating disorder?

Have you ever had a stress fracture?

Have you ever been told you have low bone density (osteopenia or osteoporosis)?

Risk Factors	Magnitude of Risk		
	Low Risk = 0 points each	Moderate Risk = 1 point each	High Risk = 2 points each
Low EA with or without DE/ED	☐ No dietary restriction	☐ Some dietary restriction‡; current/past history of DE;	☐ Meets DSM-V criteria for ED*
Low BMI	☐ BMI ≥ 18.5 or ≥ 90% EW** or weight stable	☐ BMI 17.5 < 18.5 or < 90% EW or 5 to < 10% weight loss/month	☐ BMI ≤17.5 or < 85% EW or ≥ 10% weight loss/month
Delayed Menarche	☐ Menarche < 15 years	☐ Menarche 15 to < 16 years	☐ Menarche ≥16 years
Oligomenorrhea and/or Amenorrhea	☐ > 9 menses in 12 months*	☐ 6-9 menses in 12 months*	☐ < 6 menses in 12 months*
Low BMD	☐ Z-score ≥ -1.0	☐ Z-score -1.0*** < - 2.0	☐ Z-score ≤ -2.0
Stress Reaction/Fracture	☐ None	☐ 1	☐ ≥ 2; ≥ 1 high risk or of trabecular bone sites†
Cumulative Risk (total each column, then add for total score)	_____ points +	_____ points +	_____ points = _____Total Score

Fig. 24.1 Female athlete triad: cumulative risk assessment. With permission from De Souza MJ, Br Sports Med 2014;48:289. Copyright © 2016 BMJ Publishing Group Ltd. & British Association of Sport and Exercise Medicine (2)

---

[1] The Triad Consensus Panel recommends asking these screening questions at the time of the sport pre-participation evaluation. With permission from De Souza MJ, Br Sports Med 2014;48:289. Copyright © 2016 BMJ Publishing Group Ltd. & British Association of Sport and Exercise Medicine (2).

	Cumulative Risk Score*	Low Risk	Moderate Risk	High Risk
Full Clearance	0 – 1 point	☐		
Provisional/Limited Clearance	2 – 5 points		☐ Provisional Clearance ☐ Limited Clearance	
Restricted from Training and Competition	≥ 6 points			☐ Restricted from Training/ Competition-Provisional ☐ Disqualified

Fig. 24.2 Female athlete triad: clearance and return-to-play (RTP) guidelines by medical risk stratification. Cumulative risk score determined by summing the score of each risk factor (low, moderate, high risk) from the cumulative risk assessment. With permission from De Souza MJ, Br Sports Med 2014;48:289. Copyright © 2016 BMJ Publishing Group Ltd. & British Association of Sport and Exercise Medicine (2)

Physical Examination

On physical examination, body mass index should be measured. The initial assessment includes the following key features:

1. *Pain with weight bearing* or single leg hop
2. *Tenderness with direct palpation* over the bone
3. *Pain with direct or indirect percussion* over site of injury

   Clinical judgment should guide the examination. A patient with suspected BSI should not be requested to perform a single leg hop if there is concern for a fracture that could worsen or progress to more severe injury with overload.

   Additionally, special tests focused on specific areas of the anatomy may be added to the assessment for BSI.

4. *Hip Internal Range of Motion*

   Femoral neck BSI may have pain with range of motion of the affected hip, including at the end range of internal rotation. Additionally, a patient may complain of pain with resisted hip flexion given that hip flexor tendinopathy may be associated with BSI of the lesser trochanter (Nguyen et al. 2008).

5. *Fulcrum Test*

   Femoral shaft BSI can be difficult to evaluate on physical examination as tissue limits the ability to directly palpate or percuss the femur. The fulcrum test is commonly used to evaluate for a fracture (Johnson et al. 1994). This test is performed with the patient seated. The examiner places one forearm beneath the thigh. With the other hand, the examiner presses in an anterior to posterior force to the thigh. The examiner uses the forearm as a fulcrum and can be moved along the length of the femur to stress the bone. Pain localized to the site of the fulcrum may represent an underlying BSI at this location.

6. *SI Joint Maneuvers*

   BSI to the sacrum or pelvis may be evaluated using sacroiliac joint provocative maneuvers, although these examination findings are typically insensitive for pelvic BSI.

7. *Lumbar Extension*

   Pars interarticularis fractures are overuse injuries localized primarily to the lumbar spine and may occur at the most distal vertebral segments including the fifth lumbar vertebrae. These fractures are due to repetitive extension-based activities in sport, such as with rowing or gymnastics. The injury is typically evoked with extension-based stress to the spine, including instructions for the patient to stand on a single leg and then go into lumbar extension (known as the stork test).

8. *The Calcaneal Squeeze Test*

   This test can be helpful to identify a fracture in the calcaneus. The examiner places both hands on the calcaneus and applies a compressive force to evaluate if this reproduces bone pain.

Differential Diagnosis and Suggested Diagnostic Testing

The differential diagnosis for BSI is based on the location for injury. When imaging is required to confirm the diagnosis, magnetic resonance imaging (MRI) is typically recommended as this is the most sensitive test to evaluate for BSI, may exclude other regional soft tissue etiologies, and uses non-ionizing radiation. In addition, MRI can be used to grade the severity of BSI and guide return to play for sports (Nattiv et al. 2013). Given that in certain instances MRI may not be practical due to high costs, this imaging modality should be considered more strongly in high-risk fracture locations (see below). Plain film X-ray is less expensive and reasonable for initial evaluation of a suspected BSI in non-spine locations. However, X-ray may have a high rate of false-negative findings, especially in early stages of injury, and does involve ionizing radiation. Although ultrasound may demonstrate the presence of a cortical step-off or hyperemia and can evaluate for soft tissue pathology, it typically has low yield for detecting most forms of BSI.

Pars Interarticularis

Differential diagnosis includes common causes of axial low back pain (such as zygapophyseal joint-mediated arthropathy and discogenic low back pain) and sacroiliac joint-mediated pain. Visceral referred pain should also be considered. In females, obstetric and gynecological sources of pain and symptoms must be considered, including pregnancy.

Diagnostic testing for spinal BSI has traditionally included plain film radiographs with anterior/posterior, lateral, and oblique views. Computed tomography

(CT) of the lumbar spine with thin slices oriented through the pars can evaluate for presence of fracture. However, one must consider alternatives to CT given that it involves exposure of large amounts of ionizing radiation, especially in patients of reproductive age. As an alternative, clinician can obtain MRI of the lumbar spine, using STIR sequence, oriented with thin slices (2–3 mm) through the pars interarticularis to evaluate for presence of BSI. Additionally, MRI of the lumbar spine is also useful to evaluate for presence of spine-related conditions.

Sacral/Pelvic BSI

Differential diagnosis includes tendinopathy, referred pain from primary hip pathology, spine referred pain (including discogenic low back pain or S1 radiculopathy), piriformis strain/syndrome, and sacroiliac joint-mediated pain.

Diagnostic testing for a suspected BSI typically requires the use of MRI. Most sacral BSI are high-grade injuries and thus important to identify early. Sacral and pelvic BSI occur in the bone that is more cancellous in composition and hormonally sensitive to low sex hormones. Therefore, in athletes of both sexes, presence of a pelvic BSI should prompt a more extensive endocrine workup and consideration for DXA to measure bone density.

Femoral Neck

Differential diagnosis includes hip-related pathology including femoral acetabular impingement and iliopsoas tendinopathy.

Diagnostic workup may initially include plain film X-ray to evaluate for presence of a displaced fracture and to provide information on bony anatomy, including presence of femoral acetabular impingement. MRI is more expensive but is important to obtain if there is concern for a proximal femur BSI due to the high risk of injury progressing to a full fracture requiring surgery if not detected early. Presence of bone marrow edema involving the lesser trochanter is important to identify and should also be treated as high-risk fracture, as case series have shown progression of this injury to femoral neck BSI (Nguyen et al. 2008).

Femoral Shaft

Differential diagnosis includes spine referred pain; hip referred pain; quadriceps, hamstring, or adductor tendinopathy; or myofascial pain.

Diagnostic testing includes X-ray of the femur that may reveal fracture; however, MRI should be ordered if fracture is not visualized.

Lower Leg

Differential diagnosis for exertional leg pain is broad. Causes of leg pain include medial tibial stress syndrome (MTSS)/shin splints, chronic exertional compartment syndrome (CECS), peripheral nerve entrapment, and vascular etiologies (including popliteal artery entrapment syndrome or vascular claudication).

Diagnostic testing for fractures of the tibia or fibula includes X-ray or MRI. The typical location for a tibial BSI is the posterior distal third of the tibia. However, a BSI localized to the anterior tibia warrants special mention. This injury is considered high risk due to the tensile stress that is typically associated with development of an injury at this location. Presence of "the dreaded black line" on X-ray, defined as radiolucency extended horizontally through the anterior tibial cortex, requires close evaluation to ensure fracture healing. MRI may reveal presence of MTSS. The workup for other causes of exertional leg pain, including vascular, neurological, and CECS, is beyond the scope of this chapter and should be guided by experienced medical providers.

Foot/Ankle

Differential diagnosis is anatomically based and broad. For hindfoot fractures, primary ankle joint pathology (including ankle impingement or intra-articular pathology including osteoarthritis), insertional Achilles tendinopathy, plantar fasciopathy, ankle sprain, chronic ankle instability, peripheral nerve entrapment, and presence of tarsal coalition are more common causes of pain. Midfoot pain may be caused by metatarsalgia, ligament injury including Lisfranc ligament sprain, or neuroma. Forefoot pain may be present in cases of tendinopathy, arthritis, neuroma, or sesamoiditis.

Diagnostic testing should start with weight bearing X-ray of the foot or ankle for initial evaluation, which provides information on bone alignment, presence of fracture, and joint disease. MRI can identify and grade BSI and also exclude soft tissue etiologies of pain, including presence of ligament sprain, osteochondral defect, or neuroma.

Nonoperative Management

Physical Activity

Most BSI responds favorably to nonoperative management. An initial period of rest including non-weight bearing should be prescribed if the patient experiences pain with ambulation or in the presence of a BSI at high-risk locations (see following section). Once pain-free, the patient may progress to low-impact aerobic activities including elliptical trainer or use of treadmill with partial weight bearing. For running sport athletes, deep water running may help maintain aerobic fitness without impact loading. Time for return to full sports participation is determined by severity of BSI, anatomical location, and addressing the underlying etiology of the injury to reduce risk for recurrence.

Diet

Calcium and vitamin D are both important for overall skeletal health. In the absence of food allergy, milk and dairy products provide an excellent source of dietary calcium. Additionally, calcium-rich foods often contain nutrients that promote bone health including protein and phosphorus and may be fortified with vitamin D. An additional benefit of athletes obtaining calcium from food includes increased energy intake and energy availability. Vitamin D supplementation is reasonable to ensure targeted intake of 600 IU daily based on the Institute of Medicine 2010 guidelines.

Female athletes with Triad risk factors should be referred to a nutritionist with experience in managing athletes with the Triad, especially those athletes classified in moderate- and high-risk categories (Fig. 24.2). In the presence of disordered eating or an eating disorder, referral to a mental health provider is critical to address the underlying disease and reduce risk for injury recurrence or other detrimental health effects. For medical providers not familiar with managing the Triad, referral to a sports medicine professional with experience managing the Triad is prudent. A workup for menstrual dysfunction is also important. The Female Athlete Triad Coalition has helpful information on physician referral network and educational materials for patients and medical professionals (www.femaleathletetriad.org).

Medications

Typically, use of analgesics is discouraged for management of BSI, as pain is a useful symptom for the patient to monitor for fracture healing. Anti-inflammatory medications including NSAIDs should be avoided due to concerns for impaired bone healing with this medication. Screening for vitamin D deficiency is reasonable by obtaining serum 25-hydroxy vitamin D level, and prescription of vitamin D should follow standard of care guidelines for vitamin D deficiency.

Physical Therapy

Physical therapy should be prescribed to address the biomechanical contributors to injury. As muscle should serve as the primary shock attenuator in impact-loading activities, ensuring symmetric and adequate muscle mass is important. The guiding

Table 24.1 Summary of bone stress injuries by location and management

Location	Presentation	Physical exam	Diagnostic testing	Management	Indication for surgery
Common low-risk injuries					
Metatarsal shaft 1–4	Foot pain localized to the metatarsal	Tenderness along the tibia with palpation, percussion, and/or weight bearing	X-ray, MRI	Modified weight bearing, use of walking boot or metatarsal pad to off-load affected metatarsal, progression with pain-free activity and physical therapy	Displaced fracture
Tibia	Leg pain localized to tibia	Tenderness along the tibia with palpation, percussion, and/or weight bearing	X-ray, MRI	Modified weight bearing, followed by progression as tolerated with pain-free activity and physical therapy	Rarely requires surgery, fractures localized to anterior tibial cortex with "dreaded black line" on X-ray may have failure to heal and require surgery
Fibula	Leg pain localized along fibula	Tenderness along the tibia with palpation, percussion, and/or weight bearing	X-ray, MRI		Rarely requires surgery
Femur	Thigh pain	Pain with fulcrum test	X-ray, MRI		Displaced fracture
Pelvis (including sacrum)	Buttock pain, occasional thigh pain from sacral nerve involvement	Nonspecific exam, may have tenderness with palpation over the sacrum or positive SI maneuvers	X-ray, MRI		Rarely requires surgery
Pars interarticularis	Low back pain in extension-sport athlete	Pain with extension, may have pain with stork test and other extension-based exam maneuvers	X-ray, MRI with thin slices oriented to pars interarticularis	Modified activity away from extension-based activity or sport, back brace may be prescribed to encourage activity modification for 6 weeks	Rarely requires surgery

Common higher-risk injuries

Tarsal navicular	Foot pain along medial arch	Tenderness over navicular tuberosity, focal bony tenderness, may have associated reduced ankle dorsiflexion	X-ray, MRI. Occasionally CT may be required if concerns for nonunion	Walking boot and crutches for 4–6 weeks with clinical check prior to progressing to weight bearing, PT, bone stimulator for failure of initial healing	Nonunion or recurrent fractures
Fifth metatarsal diaphyseal fracture (Jones fracture)	Lateral foot pain	Tenderness to palpation of the fifth metatarsal at metaphyseal-diaphyseal junction	X-ray, MRI	Consider casting vs. walking boot and crutches for 4–6 weeks with clinical check prior to progressing to weight bearing in athletic shoes, PT, bone stimulator for failure of initial healing	Nonunion, recurrent fractures, or elite athletes to reduce risk for nonunion and result in predictable return to play
Base of the second metatarsal	Forefoot pain	Tenderness to palpation at base of the second metatarsal, may see associated elongation of the second metatarsal (Morton's toe)	X-ray, MRI	Consider casting vs. walking boot and crutches for 4 weeks with repeat X-rays to ensure bone bridging and with clinical check prior to weight bearing, PT, bone stimulator for failure of initial healing	Nonunion
Femoral neck	Hip or groin pain, occasional thigh pain	Pain localized to the hip, especially with internal range of motion. May have pain with single leg hop test. Femoral-acetabular impingement can be associated	X-ray, MRI	Crutches for 6 weeks with clinical check for pain-free walking and no pain with internal range of motion of hip prior to progressing weight bearing and PT	Displaced fractures; tension-sided bone stress injuries may require surgery

MRI magnetic resonance imaging

principle for management of BSI is for physical therapy to be focused on helping the patient develop a softer and well-aligned landing during their sport activity. As isolated strength programs may not result in a change in movement pattern, a comprehensive gait retraining with faded feedback design is desirable to reinforce and develop durable athletic movement patterns. Foot strike pattern has been associated with force distribution during running. In general, running with a forefoot strike pattern has been shown to reduce average and instantaneous load rates compared to rearfoot strike, and these benefits can be durable (Fig. 24.3) (Davis 2016). Prospective research investigations have demonstrated increased vertical load rate in runners who sustain a BSI compared to runners with no injury history.

Specialist Referral

Referral to a bone endocrinologist should be considered for athletes of both sexes who present with a fracture in a cancellous site, including the pelvis, or with recurrent BSI. The workup and management of BSI is sex-specific. Female athletes with menstrual dysfunction require a full workup, as functional hypothalamic amenorrhea is a diagnosis of exclusion. Male athletes may require screening for low sex steroids and other endocrine conditions such as thyroid disease, hyperparathyroidism, malabsorption syndromes, or renal disease. Referral to an orthopedic specialist should be considered for athletes with atypical presentations of injury or those who sustain a BSI at a high-risk location.

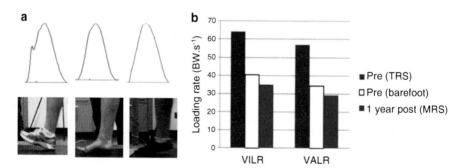

Fig. 24.3 Long-term follow-up on a patient who underwent a supervised transition to running with a FFS pattern using foot and ankle strengthening and gait retraining. (**a**) Foot strike pattern and associated vertical ground reaction forces: (left) baseline with shoes (RFS); (middle) baseline, barefoot (FFS); and (right) 1-year follow-up, minimal shoes (FFS). (**b**) VILR and VALR at baseline (Pre) when the patient was running with shoes (red), barefoot (white), and, 1 year after, when running in her minimal shoes (blue). Note the reduction of her load rates when barefoot at baseline and in her minimal shoes at 1 year after. *BW* body weight, *MRS* minimal running shoe, *TRS* traditional running shoe. With permission from Davis and Futrell. Gait. *Phys Med Rehabil Clin N Am.* 2016;27(1):339–355 Copyright © 2013 Elsevier B.V. (6)

Indications for Surgery and Operative Management

Rarely does a BSI require operative management. Exceptions include displaced fractures, some fractures localized to high-risk locations, or BSI that recur depending on clinical context.

High-risk fractures in the following locations should be evaluated by an orthopedic specialist: femoral neck (particularly tension side), lesser trochanter, anterior tibial cortex, medial malleolus, talus, tarsal navicular, fifth metatarsal diaphyseal fracture (also known as Jones fracture), base of the second metatarsal, or sesamoids of the forefoot.

Surgical management may require use of rods, pins, or screws to approximate the bone and ensure bony union. Additionally, high-risk locations with excess biomechanical forces may fail to respond favorably to nonoperative management and may recur if the athlete returns to the same activity levels prior to injury. For this reason, orthopedic surgeons may sometimes offer early surgical management to select patients who sustain injuries such as a Jones fracture, given predictable healing response and in order to hasten return to sport.

Expected Outcome and Predictors of Outcome

Most patients will be able to recover from BSI with nonsurgical management including in both high- and low-risk injury locations. However, providing patient education regarding the underlying etiology of the injury is important to reduce risk for recurrence. This includes management of biological risk factors including the Triad. Biomechanical contributors including appropriate strength and conditioning exercises should be encouraged prospectively to reduce risk for future injury. Finally, prevention strategies should be employed to reduce future risk of injury.

Prevention

Prevention of a BSI includes optimizing biological and biomechanical risk factors while also promoting optimal nutrition and sleep.

Biology

Knowledge of the Triad is important in best addressing these risk factors at a young age. In addition to developing healthy attitudes about diet, exercise, and body image, childhood and adolescence are a time of growth and peak bone mass accrual. All female athletes should be screened for Triad risk factors during their annual pre-participation physical examination (PPE) and managed appropriately prior to sports participation (De Souza 2014). The PPE is the first line of defense against developing a BSI.

Biomechanics

Bone loading during childhood and adolescence in sports and activities that encourage multidirectional jumping may result in stronger and more fracture-resistant bones. Review of the literature suggests that early participation in ball sports or jumping activities may improve bone quality and reduce risk for future fractures, even upon discontinuation of the activity (Tenforde 2015).

In contrast, encouraging softer and well-aligned landings during sport activities is a desirable goal to reduce risk for running injuries and other injuries associated with malalignment in the lower extremity, including anterior cruciate ligament injuries. Running with a forefoot strike pattern may be augmented with use of minimalist footwear to reduce the impact loading associated with risk for BSI.

Sleep

Sleep quality is important for overall health. Although the role of sleep in BSI has not been determined in athletes, compelling evidence for the importance of sleep to promote bone health comes from military investigations. In one study, a subset of subjects was randomly assigned to sleep upright or in sleep-deprived conditions, noting elevated bone turnover markers and a 5% loss of bone mass over a 7-day period (Ben Sasson 1994) .

Nutrition

Ensuring adequate energy availability is critical to promote bone health for both sexes. All athletes and active individuals should be encouraged to meet the calcium and vitamin D intake as recommended by the Institute of Medicine. For both sexes ages 9–18, calcium intake target is 1300 mg daily. Premenopausal female adults and males until age 70 should consume 1000 mg of calcium daily, whereas females aged 51 or males aged 70 or older should consume 1200 mg daily. Recommended vitamin D dietary intake is 600 IU daily for ages 9 and older.

Summary

In conclusion, BSI is a common form of overuse injury in athletes and active individuals. Evaluation of risk factors for BSI is obtained by history and physical examination. MRI is the most useful diagnostic test given high sensitivity, ability to visualize soft tissue, and enabling the provider to grade the severity of injury. Injuries in low-risk locations may be managed without advanced imaging based on repeat clinical examination to ensure bone healing. Management of injury includes activity modification, addressing underlying biological risk factors (e.g., the Triad), physical therapy to address biomechanical contributors to injury, and optimizing nutrition. Prevention includes screening and managing the Triad, addressing faulty sports biomechanics, promoting osteogenic bone loading activities at a young age, and nutrition that includes a diet with adequate energy availability and foods rich in calcium and vitamin D.

Suggested Reading

Barrack MT, Gibbs JC, De Souza MJ, et al. Higher incidence of bone stress injuries with increasing female athlete triad-related risk factors: a prospective multisite study of exercising girls and women. Am J Sports Med. 2014;42(4):949–58.

Ben Sasson SA, Finestone A, Moskowitz M, et al. Extended duration of vertical position might impair bone metabolism. Eur J Clin Investig. 1994;24:421–5.

Davis IS, Futrell E. Gait retraining: altering the fingerprint of gait. Phys Med Rehabil Clin N Am. 2016;27(1):339–55.

De Souza MJ, Nattiv A, Joy E, et al. Female athlete triad coalition consensus statement on treatment and return to play of the female athlete triad: 1st international conference held in San Francisco, California, May 2012 and 2nd international conference held in Indianapolis, Indiana, May 2013. Br J Sports Med. 2014;48(289):2014.

Ihle R, Loucks AB. Dose-response relationship between energy availability and bone turnover in young exercising women. J Bone Miner Res. 1994;19:1231–40.

Institute of Medicine. Dietary reference intakes for calcium and vitamin D. National Academy of Sciences; November 2010, Report Brief. 2010. http://wwwiomedu/w/media/Files/Report Files/2010/Dietary-Reference-Intakes-for-Calcium-and-Vitamin-D/Vitamin D and Calcium 2010 Report Brief.pdf.

Johnson AW, Weiss CB Jr, Wheeler DL. Stress fractures of the femoral shaft in athletes more common than expected. A new clinical test. Am J Sports Med. 1994;22(2):248–56.

Nattiv A, Loucks AB, Manore MM, Sanborn CF, Sundgot-Borgen J, Warren MP. American College of Sports Medicine position stand. The female athlete triad. Med Sci Sports Exerc. 2007;39(10):1867–82.

Nattiv A, Kennedy G, Barrack MT, et al. Correlation of MRI grading of bone stress injuries with clinical risk factors and return to play: a 5-year prospective study in collegiate track and field athletes. Am J Sports Med. 2013;41:1930–41.

Nguyen JT, Peterson JS, Biswal S, et al. Stress-related injuries around the lesser trochanter in long-distance runners. Am J Roetenol. 2008;190:1616–20.

Tenforde AS, Sainani KL, Sayres LC, et al. Participation in ball sports may represent a prehabilitation strategy to prevent future stress fractures and promote bone health in young athletes. PM&R J. 2015;7:222–5.

Index

© Springer International Publishing AG 2018   399
J.N. Katz et al. (eds.), *Principles of Orthopedic Practice for Primary Care
Providers*, https://doi.org/10.1007/978-3-319-68661-5

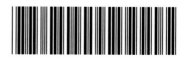